I0029610

AṢṬADAḶA YOGAMĀLĀ

AṢṬADAḶA YOGAMĀLĀ

(COLLECTED WORKS)

B.K.S. IYENGAR

Volume 4

Interviews

ALLIED PUBLISHERS PRIVATE LIMITED
NEW DELHI MUMBAI KOLKATA CHENNAI NAGPUR
AHMEDABAD BANGALORE HYDERABAD LUCKNOW

ALLIED PUBLISHERS PRIVATE LIMITED

Regd. Off. : 15 J.N. Heredia Marg, Ballard Estate, **Mumbai**–400001
Ph.: 022-42126969 • E-mail: mumbai.books@alliedpublishers.com

47/9 Prag Narain Road, Near Kalyan Bhawan, **Lucknow**–226001
Ph.: 0522-2209942 • E-mail: lko.books@alliedpublishers.com

F-1 Sun House (First Floor), C.G. Road, Navrangpura,
Ellisbridge P.O., **Ahmedabad**–380006
Ph.: 079-26465916 • E-mail: ahmbd.books@alliedpublishers.com

3-2-844/6 & 7 Kachiguda Station Road, **Hyderabad**–500027
Ph.: 040-24619079 • E-mail: hyd.books@alliedpublishers.com

5th Main Road, Gandhinagar, **Bangalore**–560009
Ph.: 080-22262081 • E-mail: bngl.books@alliedpublishers.com

1/13-14 Asaf Ali Road, **New Delhi**–110002
Ph.: 011-23239001 • E-mail: delhi.books@alliedpublishers.com

17 Chittaranjan Avenue, **Kolkata**–700072
Ph.: 033-22129618 • E-mail: cal.books@alliedpublishers.com

60 Shiv Sunder Apartments (Ground Floor), Central Bazar Road,
Bajaj Nagar, **Nagpur**–440010
Ph.: 0712-2234210 • E-mail: ngp.books@alliedpublishers.com

751 Anna Salai, **Chennai**–600002
Ph.: 044-28523938 • E-mail: chennai.books@alliedpublishers.com

Website: www.alliedpublishers.com

First Published 2004
Reprinted 2005, 2008, 2010, 2012

© Allied Publishers Private Limited

B.K.S. Iyengar asserts the moral right to be identified as the author of this work.

ISBN : 81-7764-578-1

No part of the material protected by this copyright notice may be reproduced or utilized in any form or by any means, electronic or mechanical including photocopying, recording or by any information storage and retrieval system, without prior written permission from the copyright owner.

Cover design : The Author
Artwork : S.M. Waugh

Published by Sunil Sachdev and printed by Ravi Sachdev at Allied Publishers Private Limited, Printing Division, A-104 Mayapuri Phase II, New Delhi - 110064

Invocatory Prayers

ॐ

Yogena cittasya padena vācāṁ
Malaṁ śarīrasyaca vaidyakena
Yopākarottaṁ pravaraṁ munīnāṁ
Patañjaliṁ prāñjalirānato'smi
Ābāhu puruṣākāraṁ
Śaṅkha cakrāsi dhāriṇaṁ
Sahasra śirasaṁ śvetaṁ
Praṇamāmi Patañjaliṁ

I bow before the noblest of sages Patañjali, who gave yoga for serenity and sanctity of mind, grammar for clarity and purity of speech and medicine for pure, perfect health.

I prostrate before Patañjali who is crowned with a thousand headed cobra, an incarnation of Ādiśeṣa (Anañta) whose upper body has a human form, holding the conch in one arm, disk in the second, a sword of wisdom to vanquish nescience in the third and blessing humanity from the fourth arm, while his lower body is like a coiled snake.

Yastyaktvā rūpamādyaṁ prabhavati jagato'nekadhānugrahāya
Prakṣīṇakleśarāśirviṣamaviṣadharo'nekavaktrāḥ subhogī
Sarvajñānaprasūtirbhujagaparikaraḥ prītaye yasya nityaṁ
Devohīṣaḥ savovyātsitavimalatanuryogado yogayuktaḥ

I prostrate before Lord Ādiśeṣa, who manifested himself on Earth as Patañjali to grace the human race in health and harmony,

I salute Lord Ādiśeṣa of the myriad serpent heads and mouths carrying noxious poisons, discarding which he came to Earth as a single headed Patañjali in order to eradicate ignorance and vanquish sorrow.

I pay my obeisance to him, repository of all knowledge, amidst his attendant retinue.

I pray to the Lord whose primordial form shines with peace and white effulgence, pristine in body, a master of yoga, who bestows on all his yogic light to enable mankind to rest in the house of the immortal Soul.

BY THE AUTHOR

This volume of *Aṣṭadaḷa Yogamālā* published by Allied Publishers, Delhi, is the fourth volume of the second part of the "Collected Works" of Yogācārya B.K.S. Iyengar. Each part comprises several volumes which are arranged according to the following scheme:

Articles
Interviews
Question and Answer Sessions
Techniques of *Āsanas, Prāṇāyāma, Dhyāna* and *Śavāsana*
Therapeutic Applications of Yoga
Garland of Aphorisms and Thoughts
General Index and Analytical Dictionary
Addendum

Also by the Same Author

Light on Yoga
Light on Prāṇāyāma
Concise Light on Yoga
Art of Yoga
Tree of Yoga
Light on the Yoga Sūtras of Patañjali
The Illustrated Light on Yoga
Yoga Ek Kalpataru (Marathi)
Ārogyayoga (Marathi)
Light on Aṣṭāṅga Yoga
Aṣṭadaḷa Yogamālā (Vols 1, 2 & 3)
Yoga: The Path To Holistic Health
Yoga Sarvānaāṭhi (Marathi)
Basic Guidelines for Teachers of Yoga (co-authored with G.S. Iyengar)

Also on Iyengar Yoga

Body the Shrine, Yoga Thy Light
70 Glorious Years
Iyengar His Life and Work
Yogapushpanjali
Yogadhārā

CONTENTS

PLATES

FOREWORD

Interviews that have been presented here have to be read keeping in mind how the psychological background of human nature works on different mental and intellectual planes.

Articles are written to convey ideas to the readers, and the frame in which the articles are written conveys the frame of the mind of the author, while an interview covers various things in many different ways. Interviews carry a number of questions, which give form to a number of human doubts, fears, complexes, expectations and wishes to the interviewer. The answers of an interview have to cover directly or indirectly the answers to the doubts and fears that are hidden in the questions.

Not only that, a valuable interview means that the interviewee should think emotionally and intelligently in order to answer to the general doubts and fears of human psychology as they pertain to each question. The mind of the interviewee should go beyond the mind of the interviewer to identify the deep doubts, fears and hopes of the human being. This has always been my state of mind while giving any interview.

The psychological background of humanity goes on changing as the world changes and the challenges to be faced are different. The psychological background of yoga practitioners also goes on changing as stability sets in as they go on improving in their practices. Sometimes an interview might have been given for a country with less understanding in the field of yoga. Sometimes certain replies are made under particular situations and circumstances. I thought that I should also consider these changes and present day conditions. Keeping this present state of man's intellectual development, I decided to edit my own interviews. This is the reason why you may find small differences between the interviews published at those moments and the edited interviews you have at present in your hands.

B.K.S. IYENGAR

THE INTERVIEWS

IS YOGA FOR BEAUTY AND POWER?*

Q.- In our country, it is said that a handsome body and supernatural brainpower can be obtained by *yogābhyāsa*. Is it true? Are there any yogis at present with such faculties?

Before answering this question, it is worth knowing what yoga means, so let me define what yoga is. See, Sage Patañjali defines yoga as *yogaścittavṛtti nirodhaḥ* (*Y.S.*, I.2). "Yoga is to control or still the mind of its thought currents". Man is a trinity of body, mind and self. Practice is done to integrate the three sheaths of man. Mind is the king of all our emotions and physical changes. Mind is the cause and the body is the effect. According to the emotions of the mind the body is moulded. Thus unless the mind is brought to a state of quietude, is it ever possible to have a handsome body and emotional power and beautiful poise?

Secondly, handsomeness is a gift from the creator. One might be handsome but diseased, physically as well as mentally. There are so many saints and yogis who are not physically handsome but spiritually handsome. For example, Louis Fischer, who wrote on Mahatma Gandhi called him as the ugliest man of Asia.[1]

In spite of the advancement of science and knowledge of body and mind, diseases and unhappiness are on the increase. Practice of yoga, composed of physical, ethical, mental, intellectual and spiritual aspects, affects one to subjectively experience rather than to infer by mere observations. Health is an asset to be gained by sheer hard work. In fact, complete forgetfulness of the physical consciousness and mental happiness is definitely a positive dynamic beauty and power. When one is free from physical disabilities and mental distractions, naturally, one is led to gain knowledge and wisdom and to live in the kingdom of the self. When this is achieved, does it not mean that one possesses not only a healthy, strong and handsome body but also a tranquil benevolent state of mind?

---

* Broadcast by All India Radio on 9th May, 1958.

[1] "Life of Mahatma Gandhi", *Bhavans Book*, Bharatya Vidya Bhavan, Mumbai, 1953.

Coming to the other part, namely of spiritual powers, it may well appear for an ordinary person that the natural powers of a yogi appear as supernatural, but certainly not to himself. For him the consciousness is one and unique, whether it is in a state of subconscious or superconscious. Anxieties and worries of the mind and disabilities of the body are conquered by different stages of yoga, coupled with right living, right understanding and right knowledge. When so much is achieved, naturally the intelligence becomes clear and sharp; and memory power as well as the will power are so exalted that these appear super natural to others.

Lastly it is not uncommon to find yogis with such powers and *siddhi*. Their *siddhi* or powers are meant for learning the philosophy of non-attachment so that they can proceed towards advanced spiritual practices.

DOES YOGA BUILD PERSONALITY?*

Q.- Well, Mr. Iyengar, I am very happy to have this opportunity of discussing certain aspects of yoga with you. We all know that yoga can play an important role in building the body, but this evening I have a very fascinating aspect of yoga to discuss with you. The subject is: "Does yoga help in building personality also?"

Thank you very much Mr. Pocha. The subject is indeed fascinating but first of all for my benefit could you tell me what you mean by personality?

Q.- Well, I think I shall have to give you a very common definition of personality. By personality I mean that attractiveness in an individual which commands attention and respect of the people towards that individual. The man or the woman may not be beautiful or handsome but he or she would attract attention. You know, it does not necessarily mean beauty.

Thank you. I take it that your definition of personality does not mean external appearance only. The personality is thus an integrated whole. If so, I can say with confidence that yoga plays a very important role in developing such a personality. Here I might say a few words about what yoga is. Patañjali, the father of yoga in the *Yoga Sūtra* says, *yogaścittavṛtti nirodhaḥ* (*Y.S.*, I.2), which means controlling the activities of the mind and bringing them into a single pointed attention is yoga. It is a science dealing with the mind. Mind is the mirror of the soul, because the soul is reflected through the actions of the mind and the body. You will agree that it is more difficult to control the mind than the body because the mind is subtler compared to the body. The mind is easily attracted towards external objects. Therefore, I might say, to draw the mind back into internal thought or internal world for the growth of mental personality is yoga.

---

* Interview by Mr. Pocha, broadcast on *Akaśavāṇi,* 1958.

Q.- Mr. Iyengar, before you proceed further may I ask what you mean by internal thought or internal world?

By internal world I mean the knowledge one acquires as to what is happening inside our system, which is the internal universe or you might call it "knowledge space". The consciousness composed of mind, intelligence and 'I'-consciousness is the internal body world. Man has higher aspects in life besides material achievements. In spite of advancement of science and knowledge, material satisfactions alone do not lead us towards happiness and joy from within. The mind always holds on to the senses for pleasures and pains. It is easily absorbed towards the external objects through the senses. To draw in the senses and the mind to study one's reactions to one's own thoughts, words and deeds is the internal world.

Our senses are like horses, the body is the chariot, the mind, the reins and the charioteer is the soul or the Self. If the reins are loose, the horses run wild and end up with a disaster. Similarly, the undisciplined mind wanders towards the attractive objects of the world. To discipline the mind and control it is what the *yogaśāstra* or the science of yoga teaches. By such discipline, the energy is saved which is used for right living, right thinking and right understanding of oneself. In short I say that it teaches the true ART OF LIVING. This is the internal thought.

Q.- Well, I think I get some idea. But then how does yoga influence our minds and where does our personality come into it?

The body is the temple of the soul. The body and the mind are interrelated. They are the cause and the effect of each other. If the cause is in the right path, the effect also is in the right line. For example, if the body is healthy, the mind also becomes healthy. If the mind is not healthy, the body does not function properly. Watch when a person gets annoyed or irritated, his nerves very easily get disturbed, and this disturbs his bodily activities. Take the case of a sick person, he is more irritable, has less poise than a physically fit individual. So developing the body is a means towards disciplining the mind. But both these disciplines help one to develop personality, as personality is nothing but unification of physical, psychological, emotional and intellectual characteristics of a person.

Q.- Do you mean to say that if I have a very strong mind I can develop my body without the exercises?

That is possible for those who can control the body through their mind, but this would be possible only for very few individuals. What we are interested in at present is that the average man should develop his body and through this development, he should move towards the mind and his soul. The common man has more of the animal instincts in him whereas the other instincts such as humanity and divinity remain dormant. Patañjali, the codifier of the science of yoga, though he started his text with the control of the mind directly, realised the weakness of the average man and elaborated the *kriyā yoga,* the yoga of action, in the second chapter. It is termed as *yama, niyama, āsana, prāṇāyāma, pratyāhāra, dhāraṇā, dhyāna* and *samādhi.*

These are again formed into five categories as ethical, physical, mental, intellectual and spiritual. For an average man to curb his animal instincts, he has to build up a healthy frame of body and mind through the practice of *āsana* and *prāṇāyāma. Āsana* is the various positionings of the body, and *prāṇāyāma* the regulations of breath. There are varieties of *āsana* and several types of *prāṇāyāma.* By these the body and mind are kept in a healthy state for higher aims in life, i.e., righteous and virtuous life *(dharma* and *mokṣa).*

Also it is not considered possible to have a healthy frame of body and mind without the moral character. So *yama* and *niyama* are made essential to begin with. To follow the principles of *yama* is non-injury to others by thought, word and deed, to be honest to oneself, non-covetousness, chastity and fear of the future and of death. These are s ocial virtues. By *niyama* I mean the individual virtues such as purity from within and without, tolerance, contentment, religious zeal, studying of holy scriptures which deal on evolution of life and surrendering of all our activities to God.

Q.- Thank you Mr. Iyengar, but you have not mentioned anything about the development of the mind or the exercises that lead to it?

Well, Mr. Pocha, now let me come to the point. In yoga it is called *pratyāhāra,* that is restraining the senses. We should know the causes for the afflictions of the mind. Sage Patañjali has analysed this in two of his *Yoga Sūtra.* One is: *vyādhi styāna saṁśaya pramāda ālasya avirati bhrāntidarśana alabdhabhūmikatva anavasthitatvāni cittavikṣepāḥ te antarāyāḥ* and the second is: *duḥkha daurmanasya aṅgamejayatva śvāsa praśvāsāḥ vikṣepa sahabhuvaḥ* (see *Y.S.,* I.30&31). The weakness of the body and mind, dullness, indecisiveness, carelessness, illusions, laziness, instability, suffering from aches and pains, diseases and despair, even very shallow, hollow and un-rhythmic breathing are, he says, distractions of the mind. So, in order to keep the mind in a state of well being, the *sādhaka* cultivates friendliness towards people, compassion towards inferiors, joyfulness towards those who are better of in life and indifference towards vice and virtue, pleasure and pain – *maitrī karuṇā muditā upekṣāṇāṁ sukha duḥkha puṇya apuṇya viṣayāṇāṁ bhāvanātaḥ cittaprasādanam* (*Y.S.*, I.33). In this way, when the mental attitude is gained, will he not have a balanced mind?

When the body is healthy, is one conscious of it? Are you conscious of your tip of the ear or tip of the nose unless there is a wound? So also when the mind is brought to a state of stillness, what remains? The 'I'-ness. Is it not? When the fuel is extinguished from the fire, do you still see the fire or the flame? So also when the *vāsanā* or the fire of desires are extinguished, the mind is transformed towards knowledge and illumination. When you achieve such a state, there can be no greater glory or greater joy. It is a state where the body, the mind and soul are one. That gives the personality the power to attract. Here, the external beauty is not considered at all. When you are aware in that state there is no place for dualities.

Q.- Mr. Iyengar, I do understand now that by developing a healthy body one builds up a subtle and a healthy mind. I can quite see your point that the mind and soul will reflect through one's body and naturally that is your personality but now I would like to know how long does a man require to practise these yogic exercises to develop such a personality.

This doubt is as old as civilisation itself. Realising that this very same doubt would recur to one and all, Sage Patañjali explains, *sa tu dīrghakāla nairantarya satkāra āsevitaḥ dṛḍhabhūmiḥ* (*Y.S.*, I.14) – if long non-stop practice without any disturbance, with a single minded effort and determination is done, then you are the master of yourself.

Actually the progress depends upon individual ability, practice and persistent perseverance. Some can develop very quickly. Then there is the other class of people whose progress is slow, because they are not mentally matured enough. But when the mental attitudes are cultivated and practice is intense, the progress is bound to be quicker.

One thing that is certain, Mr. Pocha, no labour is lost for whatever is gained is a permanent gain.

Q.- Is it possible for a man to learn these exercises without a teacher?

It is possible but not very advisable. Let me not call them exercises, these are *āsana*. There are certain *āsana*, which cannot be done without an instructor and if undertaken without a proper knowledge may injure the body as well as the mind. For instance, though it is possible for children to learn from books, do we not send them to school and engage a teacher to teach at home? Why? So that they can learn quick and follow the right method. This also holds well in other fields.

Let me tell you how it may endanger the system. Take for example *prāṇāyāma*. These are not breathing exercises, but the tuning of the breath. Breath is an indirect method of controlling the mind. If the breath is rhythmic, the mind is in tranquillity. When a person loses his temper, he breathes fast, while he is in a state of joy, his breath is controlled and deep. I am telling you this as an example to show how closely these two are interconnected. Even the authorities say, *yathā siṁho gajo vyāghro bhavedvaśyaḥ śanaiḥ śanaiḥ* (*H.Y.P.,* II.15), as you tame a lion, an elephant or tiger by degrees, tame the breath in the same way. Still further Svātmārāma says,

prāṇāyāmena yuktena sarva roga kśayo bhavet /
ayuktābhyāsayogena sarvaroga samudbhavaḥ //
(*H.Y.P.,* II.16)

i.e. if breathing techniques of *prāṇāyāma* are properly done, diseases will vanish, otherwise they are unknowingly invited. By reading books one may do things wrongly or go beyond one's capacity and invite danger. Even walking in the street carelessly brings misery. So is it not better to have the guidance of a teacher?

Q.- I see yoga being a special type of exercise, is it possible for a teacher to teach more than one person at a time?

I think so. In my opinion it is possible for a teacher to give mass training. As a matter of fact I introduced yoga in the mass for I have trained students of different colleges and schools.

Q.- What time is it necessary to devote to these exercises every day or every week for acquiring this knowledge? Once one becomes perfect, is it necessary to continue these practices?

If you are practising casually, the effects too will be casual. If you practise regularly, the effects will grow subtler and subtler, hence, regular practice increases the quality of presentation and the effects too would be finer. So one has to practise every day regularly. One can practise according to the availability of the time, either in the morning or evening, but to divide the sequences, complicated *āsana* can be done in the morning, while soothing, calming *āsana* can be done in the evenings.

Patañjali says, *yogāṅgānuṣṭhānāt aśuddhikṣaye jñānadīptiḥ āvivekakhyāteḥ* (*Y.S.*, II.28). Through practice of yoga the impurities of the body and mind are destroyed and the light of knowledge and wisdom dawns. Is there an end to knowledge and understanding? As it is not possible to demarcate the end in knowledge, continued practice must go on.

Does a musician who projects himself in the art of music give up? How can one decide what is perfection? Continuity in the practice refines the *sādhanā*. So how can one stop? The moment you stop there is going to be a downfall from perfection. And again, perfection cannot be gauged until flawlessness is experienced. The perfection in *āsana* is when the consciousness engulfs the entire body without taint.

Q.- What is the age limit? At what age one may start to learn yoga? Can a man or a woman start at any age? Do the exercises differ for men and women?

Yuvā vṛddho'tivṛddho vyādhito durbalo'pi vā /
abhyāsāt siddhimāpnoti sarvayogeṣvatandritaḥ //
(*H.Y.P.*, I.64)[1]

Yoga can be practised by men and women of any age, whether weak or strong, young or old. In my own experience I have taught yoga to children from the age of five and to men and women of eighty. I recently taught yoga to the Queen Mother of Belgium who is eighty-four. In my class here there are people in their late eighties and nineties. This proves that yoga can be done by one and all. Only it had to be done according to one's age, constitution and circumstances. There is no different method for women. Only a few things are not permissible which have to be known by the teachers. That is all.

---

[1] Any person who practises all aspects of yoga untiringly attains success even if he is young, old, very old, sick or weak.

YOGA FOR EQUIPOISE*

Q.- *Guruji*, acrobatics have taken an art form in foreign countries. What is the difference between that and yoga?

We have the body and the mind. These are like light and darkness, sorrow and happiness. Often we see that the body may be strong but the mind remains weak. Or the body may be weak and the mind may be strong. How can we distinguish this and balance them? There is no body without mind and no mind without body. Hence, both are very important for our spiritual evolution.

Citta vṛtti nirodhaḥ does not mean ignoring both the body and the mind. Actually this word conveys to have a grip on both the body and the mind to develop a balanced state of equipoise in the *citta* – consciousness. Further we always feel that the body and the mind struggle with each other, oppose each other, and overwhelm the *citta*. Putting an end to this struggle and opposition between body and mind, and proceeding to equilibrium is yoga. If we are able to solve this struggle between body and mind, we will be able to attain stability and peace within ourselves. Yoga involves living in tranquillity in body as well as in mind.

There is a difference between acrobatics and yoga. Acrobatics only flexes the body and gives it shape. It is just a conative movement. However the involvement of the mind is only on the body. In acrobatics there is no awareness of the breath. Thus acrobatics is like *āsana* minus *prāṇāyāma* and mind control. In acrobatics the body is the main instrument, in *āsana* body, breath and mind are equally treated and used as important instruments. Without *prāṇāyāma* there is neither yoga nor are there *āsana*. Yogic practice covers body, breath, mind, intelligence, consciousness and self to intermingle and interact. When we practise a particular *āsana* we have to move the body to achieve the right required position. For that we have to bring to bear our mind and intelligence to execute it and then observe the specific effect of that particular action. There should be perfect co-ordination of body, mind, energy-flow and intelligence. Then only can we say that we made our body listen to our mind and intelligence in order to perfect the *āsana*.

---

* Interview by Dr. Ramachandra, published in *Andhra Patrika* on 8th May, 1966. (translated from Telugu)

Our efforts to remove the struggle between the attitudes of body and mind and bring them to a state of equilibrium are what yoga is about. As a result we feel that body and mind are absent though they are present in reality. This feeling is known as *samādhi sthiti*. To reach this feeling, the practice of *āsana* is one of the ways. We have to perform almost all the *āsana* and bring unity between body and mind as the main aim in *sādhanā*, so that they act as one force, one entity, though both are present in separate form, with the feeling of coming close to the soul which is an eternal entity.

Q.- How can we know the mind and keep it peaceful?

Our minds get disturbed for various reasons such as work factors, emotions, our relationships with each other. We need to know the inner depth of our body and find out what we can do with it. To know this depth we have to work with our body and mind while practising the *āsana* so that we know their intricacies. Each *āsana* has a purpose and a result. This purpose and result affect the mind. Both have their own *dharma*. With a particular refined *āsana* we can make our mind travel in its own place - the body - we can bring steadiness to the body through *āsana* and attain peace of mind. It means we have to endeavour to keep the cells of the body and wanderings of the mind in a balanced state. *Āsana* helps to minimise the disharmony between body and mind.

Q.- Is yoga only beneficial to the individual, a select group of people or society?

Yoga begins with oneself and is done for one's own self. Unless society begins yoga, it has no benefit on society. Only the individual who does yoga enjoys the pleasure of yoga practice. This joy can only be passed on or shared with others if they consent to do it. The individual alone derives the fruits and these effects cannot be shared or sold for others in the market place. After all, society is made up of individuals. If individuals shake hands, work together, and improve themselves, then society is sure to benefit.

Q.- Is it possible to attain the *siddhi* spoken of by Patañjali in our day and age?

All efforts culminate with some effects and effects are nothing but *siddhi*. This is experienced by all of us. Similarly, *siddhi*, which appear as super-normal to us, are just normal to a yogi. Due to change of time and circumstances as well as change in the way of practice of *sādhanā*, the *siddhi* have to be looked at differently. In olden days, the teaching of *āsana* and *prāṇāyāma* used to begin before the thread ceremony was performed, and *brahmopadeśam*[1] was done through this thread ceremony at the age of five or seven for both girls and boys in all the three *varṇa*. Obviously after the thread ceremony the *brahmacāri* or the *brahmacāriṇi* stayed in the *gurukula* to practise both physical and spiritual *sādhanā*. Nowadays we only know about yoga but do not practise as it has to be practised. If we practise yoga the way the texts proclaim, then we cannot say that the *siddhi* do not come. If one has to aim at them, then the supreme effort is required. The joy obtained by practice is also a kind of *siddhi*. *Siddhi* are real and are possible with intense efforts but do not come easily for everyone.

Q.- Does yoga enlighten? Can one have *darśana* of the Lord[2] by perfect alignment of the body and the mind? Have you had it?

Enlightenment is the essence of yoga. First of all, the temple of the soul – the body – has to be aligned with the mind and then with the self. The aphorist Patañjali has given detailed explanations with methodical disciplines on achieving this state. If his explanations are put religiously and devotedly into practice, it is definitely possible to experience that state.

Whatever way I express my felt experiences I am afraid that it is not going to satisfy you at all. For me, the alignment in my body is the enlightenment of my mind and self. Let me go a little deeper into this aspect.

The word enlightenment or realisation connotes almost the same meaning. When you throw the light on the object, the object reveals itself and you realise what the object is. Similarly, with the practice of yoga you throw the light on your body, mind, intelligence and consciousness and in turn they reveal themselves. Otherwise, all these are dark.

Yoga has many connotations. They are essential to associate, to unite, or to yoke all the evolutes of *prakṛti*, for them to dissolve in the Soul. Unless one experiences this state, there is no vision of God.

When I say that the practice of yoga throws light, it may not be a right expression. As we practise yoga, our belongings, namely, the evolutes of *prakṛti* such as the elements – earth, water, fire, air and ether, and their atomic qualities like odour, taste, shape, touch and sound; organs of action – *karmendriya;* senses of perception – *jñānendriya;* mind – *manas;* intelligence

[1] *Brahma* means the Universal Supreme Soul. *Upadeśam* means instructions and guidance in spiritual knowledge. The *Brahmopadeśam* (the thread ceremony) is the beginning of guiding the student in spiritual knowledge. Later, the pupils are taught *Veda* and *Upaniṣad* to have *brahma jñana*.

[2] *Darśana* of the Lord = Sight or the vision of God.

- buddhi; I-ness *- ahaṁkāra;* consciousness *- citta;* and conscience *- dharmendriya,* become clear, clean and pure. In fact, they are the caves, one behind the other covering the soul. Each cave becomes darker and darker to penetrate. Like an archaeologist we have to excavate by intense penetration the internal sheaths of the self, in our practice of yoga. This helps to remove the caves of darkness of the sheaths for the self to shine on itself. This is enlightenment, for one to experience what the real self is like.

Enlightenment in body, mind, intelligence and consciousness leads towards the conception of the Self. In yogic terminology this is known as *ātma-sākṣātkāra* or *Brahma-sākṣātkāra* as perception of the Self or the perception of the God.

Darśana means to look, perceive or behold clearly, thoroughly and completely. If the mirror has to reflect the object accurately, the mirror needs to be clear and clean. In the same way the body, with its components mind, intelligence and consciousness, also needs to be crystal clear and clean in order to have a clear reflection of the Self.

Body, organs, senses, mind, intelligence, ego, *citta* and conscience influence the self a great deal. Practice of yoga helps to minimise their influences and later when maturity dawns, one gets dissociated from their influences in order to sight the Self. This achievement is possible only through the track of practice *- abhyāsa -* and desirelessness *- vairāgya -* of the yogic *sādhanā.*

Here comes the question of alignment of the body and the mind with the self. Unless all these are aligned, cleansed and purified, divinity *- śuddhi sāmyatā -* seems a mirage.

This pure Self alone can equate itself with God. At that state one is at the peak of enlightenment and the light of the Self graces and spreads evenly from soul to sole and from sole to soul. At this stage the *darśana* of the Lord may be possible.

Let me not boost myself or be proud, but let me admit with humbleness that I had the sight of the Self, that remains fresh in my heart.

Q.- Is it possible to practise yoga with the diversification of the mind in daily life?

Yoga helps us to control our mind and emotions to a great extent. By regular practice of *āsana,* chronic diseases that are incurable by medication, can be healed or minimised. Excessive sexual desire can be controlled and energy can be diversified. Memory improves. Individuals with physical or mental problems are helped by regular practice of *āsana* and I have seen the changes. However what to practise is not the same for everybody even with problems that are the same. I decide on the sequence of *āsana* to be practised by the afflicted by assessing his/her capability.

As modern life has changed compared to ancient life, we are constantly under stress and strain. Speed has become a silent killer. The outer environment is affecting not only the human body but the mind too. Advertisements, movies and so forth distract the mind. All these cause diversification of the mind. The question is not only whether it is possible to do yoga in such circumstances. On the contrary it appears to have become necessary to do yoga so that one withdraws the mind from the above mentioned diversions and focuses within. By yogic practices, the scattered energy of the mind is brought into focus and then stored, channelled and directed in a right direction to lead a better life.

Yoga as scientifically codified by Lord Patañjali, in truth, is a wonderful way to live healthily as it helps to relieve physical and mental problems and builds up emotional stability.

A person can benefit from yoga in terms of physical balance – *śārīrika santulana,* right balance between the organs of action and the senses of perception – *eindriyaka santulana,* rhythmic movement of the breath – *prāṇika santulana,* mental balance – *mānasika santulana,* intellectual balance – *bauddhika santulana* – and equipoise in the Self, the soul – *ātmika santulana.*

Sir Yehudi Menuhin realised that if he wanted to improve his violin playing, he should learn some particular holistic method and the thought struck him to take to yoga. After completion of my course of *āsana* and *prāṇāyāma* he told me: "Sir, earlier I knew what to play on the violin and now, after practising yoga, I know how to play on the violin." He did not merely play the music as on the pages but played with renewed life. By practice of yoga one learns how to balance oneself with proper pressure in the various muscles, tissues, tendons and organs. This helped Menuhin to use his fingers and nerves with the required pressure to play the violin with ease, with effortlessness and in a natural way. With this yogic technique he conquered the world of music in a lively manner and reached the ultimate *siddhi* in his profession.

YOGA IN EDUCATIONAL INSTITUTIONS*

Dear Friend,

The government of Maharashtra has shown interest in introducing yoga as a form of instruction in educational institutions. As a valued personality in the field of yoga, your co-operation is earnestly solicited in framing the guidelines for submission to the Government for ultimate implementation.

This measure is taken as it is felt by me that your valued opinion in this regard may help to form a uniform course throughout the state of Maharashtra.

A special symposium for discussion on Yoga Education is to be held in the month of April '71 by the Friends of Yoga Society, on behalf of the Government of Maharashtra, where the subject of yoga will be discussed.

A questionnaire is furnished below for knowing your opinion on various relevant matters. It is also requested that you may give your suggestions, if any, separately.

It will be appreciated if the completed form of questionnaire is returned to me by the 1st of Feb. 1971 or earlier if possible.

Thanking you,

Yours in Yoga
(HANSRAJ YADAV YOGACHARYA)
FRIENDS OF YOGA SOCIETY – PUNE, Box No. 481

G.P.O. Bombay 1.

---

* Symposium of Yoga Education, April 1971.

QUESTIONNAIRE

Q.- What should be the aim and objective of teaching yoga in education?

The first aim and object of teaching yoga in educational institutions for me is to inculcate good, robust physical and mental health, healthy relationships with co-students and interest in the art.

Q.- Of what minimum age should the student be for receiving yoga education?

The minimum age to begin yoga as a play-game is seven years and above. For a serious process in practice they should be above fifteen or sixteen. However, simple, easy *yogāsana* can be taught at seven years of age to keep up the zeal in the art of yoga.

Q.- To whom should the teaching of yoga be entrusted: the PT[1] teacher, general teacher, or a special yoga teacher?

Initially, when yoga is to be introduced in the institutions, yoga practitioners alone have to take the responsibilities so that the subject is taught in the right perspective. However, the PT instructor or the teachers who have already acquired knowledge in the art of teaching and interested in yoga can be trained for three to six months under the able guidance of a yoga teacher so that they take the initial responsibilities for conducting such classes in their respective schools. However, they should be in touch with the yoga teachers, so that if any doubts arise, they are met and go back to teach with further confidence. As they are already well equipped in the art of teaching which is an advantage, training them as yoga teachers becomes easy. With this good background in the art of teaching the yoga teachers can build up how to start, how much to teach and give an over-all view of why they are taught.

It would be pertinent for me to mention here that since a year ago yoga is a subject approved by the London as well as the Greater London Educational Authorities under my guidance and I have taught and trained forty pupils of mine not only to practise but also how to teach other students. If I go again this year to England, I will take the PT instructors, make them undergo training themselves and guide them to teach yoga to the schoolchildren under my watchful eyes. This way they gain confidence and do not go wrong. This is for me ethics in yoga teaching.

---

[1] PT - physical training

Each year I guide them in the art of teaching the fineness that yoga demands and how a teacher is made to acquire further knowledge to go ahead with the pupils to ignite interest to become teachers later. I have also done this in the schools and colleges of Pune from 1937 to 1940.

Q.- From which class should yoga be taught?

When the child is able to understand the things that the teacher explains in simple language, then yoga can be conveniently taught. So, as far as my opinion is concerned, one can start teaching yoga to children from the age of seven. However, *āsana* has to be taught for a period of twenty minutes to half an hour just in a playful way, which can be incorporated within PT session. Later on, when they grow up, the sessions can be longer.

Q.- Which topics in yoga are essentially to be taught to students?

The yogis should descend in their thinking to the level of the children's intellectual calibre and then teach what the child needs. Children cannot accept serious yoga. This type is for adults. Children should be taught yoga that is congenial to them. They like quickness and variety. This not only builds will power but also memory and a state of healthy competition. My main aim is to create interest before I leap for higher status in yoga.

Q.- Should there be any gradation in teaching, like a special course for a certain standard and onward?

Yes, gradations have to be formulated. The institutions which engage teachers have to keep the candle of yoga burning by giving advanced courses when the pupils show improvement after a year or so. The syllabus[1] of yoga should be formulated according to the gradations so that it is taught accordingly during the class hours and that it advances progressively. For those who are genuinely interested to learn more on yoga and its philosophy, a special chair has to be created to impart specific philosophical thoughts on yoga, or allied subjects, as a way of life. In the universities, these special courses, with an educative syllabus on yogic philosophy, may be framed so that they can make a career in this field.

[1] Now I have formulated the syllabi, which are applicable from standard 5 to 12 in junior college. These syllabi are followed by Doon School, Welham School and St. Ann's School in Dehra Doon.

Q.- Which is the ideal time when yoga should be taught during teaching hours?

The best time to teach yoga is in the evenings. If it is during the class periods, it should be the last two periods. If the schools are in the mornings, it is better in the early mornings. It should be at least three hours after meals and a half-hour before meals. This is concerned only with the practical aspects of yoga.

Q.- How many hours should be devoted in a week to yoga lessons?

Three days a week or twice a week, with forty-five minutes to one hour duration, is quite sufficient to make boys and girls yoga-minded. This will keep them physically healthy and mentally alert.

Q.- How many students in maximum should be taken by a yoga teacher at a particular time?

One can begin with twenty students to start with. Along with the twenty students a few can be added later to learn the art of looking to one and all needs. Later more may be added. I have taken forty to fifty pupils at a time in a class when I was asked to teach by the educational authorities from 1937 to 1940, giving attention to one and all. It depends on the teaching calibre of the yoga teacher. He should be able to keep all the students alert while teaching.

However, these days one finds a class consisting of sixty to seventy students or even more. In that case the class can be divided into two groups with two teachers or two periods can be given alternatively to the groups with one day as PT and one day as yoga.

Q.- Could yoga be taught as co-education or should it be separate for boys and girls?

I have taught mixed classes to boys and girls in the co-educational schools as well as separately in girls' schools and boys' schools, I have also conducted classes for men and women separately and in clubs. Though I prefer teachers to teach separately for boys and girls, the days have changed and one has to be equipped to teach them jointly. Only the teacher should be clever, clear, clean in character and have a strong mind to keep the group under control and to win over mischief-mongers. I have conducted mixed classes as well as separately for girls and boys. If the girls want to practise separately, then provision should be made for separate classes.

Q.- Apart from *āsanas* what other parts of yoga should be taught?

For youngsters of school and college, *śarīra vidyā* – knowledge of human body – and *yogāsanas* are to be taught; as they grow, I am convinced that they will automatically take to the higher aspects of life.

Prāṇāyāma, dealing with ordinary correct deep breathing, can be introduced for secondary high school and college students. Retention of breath in *prāṇāyāma* can make the faces of youngsters grow old, so it is advisable not to teach until they reach the age of twenty to twenty-two years. Ethical discipline can easily be explained while the teacher is conducting *āsana* classes through stories so that the ideal background is cultivated to be followed in later years.

Q.- Do you think that *yogāsanas* can be taught under a general classification? If yes, what are the various classifications?

The classifications are to be made in such a way that children perform with ease and grasp the effect on their bodies and minds. They are to be sequenced according to the classification. However, while teaching, the *āsana* have to be chosen and graded from simple to complicated ones. For example the classifications may be made first with:

1) Standing *āsana* – *Uttiṣṭha sthiti*,
2) Sitting *āsana* – *Upaviṣṭha sthiti*,
3) Forward extension – *Paśchima pratana sthiti*,
4) Backward extension – *Pūrva pratana sthiti*,
5) Lateral twisting – *Parivṛtta sthiti*,
6) Inversions – *Viparīta sthiti*,
7) Body knotting *āsana* – *Grathan sthiti*,
8) Supine *āsana* – *Supta sthiti*,
9) Balancing *āsana* – *Bhujatolana sthiti*,
10) Resting *āsana* – *Viśrānta kāraka sthiti*.

The *āsana* from all these classifications are chosen from the simple to the complicated.

Q.- Should yoga be made compulsory or should it be optional?

When yoga teachers are not available, how can one think on lines of compulsion? To prove the efficacy of yoga, if I am in charge I will take those students who do the present-day physical training (PT) to try yoga also. I can prove that the efficacy of yoga is far greater than PT exercises.

I build up in students the alertness as well as the physical ability to endure the strain with ease. When the students feel that the effect of yoga is greater than PT, then I am sure that the demand to introduce yoga in the educational institutions will come not only from students but also from parents. Then the authorities have no other option but to accept the introduction of yoga in their schools and colleges.

Q.- What facilities should be provided in the campus for teaching yoga?

Facilities should consist of a clean room with an even floor and a big thick non-slippery carpet. Blankets should be provided for the comfort of the children. One or two schoolteachers should also join and learn to be able later on to take over the classes from the yoga teacher.

Q.- Do you suggest any follow-up like examinations, tests, evaluation, etc. If yes, please specify.

Tests on their progress should be conducted and the best student should be awarded a prize to keep up the interest in yoga. More prizes should be introduced as in other activities.

The examinations can be taken provided the subject is recognised and the marks are included in the totalling.[1]

Q.- Till such time as yoga is introduced in the teaching institutions, could a short-term course of yoga be introduced?

For me yoga teachers are not enough in abundance to introduce yoga at one stroke of the pen as a compulsory subject. A beginning has to be made and a short-term course of six months or one term is to be gladly accepted by yoga teachers. If the same pupils like to continue further for the second term, then qualitative training in what they were practising, should be added. It can also be introduced for ten or fifteen days during vacation as a vocational course, which may create interest in students. Youngsters want power, quickness in movement, lightness of body and mind, and yoga teachers should keep the youngsters active throughout the yoga class. For

---

[1] Now, yoga is recognised in the Indian Council for Secondary Certificate (ICSC) and they are examined from year 1998.

that reason the style of yoga to be taught has to be revolutionised to suit the present-day demand, i.e., short and sweet but firm and determined effort. I have taught for years in the National Defence Academy for the cadets as well as for the officers, and I feel that yogis have to change their methods to meet the demand of the present-day generation. Then only can yoga become a clear signal for introduction as part and parcel of the educational curriculum.

UNIVERSAL SUBJECT WITH MULTI-EFFECTS*

Q.- Is yoga a science or art?

Yoga is both, a science as well as an art. Where there is a "technique", there is science and where there is expression of form, beauty and grace, it is art. Yoga has its own technique of physiological, psychological and supramental well being of man. So it is a science. Like a musician who plays with his instrument, a student or an adept in yoga plays with his body, like music, depicting different forms of nature presenting Universal Consciousness. Or like a sculptor, who sculptures with his chisel and hammer, the yogi chisels with his body and mind and expands the consciousness.

For me, there is no art without philosophy and yoga is a live philosophy showing the right type of living with character building, in which the practitioner is drawn towards the shrine of divinity within himself. Truly it is indeed the art of living. Yoga does not express a view on life but shows the way of right living. Hence it is a science, an art and a philosophy.

Q.- Do you think that a scientific approach to yoga will lead to a better understanding among mankind?

It is not just by a scientific approach, but its application to live a better life certainly helps mankind to build up a good society and community.

Science, no doubt, is a boon to mankind. Its advancement has resulted in a great deal of benefits. Nevertheless, speaking on the domain of intellect, mind, consciousness, it has no limitations. It is here that the importance of yoga lies. The world of mischief and mistrust belongs to the tricky-mind. Hence I feel the necessity of a scientific approach and research to yoga as it has a vital contribution to make towards the creation of a climate for better friendliness, compassion and correct understanding of one with the other. Then the far more important application of yoga in daily life will definitely help mankind to a happier and healthier life.

---

* Interview by Arvind Mulla. Published in *Bhavan's Journal*, 15th April 1973.

Q.- But, Sir, to an ordinary mind, yoga means swallowing nails, drinking acid, gulping down snakes, walking on water, etc. Do you subscribe to this view of mysticism, magic and miracles?

Like anatomy and physiology, yoga is a practical science concerned with the subject of human development. There is no question of miracles. What appears as a miracle to an ordinary person, for a yogi is only the subtle manifestation of a well-established law in the realm of nature. For example, what seems as *samādhi* or super-conscious state of mind for a lay man, for a yogi it is but a different state of mind or consciousness in which death and life are experienced as one indivisible unit. To arouse the curiosity of men, miracles have their own value. However, the yogic texts warn the student of yoga of the dangers of the *siddhi* or the power to work miracles.

Walking on water, swallowing acids, nails, and so forth are possible.[1] It is not an impossibility. These powers are the result of certain specific *sādhanā*. A person after some practice in yoga acquires certain powers that he is tempted to use on a lay person either to impress him or to arouse faith in him. While attempting to be free from the control of the elements, he is unintentionally caught in the whirlwind. It is like a man who in order to escape a strong gust of wind rushes headlong into a cyclone. Such a practitioner is neither enlightened nor can he come back to his original state of that innocence he had while he was practising before he acquired the power.

A true aspirant must remember these are passing phases in the process of one's development to become an integrated whole person. It is the maturity of body, nerves, emotion and intellect which are important in order to acquire perfect consciousness.

Q.- Are you a *haṭha yogi* or a *rāja yogi*?

I am neither a *haṭha yogi*, nor a *rāja yogi*. I am only a yoga practitioner. It is not correct to demarcate yoga into artificial divisions, such as *haṭha yoga* or *rāja yoga*, except for theoretical purposes. Otherwise yoga is one.

The word *haṭha* is composed of two letters, *ha* and *ṭha*. *Ha* is the sun or positive electricity and *ṭha* is the negative electricity or moon. The union of the two generates bio-energy – *prāṇa śakti*. *Haṭha yoga* is a science that studies this subject of *prāṇa*. Just as electricity is felt or known

---

[1] Patañjali in *sūtra* III.40, *(Vibhūti Pāda)* says that by conquering the *udāna vāyu* a yogi can walk over water, mud and thorns since he can levitate easily. So walking on water is because of *udāna-jaya*. In III.41, he says that by conquering the *samāna vāyu*, a yogi gets control over the fire element. If the gastric fire which causes digestion is stoked, then a yogi can digest nails, snake venom, acid or anything. However, in spite of having *siddhi*, a yogi with the disciplines of *yama* and *niyama* would not attempt such ghastly things.

only when we switch on a light or a fan whereas for all practical purposes we are unaware of its existence, likewise bio-energy is also felt when *haṭha yoga* helps us to become aware of it. *Haṭha* also means will and *haṭha yoga* requires relentless practice, it is the triumph of will over matter.

Rāja means king. In *rāja yoga* the practitioner has to assiduously cultivate his nature and character by transforming the lower self into higher Self – the *rāja* or the Self. The body is the *kṣetra* or field. Just as a farmer cultivates his field, man needs his intelligence to cultivate and culture the body. The farmer is the *kṣetrajña* – the knower of the field or *puruṣa* who cultivates his *kṣetra* or field. This cultivated state is the state of a balanced personality in which the intelligence and emotion are well poised at all times without oscillation. This state of experience is called *rāja yoga;* while *haṭha yoga* treats *prāṇa* as a motivator for the consciousness to function and pays importance to control this energy so that the oscillating consciousness is quietened.

Hence the *sādhaka* has to follow both principles of *haṭha-yoga* and *rāja-yoga* to reach the Ultimate – *ātma-sākṣātkāra* – as both are intermingled and interwoven. Know that there is no *haṭha yoga* without *rāja yoga* and no *rāja yoga* without *haṭha yoga.*[1]

Q.- What are the basic requirements for the practice of yoga?

While Patañjali speaks of *śraddhā* – faith, *vīrya* – courage, *smṛti* – memory, *samādhi* – deep penetration and *prajñā* – uninterrupted awareness, as the basic requirements (see *Y.S.,* I.20), Svātmārāma in the *Haṭhayoga Pradīpikā* mentions *utsāha* – zeal, *sāhasa* – venture or enterprise, *dhairya* – courage, *tattva jñāna* – self-knowledge and *janasaṅga parityāga* – to remain aloof from the crowd as well as their comments regarding yoga, as essentials to practise yoga (*H.Y.P.,* I.16).

The will to do is the summum bonum of yoga. With progress in yoga, the senses are refined, the intellect becomes firm and the refineness develops. Fundamentally what is required is tenacity of purpose, "relentless practice" and complete faith in what one does.

Q.- Is it necessary to lead a celibate life in order to practise yoga? What I mean is, should one remain unmarried in order to practise yoga?

Sir, I am myself a married man and am a father as well. That should answer your question. It is we, as householders, who are in the midst of emotional temptations and are subject to the stresses and strains of family life who need yoga.

---

[1] Read *Aṣṭadaḷa Yogamālā,* vol. 2, sections II and III.

What about a *sannyāsin?* He may have renounced the family and the world. But to develop *vairāgya* – total renunciation – he knows that he too needs to practise yoga.

Celibacy does not mean just to remain unmarried. It implies overcoming desires and temptations. Therefore one needs yoga to control the mind.

Whether one is a *sannyāsi*, celibate or married, yoga ultimately is meant to control and sublimate the senses and mind of the aspirant. Yoga helps one to lessen one's desires and minimises attachments towards pleasant objects. Therefore, yoga is meant for one and all. Weakness and indulgence is human nature. No doubt, practice of yoga helps one to overcome one's weaknesses and indulgences.

Q.- What about dietetic discipline?

Diet is mainly determined by geographical conditions, such as climate, altitude, flora and fauna of a place. But my advice is – do not eat if the saliva does not spring from the mouth when food is brought before you. When the brain speculates with choice, it means the body does not need that food and if you persist in eating according to the choice of the tongue, it is an abuse of food and so non-nourishing.

As the saying goes, "As you sow, so shall you reap", what we eat influences our mind.

A non-vegetarian diet is not conducive to development of the mental and spiritual aspects of yoga. When an animal is lead to a slaughterhouse, does anyone study the terror, fear and anguish before it is slaughtered? This consequently changes the chemical composition of the animal's body, which is very disturbed. One eats this disturbed, perturbed, frightened and chemically changed flesh of the animal, naturally it affects the system and disturbs the harmony of one's body and mind.

The beauty of yogic practice is that if one practises regularly, with a right religious attitude in mind, one cannot relish non-vegetarian food at all. The body and mind both refuse impure food since the system does not accept it. Not only does it upset the chemicals of the body but also the thinking process of one's mind.

Q.- Is a belief in God essential for the practice of yoga? Have you seen God?

If I say yes, it is not going to remove your doubt about the belief in God. As regards belief in God, for me the very act of doing, and the art, is God. Hence, there is no scope for belief independent of action. I had the sight of God as I pray to Him in *saguṇa*[1] form.

[1] God, who is the treasure house of good, auspicious and divine qualities is considered as *saguṇa*. By worshipping such a God one's mind gets purified, since the consciousness imbibes such qualities.

Also know that seeing God is something like seeing one's own back. You can see your own back only in a mirror, and that too only a reflection of the back and not the actual back. The yogi says to feel the movements on the back while doing yoga. This in turn takes one to look within the mirror of one's own relationship, both with the external world of physical and psychical realities as well as one's own inner world – *cidākāśa*.

Yoga philosophy believes in God, Patañjali explains the splendour and geniusness of God. But he does not insist that the *sādhaka* should believe straight away in God and come to him for yogic knowledge. He asks the aspirants to develop faith in God so that they begin to realise and feel the existence of God. The question of essentiality of belief does not come first. It is a process of realisation. His very approach is to have God-realisation through Self-realisation.

Q.- Mr. Iyengar, you must have been practising yoga for the last thirty-five years, at least. May we know the circumstances under which you took to yoga?

For my present position in relation to yoga two factors are responsible. First my ill health, and secondly the challenge that my body refused to take up due to stiffness and aches, and my mind due to its incapacity. However I had a very strong will power in my weak body and feeble mind.

Since 1934, with the blessings of my *guru*, Shri T. Krishnamacharya of Mysore, I began for gaining health and am practising yoga now as my *dharma* and at the same time helping people who were affected with diseases but also guiding on its philosophical aspects. I used to practise for ten hours every day. Now I get so completely absorbed in yoga that I and yoga have become inseparable.

Q.- During your practice of yoga, you must have come across different physical maladies and mental illnesses. Would you name a few, giving duration of time taken to effect the cure? What psychological changes do you find amongst your students as a result of practice of yoga?

I mentioned earlier that I was the patient of tuberculosis, malaria, jaundice, and so forth. This weak body could not take the vigorous discipline and rigorous practice introduced by my guru. I suffered from severe body ache, backache, restlessness, heavy anal bleeding, constipation and so on. I overcame these physical problems as the practises became well established. However, I had a very strong will power though my body was weak and my mind feeble.

I have to thank God that I had no mental illness. As my will power was strong, I never surrendered myself to human weaknesses. God protected me throughout.

To mention but a few of the ailments cured by me through yogic practices, I would say arthritis, slipped-disc, polio deformities, injuries due to war or accident, insomnia, glandular mal-secretion, appendicitis, heart-troubles, nervous break-down, nephritis, viral infection of the spine, and so forth. I have treated these ailments in India and abroad. During my recent visit to Mauritius, I had a case of cancer. The doctors were amazed. After the operation the doctors insisted that the patient continue the yoga exercises under my direction and thereby she was able to regain control of her bladder. I treated a similar case in London, doctors also referred this case to me.

In Pune a very well known doctor brought to me a patient suffering from spinal fluid in the lumbar region. I am happy to state that the patient is now completely cured. A few years back I treated a case of multiple fractures of the elbow. After the operation the elbow remained at a right angle. She came to get back her mobility and movement and by the grace of yoga got what she wanted. Now she conducts yoga classes not only in Bangalore but also in the West. Her surgeon who operated on the elbow too, referred her to me.

As regards duration, it may be one month or one year depending on several factors, especially the constitution of the patient and the degree of co-operation the patient gives.

The last part of your question should be addressed to the students themselves. In my own case the refinement is so marked that words fail to express the benefits. The mental changes that have taken place in me are immeasurable. If you ask some of my senior pupils who studied under me twenty to thirty years back, they will tell you of the changes that have taken place not only in me but in them also.

Q.- Then, according to you, yoga has a therapeutic value. How far is this contribution of yoga recognised in the world of medicine?

As I have already told you in my reply to your last question, doctors in the West have already recognised the therapeutic value of yoga, mainly because there the patients as well as the doctors have a scientific bent of mind and give me complete co-operation.

Unfortunately in India the concern is more with the supernatural rather than the therapeutic effects of yoga. But a beginning has been made and some experiments are going on at several Institutes.

Q.- Is yoga your mission or a vocation?

It is neither. I am attached to yoga and I am still at the experimental level, trying better in *āsana, prāṇāyāma* and *dhyāna* practices in their minutest detail.

Q.- I think your book *Light on Yoga* mentions different types of diseases and the curative *āsana* for these diseases. Don't you feel, a cheaper edition would enable more people to benefit by your book?

It is true that the price is rather high, mainly because of over six hundred photographs. In order to meet the popular demand a paperback edition has been released which is reduced by thirty-three per cent and an abridged edition is expected to be out soon.[1]

Q.- Please tell us the technique of Transcendental Meditation.

Meditation is one. There is no such thing as transcendental meditation. Do you think meditation is like a trans-world airline? The raising of consciousness from one set of conditioning to another is the objective in meditation. This process is itself transcendental. When all conditioning ceases to operate for the meditator, then there is no meditation separate from the object of meditation or the meditator.

For the practice of meditation the best *āsana* is either *Padmāsana* or *Svastikāsana*. One has to sit straight aligning the central line from the perineum to the middle of the throat and the crown of the head. The eyes are closed and drawn in towards the seat of the mind, i.e., heart-intelligence, or *manas cakra*.[2] The spine must be absolutely erect and alert, but the brain must be made to remain quiet. The eyes, being nearer to the brain, are like the windows of the brain as they reflect all the activities of the brain through their expressions. Ears are the windows of the mind, which is the dwelling house of consciousness. Movement of consciousness is felt only through sound. Sound is in space. *Cidākāśa* is the inner space, the space of consciousness and ears have the faculty of listening to the sound of consciousness.[3]

---

[1] The new edition of the *Illustrated Light on Yoga*, Harper Collins, London, is now available.
[2] Please see vol. 2, pl no. 6. In that diagram the *manas chakra* is situated just below the *anāhata cakra*.
[3] See the author's *Light on Yoga*, p. 461, and *Light on Prāṇāyāma*, chapter 29, pp. 224-231.

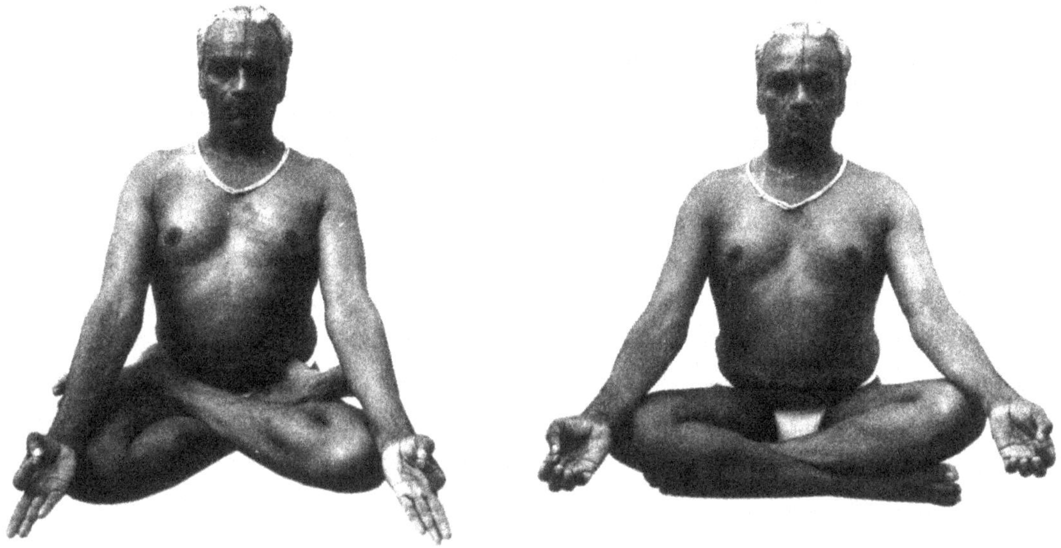

Plate n. 1 – *Padmāsana* and *Svastikāsana*

To still that sound, the movements of consciousness must be stilled. The ears must be deliberately withdrawn from the external sound and directed inwards, to listen to the sound within. The moment the ears are drawn inwards to listen to the vibration of consciousness, the consciousness gets disciplined and quietness sets in and stillness is secured. From that stillness, silence is brought in, which Patañjali describes as *citta vṛtti nirodha*. To attain this state is meditation. You may call it transcendental or whatever you prefer.

Q.- Do you have hippies as your followers?

No. Often they come to my class to join, but they see the discipline I demand and they never come back. For them freedom is misunderstood. They think freedom is licence to act as they like. Whereas freedom comes after discipline, it is the end of discipline, which later urges one to action from the inner voice. Freedom comes when the disciplined action is converted with rigorous discipline into a natural action.

Q.- What is your opinion about teaching yoga in schools and colleges in India?

It is an excellent idea. But unfortunately Indians live in their past glory. Brawn is ignored. Consequently we have imbalance in development and bad health results. I think yoga should form an essential part of education. I would add that no University degree be given to the coming generation, unless they have a perfectly healthy body and mind. But of course all this depends upon the Ministry of Education.

Maj. General Habibullah, whom I had cured of amoebic dysentery, also made me teach yoga to cadets and officers of the National Defence Academy, Khadakwasla, for three years.

It is also necessary to distinguish between yoga and other types of physical education, mass drill, etc. I had the pleasure of introducing yoga for the first time in schools and colleges in 1937. I taught in several schools in the early days of my career. In those days many yogis opposed me, but school authorities recognised the importance of yogic education. Basically the syllabus of yoga for school children has to be thought of carefully.[1]

Q.- Then why was yoga discontinued at the Defence Academy?

After Maj. General Habibullah's transfer I was informed that due to want of funds, they had to discontinue yoga classes.[2]

Q.- Could you tell us something about the teaching of yoga in foreign countries?

In 1969 the Adult Education Scheme of the Inner London Education Authority introduced yoga under my guidance and direction. Every year I train teachers to conduct classes under this scheme and I certify them to be accepted as teachers to teach yoga in these classes. In July 1971 my student in Brighton started the B.K.S. Iyengar Yoga Institute under my direction, to teach yoga and to train teachers in yoga. There are similar organisations in London, Bath, Leeds, Bristol and Manchester in England. Then there are classes run by my students in Paris, Brussels, Munich, Gstaad in Switzerland, Breda in Holland, Florence, Venice and Rome in Italy; Cape Town, Johannesburg, Pretoria and Natal in South Africa; Michigan in USA; Colombo in Ceylon, Waikato in New Zealand; Perth and Toowang in West Australia, and Mauritius.

---

[1] See *Aṣṭadaḷa Yogamālā*, vol. 3, sect VI & VII "Yoga in Schools", and "Yoga for Sports Persons and Athletes"; see also this vol., "Yoga in Educational Institutions", pp. 25.

[2] The National Defence Academy had discontinued yoga classes, but in 1973 they started again and continued until 2001.

In fact the classes conducted under the inner London Education Authority are over-subscribed. I had to divide my usual class of two and a half-hours into two classes of an hour and a quarter, in order to accommodate more and more students.[1]

This year I was also asked to prepare a syllabus for the second year to a sixteen year group; I have prepared the syllabus purely for bodily growth and poise alone, as the group is too young for philosophic considerations of yoga.

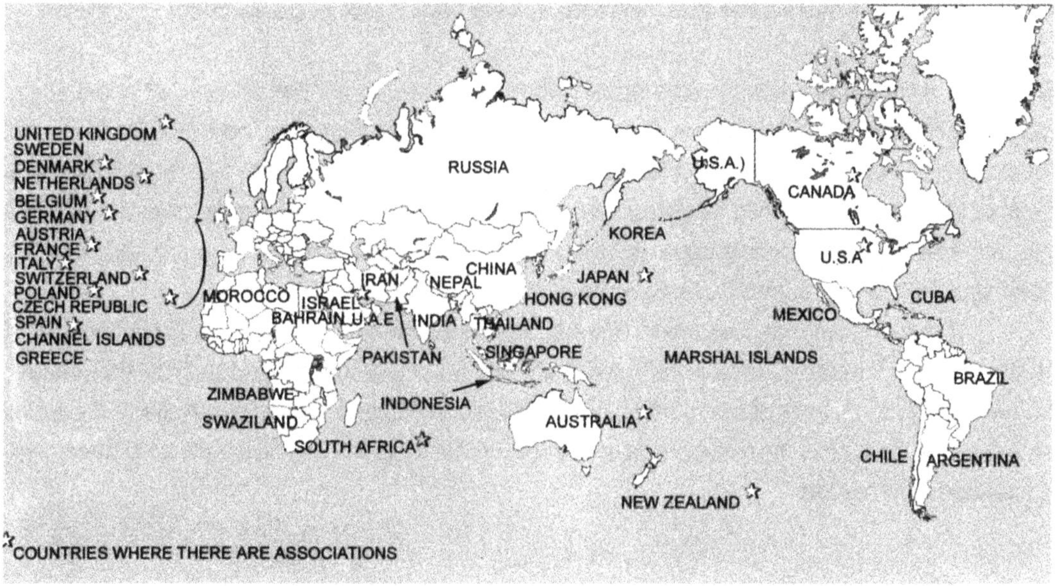

Plate n. 2 – World map of Iyengar Yoga Associations

Q.- What do you think about the World Yoga University?

Well, that is the laborious and painful birth of an institution of worldwide importance which took place in New Delhi last December. When the World Conference on Scientific Yoga was held under the presidentship of Christopher Hill, the founder of Christ Yoga Centre in London, according to the latest report, it was accepted that the University will be most probably situated somewhere in the USA. In fact enrolment of students has already started. I am the Chairman of the Committee on Yoga Teaching, Propagation of Yoga and Social Aspects of Yoga.

---

[1] Now there are many yoga institutes and centres all over the world, many countries have B.K.S. Iyengar Yoga Associations.

The University will serve a very useful purpose if all those who come to it are devoted to yoga and come with an open mind and humble heart. I do hope a true scientific spirit guides its deliberations so that a uniform approach in technique and theory will be maintained which will be clear, precise and at the same time helpful to the needy public. (But the idea fizzled out as years went by).

Q.- So yoga has entered the international sphere. But is not yoga exclusively Indian?

Sir, can a science or mathematics accept such nationalistic thinking? Are not science and mathematics universal? Is there American electricity? Or Russian cancer? Or European tuberculosis? Yoga may have originated in India but it belongs as much to a man in Moscow, Sydney, London or New Delhi. Yoga is for all men, women and children irrespective of race, class, gender, colour, country, language or religion. Yoga after all aims at a union of individual consciousness with Cosmic Consciousness.

A man's physique, nature and needs are the same whether he lives in the East, West, North or South. Therefore, yoga is definitely a Universal Culture as it helps to satisfy the needs of human beings in all parts of the world. Why should you consider it exclusively Indian? The Indian sages themselves who practised yoga and wrote about it did not intend it only for Indians. They addressed all mankind.

MY AIM IS TO SPREAD THE KNOWLEDGE OF YOGA*

He has taught yoga to Yehudi Menuhin, Clifford Curzon, Jeddu Krishnamurti, Jayaprakash Narayan and G.S. Pathak. Last January an ultra-modern Yoga Foundation was set up in Pune out of funds collected in India and abroad. Built in memory of B.K.S. Iyengar's late wife Ramāmaṇi, the Foundation will attract yoga buffs from all over the world.

Q.- How and when was your interest in yoga aroused?

I was a sickly teenager – weighing forty to fifty pounds with an eighteen to twenty inch chest and a top-heavy head – a suspected case of tuberculosis and a burden to my family. In sheer desperation, I went from Bangalore to Mysore – to my sister's husband, Shri Krishnamacharya, who was the head of the *yogaśālā* patronised by the Maharaja of Mysore. There I began to practise a few *yogāsana* under his guidance.

Q.- Did yoga help your physical condition?

It was a hard and long struggle. I had no confidence in yoga. But I persisted as I was more or less down and out financially and I thought perhaps something of a career as a performer of yoga might result from my effort. Fortunately it did. My physical condition improved considerably and I gained in confidence to live.

---

* Interview by P.R. Shinde, published by *The Illustrated Weekly of India*, May 25th, 1975.

Q.- Why did you choose Pune as your place of work?

Sheer coincidence. My *guru* and I were giving a yoga demonstration at Belgaum in 1936. Mr. V.B. Gokhale, the civil surgeon, saw our performance and was impressed. He asked us to teach students of schools and colleges in Pune at the Deccan Gymkhana. My *guru* decided to send me to Pune. The initial contract was for six months. Subsequently it was extended to three years. After the stint, I was on my own.

Q.- Why do you think yoga is superior to other systems of physical culture?

Yoga is *sarvāṅga sādhanā*. Yoga aims at developing and keeping in good order our muscles, bones and glands; our nervous system, respiratory system and circulation. The other systems aim at physical development only. Weightlifting, for example, can help develop muscles and nothing else.[1]

Q.- Why are Westerners more interested in yoga than Indians?

The popular misconception about a yogi in this country is that of a recluse or a *sannyāsi* sitting cross-legged in a mountain-cave or on the riverbank. Now yoga does not mean running away from life or its problems. In fact, yoga gives one the strength to face life squarely. Misconceptions about yoga persist in the West too. I was once asked by the custom's men at London airport if I could swallow pound coins or walk on fire! The West is now realising yoga could be the answer to the stress and strain of their life-style.

Unfortunately even Indians have forgotten that yoga was presented to us by our sages and yogis as a way of life. Secondly, our present generation is attracted to the western way of life more than our way of life. And some feel that yoga, being a philosophy, has no place in practical day to day life.

This picture will change as our people begin to know the constricting problems they face in life and how it will help them to cleanse themselves through the method of yoga.

Therefore, the question if Westerners are more interested than Easterners, is not correct. In fact both the hemispheres are interested in yoga. It is the misconception on yoga that creates confusion in them and takes them away from the practicality.

---

[1] See *Aṣṭadaḷa Yogamālā*, vol. 3, section VII.

Q.- Is yoga the answer to tensions created by modern life?

Certainly. For a relaxed and tranquil state of mind and body, there are excellent *yogāsana* like *Śavāsana*. I am glad heart specialists have started recommending this *āsana* to their patients.

Q.- When other medicines have failed them, do a lot of people seek your help as a last resort?

Quite a few come to me as a last resort – especially physical wrecks and the mentally disturbed or frustrated people. Of course, in such cases, it is first necessary to create confidence in them and help them face their problems.[1]

Q.- Do you insist on your students being vegetarians, non-smokers and non-drinkers?

Not at all. I cannot force my ideas of discipline straightaway on them. The change has to come gradually. As they keep on practising yoga, the body-system and mental thinking begins to change. But I have found that most of them voluntarily give up these things. The inner system rejects wrong food and drinks. The lungs refuse to accept the tobacco smoke. The practitioner one day has to give up either yoga or the above habits. Mostly he will stick to yoga and give up wrong things in life.

Q.- Some yogis claim to stop their heartbeat for some time and others to seal themselves in closed chambers. What is the point of such experiments?

This is not yoga and gives a bad name to the science. These tricks are meant to impress the gullible public – just as some *gurus* or *svāmis* produce ash from their hair. You know what happened to that much-publicised experiment of walking on water in Mumbai.[2] My concern is to keep an average man healthy in body and mind.

---

[1] See *Aṣṭadaḷa Yogamālā*, vol. 3, section II.

[2] This refers to a yogi in Mumbai who collected lots of money to walk on water; he sank.

Q.- Have any of your students been on narcotics?

Very few. The practice of yoga can take you to such a state of exhilaration that there is no need for LSD. In this connection, one of my students, who teaches yoga in a county school in England, narrated an experience. The school had engaged her to get rid of some of the boys' addiction to drugs. She succeeded. There was some hitch in her contract and the school authorities had to terminate her service. The boys took to drugs again. She had to be re-engaged.

Q.- What do you hope to achieve with your Yoga Foundation?

Here students from all over the world will learn yoga. Also, those who want to, will be trained to teach yoga. In general, my aim is to spread the knowledge of yoga all over the world.

Q.- Do you think if politicians were to practise yoga, our country would be a better place?

Why only politicians? The whole world would be a better place, for yoga essentially is for peace and harmony.

INTERVIEW BY GERMAN TV*

Q.- Mr. Iyengar, you are an internationally very well-known teacher of yoga. You've taught all over the world, not just in India. What exactly is yoga, in a very few words?

If you want me to condense the meaning of yoga, then, traditionally yoga is the method of stilling the movements or the inner wavering of the consciousness so that the individual self is experienced. Then yoga is to unite the individual self with the Universal Soul. In short, yoga is the union of the body with the mind, and mind with the self and then the self with God.

Q.- Now why is there all of a sudden so much interest in Indian culture and mystique? Why do all these Westerners come here to study yoga?

Well, as far as I understand, I think the technological and scientific advancement as well as modern comforts have not given what we call "inner joy", or "inner peace". Only yoga, as a subjective science, deals totally and entirely with one's own body, mind and self. Hence, people not only in the West but also in the East have turned their mind to yoga to see whether they can get that inner harmony, poise and peace.

Though India is the origin of yogic science, as a science yoga is universal. The philosophy of yoga is applicable to the whole of humanity without the basics of class, caste, creed, gender, colour or race.

Yoga is a culture of mankind. Hence, it is applicable, adoptable, attainable and adaptable to inner peace, inner joy, happiness, satisfaction and spiritual contentment.

---

* Pune, November 1977.

Q.- Is yoga something to do with magic or mystery, or some kind of occult thing?

Yoga has nothing to do with what you hear, but it is a pure discipline in order to achieve the highest pinnacle in one's life.

It is true that through the practice of yoga, when the elemental body, the senses of perception, mind, intelligence, 'I'-ness and consciousness all are trained, disciplined, controlled, tamed and transformed to that state of consciousness, super-natural powers are the result. Each of these yield special powers in the form of occult or mystical powers as each of them reaches the highest and purest state of its existence. Obviously they serve the purpose of their existence. But the aspirant has to go beyond all these to experience the real and pure state of existence.

Q.- Many people say that yoga can cure psychological and physical illnesses. Is that true?

Yes. You know, the practice of yoga is basically meant to release the physical, physiological, emotional and intellectual tensions built up in the nervous system. It helps to cure or minimise fluctuations and stress. The nerves are considered by the yogis as the "unconscious mind". Yoga plays a major role in order to keep all the systems of man in an entirely healthy state, and as such it is bound to be a curative subject also.

Q.- What is the difference between yoga and gymnastics? Or would you say it could be achieved by gymnastics too?

How can yoga, which works from the body to the sight of the soul, be achieved by gymnastics, which are just physical or conative? No. The differences between yoga and gymnastics are many: yoga is a subject where you have to think and use your intelligence to work, re-work and see how the body is used as an agent of the self, whereas in gymnastics, it is only a spectacular presentation of a muscular build, without penetrating or touching the inner intelligence or the self. Secondly, yoga is an all-round action. It deals with the body, the mind, the intelligence, the reason and the self, whereas gymnastics is treated as an exercise only on muscular aspects, beyond that there appears to be nothing. You do not see an inner evolution in gymnasts, whereas in a yoga practitioner the intelligence becomes sharp and hence evolution of growth at all levels is felt.

Q.- Now, there are a lot of secret things about yoga. We know that there are different kinds of yoga. Especially about *tāntric* yoga, why is there all this kind of mystery?

It is not a question of mystery. There is no mystery in yoga. In olden days, when this subject was taught, they used to keep this subject as a secret one, because it was treated as a sacred subject. So being a sacred subject, they wanted to keep it as far as possible for the pupils who were ripe in understanding the emotional and intellectual aspects of life. So it became a secret subject. Actually it is a sacred and not a secret subject.

Yoga is one but it has branched out into names as God is one but called by various names.

Q.- Do you feel that people from the West are capable of understanding and accepting yoga, *tāntric* yoga, meditation and things like that?

I do not think of the word *tāntric* as you think. For me *tantra* is a technique with a scientific treatise. It is a practical right royal path. See, if you demarcate yoga, then the problem of strife has to come. We cannot demarcate *dharma*. We cannot demarcate God, so we cannot demarcate yoga. But, in order to achieve, there is a tremendous discipline. There should be no demarcation of personal or emotional problems as they are the same whether it is East or West. Yoga is a subject in which you begin to feel from within your own existence, that is the Self. It is a process in which the body challenges the mind and the mind challenges the body; and then the body and mind together challenge the self. These challenges are required because there is a communication gap between the body, the mind, the intelligence and the self. Practice of yoga closes this communication gap between self and body and brings integration between the agents of the self and the Self and make them commune with each other.

If you think that *tāntric* yoga is a magical or opportunistic expedient method of rituals to charm or to influence people, then it is not yoga at all. Yoga essentially has to bring Self-realisation to the practitioner.

Q.- There are a lot of people in the West trying to exploit yoga for sexual purposes.

Is it the fault of yoga? Yoga does not proclaim to be a practice for sexual enjoyment.

You know, my friend, almost all arts, almost all sciences and all philosophies, have both sides of the coin. It may be viewed as amusement, as abuse, or as emancipation. I can say that only a very small number of *sādhaka* practise religiously for spiritual upliftment. Therefore, it depends on the temperament of a person, and hence it is not the fault of the subject but the *sādhaka*.

Q.- Would you condone this?

It is not a question of condoning it. To err is human. It happens because of human weakness, so naturally, they need training and education, which depend upon the teacher who lives and leads his life on the principles of ethical living for the practitioners to follow.

Q.- Now, yogis and *gurus*, would you consider yourself a *guru*?

Well, I do not know whether I am a *guru*, but people call me a *guru*. May be it is because of the way I teach and practise and live as far as possible in the yogic way of life, that most people call me *Gurujī*.

Q.- OK. What is a *guru* supposed to be?

First of all, the word *guru* is composed of two words: *gu* and *ru*. *Gu* means ignorance or inadvertence and *ru* means knowledge or advertence. One who brings advertence, enlightens and illuminates a pupil from his ignorance towards light and wisdom is called a *guru*.

Pupils who accept the *guru* have to rub along with the teacher. The pupils have to find out themselves. They have to live with the teacher to understand his calibre, his ways of living, his modes and so forth. Intellectuals of today are like political people. So, we should not be carried away by intellectual talks. We have to rub along with them to find out what they are preaching, what they practise and how they live. As long as one does not see what they preach is practised, they cannot be called *gurus*. People are carried away by the magnificent word of 'the *guru*'. In my *sādhanā*, I have no words but actions. Actions cannot magnify but words magnify. My teaching is from my direct practice which I experience and share with my pupils.

Q.- So you are a *guru*. There are lots of *gurus* in India. It is very famous for *gurus* and so on. In *Pune* there is a very famous *guru*.[1] What exactly is your opinion, not of the man, but of his teachings?

You know, being a student of yoga and being a student of spiritual life, it is very unfair on my part to speak against anybody. If you question me to criticise someone by my opinion, I cannot do it. If you ask about what I am doing, I think I have answered you already on this point.

Q.- How do you see the future of all this influence of Westerners coming into India? Is it a good sign of co-operation between cultures in the East and the West?

Humanity is one. We should not demarcate East and West. You are made up of similar feelings, similar emotions, whether you are from the East or West, North or South. The emotions may vary in degrees from individual to individual, but all have emotions, intelligence and a search from the finite towards the infinite. We have to adopt yoga which is akin to all mankind, without denying that it has come from the East. But, nowhere do the texts say that it is meant for only Easterners. Yoga is for the elevation of man, whether he belongs to the East, West, South or North. So one should not demarcate geographically concerning yoga.

Q.- Yoga is not a religion as such?

If you put this question of religion to me, well, I say that one should know what religion is. See, it is a very delicate question. First of all we have to realise that self-study involves religiousness in practice. No doubt yoga is a spiritual *sādhanā*, a spiritual practice. It is a way of living. The moment one starts practising, the experiences that sprout make one start living a right life and doing right duties. So the word religion comes only when a person starts living and practising in a right way, which are nothing but the signs of religiousness. So signs of religion being realisation of how to live a righteous and virtuous life and utilise one's life for the betterment of our own self-advancement, then it cannot be said that it is not a religion.

---

[1]Bhagwan Shri Rajneesh, Osho

YOGA: THE POWER FOR TURNING IMAGINATION INTO FACT*

Mr. Iyengar is regarded as the most remarkable exponent of yoga alive today. In India he has been unofficially titled Matsyendra – Shiva's own pupil, and Yogiraj – King of Yogis.[1] *His innumerable admirers and pupils throughout the world know him as an unequalled performer, a rigorously demanding teacher and also as a warm and fun-loving friend.*

He is the author of the best-selling Light on Yoga *available internationally and in many languages and he has just published his autobiography. His application of yoga technique to health problems is widely known and his patience and generosity with this help is legendary.*

It was Odyssey's *great privilege to interview him on his recent and first visit to Cape Town. The local committee of the International Yoga Teachers' Association had planned a fairly tight schedule for him and we were fortunate in being able to join Mr. Iyengar as he was about to enjoy a walk through Cape Town's lovely Botanical Gardens at Kirstenbosch.*

Q.- It's a very wonderful surprise to see you in Cape Town, and a big welcome to you. It's a suprise because the last time the issue of your coming to South Africa was raised, there was, I remember, a problem, I think from your own government, about getting permission to come. What was the story there?

When my pupils invited me to come to South Africa I requested them to mention clearly about the payment. You know that I am a family man and for the maintenance of my family in India I need money. And when that question arose they thought that being a yoga teacher, I was charging people and that would be against the international trade practice. Then I applied in writing for the visas and this dragged on for about nine years. When my pupil Joyce Stuart wrote to me saying that she would be opening the Institute I took the opportunity and the court gave permission for me to visit South Africa.

---

* Interview by Aubrey Meyer. Published by the South African magazine *Odyssey*, vol. 3, no. 6, Nov./Dec. 1979.

[1] Swami Shivananda of Rishikesh called him "Matsyendranath" and gave him the title *Yogiraj* in 1952.

Q.- That's marvellous. Was there never any difficulty from the South African side?

No, no, there was no difficulty at all from this end.

Q.- And so this particular visit was to open Joyce's *āśram?*

Yes. It was a wonderful and auspicious occasion. Now people will dedicate themselves to the art more and more.

Q.- I believe that it's modelled very closely on your own institute in *Pune.*

Not exactly 'closely'. The main hall of Pune is exactly the same as here![1]

Q.- I would like to ask you a bit about your earlier life and how yoga became for you what it is today; what were the sort of origins?

Well, when I started, I started only from a health point of view. It was suspected that I had tuberculosis and later developed typhoid, malaria and all sorts of things. Naturally I was almost a lost product to the world. Somehow or other destiny took me to the art of yoga and slowly by its practice I began gaining health, and gradually people insisted that I should teach. So my art of teaching and practice went together and there was very little interval between the two. When people started getting interested more and more, I had to work naturally hard to go into the depth of the subject, and that depth of working into the subject enlightened me.

Q.- When did you first come to the West with yoga? And what prompted that?

It was in 1952 when Mr. Menuhin, the world-famous violinist, visited India at the request of the Prime Minister. It was his first visit because he had determined that he would only visit when India got independence. Due to the heavy schedule of concerts he had given during the war he had lost some control over himself and over his instrument, and he was searching for someone who could guide him, who could help reshape his playing, and luckily a pupil of mine suggested my name and I taught him, which had a successful bearing on his playing.

[1] The Main Hall of the R.I.M.Y.I., Pune, has been extended (in 2003), and is now considerably larger than before.

Q.- Yes, I remember it was of great benefit to him – he still practises?

Yes, still practises. He invited me to teach and that was how the seed of yoga was planted on the European continent in 1954.[1]

Q.- And now twenty-five years later?

It is like a gigantic tree that has grown all over Europe.

Q.- How many people are now practising?

Well, it has grown like a Banyan tree and not less than two hundred-thousand people the world over have adopted the system that I developed.

Q.- Is there a reason, do you think, why people tend to go for yoga, and in particular for your sort of yoga?

Man's character is to find something new, something fresh, and something dynamic and revolutionary. As many took to the yoga of my way of doing, they found a change in their health and well being. As certain changes took place in them, they began telling their friends and relatives to go for yoga as it had changed them. From this point of view this was a new evolution in yoga. As they found the change from the point of physical and mental health, members increased attendance. Religion is often equated with going to the church or the temple but here, though they may not go to the churches or the temples, the younger generation had a feeling to try yoga in order to discover the essence of life. In the search for the spiritual essence many turned to yoga as yoga fulfils the aspiration of each individual, and it began gaining ground. Man thinks in terms of himself before he thinks in terms of others. So I brought to their notice this practical subject which made their consciousness develop within themselves. This later spread like a whirlwind from frontier to frontier.

Q.- Some people say that yoga is a religion, but it's almost bigger than a religion, it's more far reaching.

---

[1] Lord Yehudi Menuhin died in 1999.

First of all the word *dharma* has no English equivalent. *Dharma* is that which up-holds, supports and sustains the human race. *Dharma* is a science of duty or a way to live a righteous life. But it is termed as religion. Whatever the word may be, its meaning is to live righteously. In the same sense yoga is branded as religion, because its origin is found in India through the *Veda*. The unfortunate thing is the poverty of intelligence that brands yoga as a religion of the East. We do not say yoga is religion. For us it is a philosophy of life. Just as a coin has two sides, so has yoga. You may call yoga a religion or call it self-culture, it is a discipline for one's well being. Though it starts with the cult of the body, it is for the culture of the self. Know that one man's culture can change a civilisation. For instance, take Jesus Christ, or Mahavira or Gautama Buddha or Krishna. Each one changed the life of man according to their time. The change in civilisations does not come through a group of efforts, but through one man's effort. When one man reaches enlightenment, a tremendous change takes place in civilisation; Christ's enlightenment brought Christianity, Mahavira's enlightenment brought Jainism, Buddha's enlightenment brought Buddhism, so it is in this art of yoga.

I have worked on the alignment of muscles and balance of energy, by which the steady balance of the intelligence is brought about. This concept was lost because of the break in links, especially in the practice of *āsana*, *prāṇāyāma* and *dhyāna*. So the evolution which took place in me is providing slowly a standard as well as a direction for many people to follow. This method of one man's practice has been transforming into the system of yoga as civilisation *(Laughter)*. So yoga is not a religion in the sense you asked but it embraces everything of life. We can easily call it a religion of the universe. You and I are made up of the same stuff. You have got physical problems, I have got physical problems; you have got mental problems, I have got mental problems; you have intellectual problems, I have also intellectual problems; you are seeking the truth, I am also seeking the truth. So in this sense, I say, it is a culture of the self. And it is a universal religion as long as you do not dominate with colours. 'Colours' means: Oh, it is a Hindu religion, it's a Christian religion. Let us not give yoga a religious colour. Let it be a religion of humanity.

Q.- This was something I wanted to ask you. Is it not really a peculiarly Indian discipline?

No, no. According to our ancient texts, religion is defined as *patitam patatam patiṣchantam dhārayati iti dharmaḥ*.[1] "That which uplifts, supports and upholds a person who is falling, has fallen, or may be in a state of falling physically, mentally, morally and spiritually." In one sense this definition may hold good as religion.

---

[1] *Mahābhārata.*

Q.- Anywhere, any place . . . whatever . . .?

Yes. So if you take its meaning the way we have been advised to follow, then it has no barriers. Right thinking, right acting, right living – has no barriers. We all have different viewpoints and different ways of thinking. If you look at a mountain, at the cut of the stone, you see each side has got a different facet. But on the top there is no difference at all. Yet the facets are changing. So in all religions, some changes take place due to environment or geographical conditions. Truth is one and God is one. It is man who gives different names and forms to God. It is the same man who gives different colours to religion. But the truth, as one, cannot vary, so if understanding varies, it means it is not truth. But when you reach the state where your way of thinking and my way of thinking are the same, you have come to the pinnacle, the goal – the experience becomes the same and the truth too is felt as one.

Q.- And that's the result of the correct practice of yoga?

Yes. That cannot change or vary at all. At the perfection of *sādhanā*, experiences felt by all should be the same at the end. But if you say that according to your experience you have this, and I say, according to my experience I have that, it means that we have not reached the final state of truth at all. We are still individuals practising on our wavelengths of the mind. The moment one has reached the peak one sees surroundings around as well as everything evenly. When one reaches that highest peak, the barriers do not exist any more as individuality disappears and all become one.

Q.- I want to backtrack a little. You spoke earlier of your method being – and you used the words very carefully – the 'cult' of the body. And I think, in my small experience of the subject, there is a tremendous amount of misunderstanding on this very point. People are inclined to think that self-realisation or enlightenment is something that can be imagined, something you can create in your mind.

First of all the body, mind, intelligence, all these are the instruments for Self-realisation and they have a great role to play in this process. The *Muṇḍaka Upaniṣad* says, "A weakling cannot reach the Soul." As far as the imagination is concerned, it is the key to go ahead. Imagination has two qualities, constructive and destructive. Imagination, where no effort is made to work on the ideas, is destructive. This kind of imagination is futile thinking. Either you have to have a direct perception, or you have to work out your imagination to find out whether that imagination is a fact or not. The moment the imaginative idea, through your action, becomes a fact it is constructive and you are progressive.

Q.- So it's not enough to work only with your imagination?

How can you work? Imagination is only an idea. The idea has to be made into a fact, and the moment it becomes a fact the imagination disappears. It becomes direct perception. The idea of imagination has to be directly perceived and experienced. When you are hungry or thirsty just the imagination of taking food or water does not quench. They are quenched only by having food and water, it is the same with Self-realisation. Idle imagination has no value. It has value when you put that into practice, face trials and errors to reach where these two get automatically eliminated.

Q.- So your way of reinforcing that search to develop the original inspiration as it were, is to use the body – do I understand correctly?

No, it is not only a question of using the body. The body is part and parcel of the self, is it not? Isn't it an outer sheath of the self? So how can you differentiate when the self uses its own sheath – the body – as an instrument for progression? As I said earlier about religion, here too the moment the individual differentiates body from the self without realising its great service to the self, he creates a barrier within himself and creates a battlefield between the body and the self. Therefore, creating barriers between the body, the mind and the self does not lead towards solution. The body and mind are there to serve the self, therefore you need to culture them all.

Q.- Do you feel that people who practise yoga, who don't practise the total discipline, are bluffing themselves?

May be. Spirituality is not a discursive or theoretical subject. It is not imaginative either. It is an experiential subject. It has to be followed and practised with faith and determination. The disciplines as explained in the *Yoga Sūtra* have to be adopted and absorbed. This adoption and absorption is nothing but yoga.

Q.- All facets of yourself?

Yes, one has to work with all the aspects from body to the self. Any spark of action, any spark of imagination, starts from the very source of the being, which we call the self, and it projects to the extremities of the body. So the body has to experience that which is factual and send back to the self the knowledge as to whether your thinking is right or wrong. This outward and inward communication happens through the communion of evolution and involution processes. This is for the light of illumination to dawn, for finding out the "right". Evolution is going from the self outward and towards the skin, involution is going from the periphery of the skin towards the self. Throughout yogic practice, this communication and communing should run continuously.

I am trying with my students to dynamise both, from the self to the body and from the body to the self. I am bringing these two together like striking two stones that make light spark. Throughout practice there should be a sort of understanding between body, mind and self. In the beginning of practice the conflicts appear, but later on these conflicts disappear and harmony sets in. Only then does the body cult end and the culture of the self begin.

Q.- I would like to ask you a few questions on behalf of people who are interested in yoga, people who perhaps have had the spark of imagination to start with, as well as people who have had the example of someone like yourself to inspire them. They're doubtless going to make certain changes in their lives, it seems that a lot of people go to awful extremes very suddenly.

The reason for that is that they read books! They take ideas from someone else: "Someone experienced that, let me also try." This imaginative idea is based mostly on wrong ambition and greed. If someone has become rich, our inner greed too surfaces. We say, "Oh! Let me become rich like the other one". As material greed is dangerous, so the spiritual greed too is dangerous. The way I teach or preach takes into account my struggles in earlier life to reach this stage. But many teachers have forgotten their struggles to get where they are now and they talk from that level of achievement instead of making their followers start from where they began, so failure and grief follow. Experienced teachers like us, who do not forget the foundation upon which we build ourselves up, can remove whatever obstacles that arise in the path of one's search. In my case I have definitely not forgotten the foundation, but many do forget. They jump and that is why their practice gets un-rhythmic and in their training process the building up, the foundation, is lost. Some show the path on which they trod while some sell an imaginative ground.

Q.- So really they are in quite a dangerous position?

That's bound to happen, is it not? If you don't look at the cars and walk carelessly in the street, what happens? It may happen the same in the path of yoga. Yoga is a path, it is a way, so if you go criss-crossing without knowing what you are doing and what you have to do, naturally you will be affected not only physically and mentally, but also spiritually.

Q.- Would this partly account for the fact that you have a reputation for being extremely fierce?

(Laughter) Please do not put words like fierceness in my practice and teaching. I am no doubt intense in teaching and a keen observer of my students' presentations, but I do not consider fierceness as a bad reputation. Believe me, no one can point their finger at me about my moral, mental, physical or spiritual character. Because there is no blemish or flaw in those qualities, they have to find something to criticise me on. Today criticism is considered an intellectual growth in man and criticism is the nature of man. If I say I am 'furious', it is because I have done and experienced the real work. What I practise and experience, I teach that. I don't preach. If I had not experienced it, it would mean that I would be leading you to illusion, would I not? See the furiousness from a different angle. The moment I am soft, and lead you with imagination into illusion, it will be my dishonesty. In order to ensure that you do not fall down, I have to show 'furiousness' so that I do not misguide you and can build you up.

If a pupil has to be built up, it is a direct challenge. There should be no question of compromise. What has to be done is to be done. What has to be followed has to be followed. By preaching one does not bring about transformation. The transformation can be brought about only by direct teaching. Teaching is a straightforward process, but it is a harsh process. Preaching is a kind of advice which one may accept or reject, whereas teaching is a process of imparting the knowledge face to face.

Q.- Well, I think the fact that you have so many loyal and devoted pupils around the world is proof of your integrity.

Well, my integrity in teaching is making people to come to me, otherwise they wouldn't come at all. I do have this reputation for so-called 'cruelty' and 'furiousness'. Yet people say they come because of the sincerity of purpose and the devotion I have to the art and the affection I show after the classes. In my experience, and I have taught thousands and thousands, I have given them one good thing i.e., to practise sincerely, honestly and advertently. There are many teachers and preachers who speak fluently, they may use a language that may attract or hypnotise, but my actions, as you here said, cannot hypnotise. They are ruthless.

Q.- We've only spoken to Mr. Iyengar the teacher, but you are obviously also Mr. Iyengar the pupil.

I am a pupil to myself throughout.

Q.- Did you ever have a teacher of your own?

Well, in the beginning yes! Of course I pay my respects to my *Gurujī* who initiated me into the art, but you know it so happened for the good. After two years with him, in 1937, my *Gurujī* sent me to Pune, so I came to Pune at the request of a club for six months. When I started asking him to guide me, he said, "If you want to do it, do it. Otherwise leave it!" This was the challenge he threw at me after sending me to Pune and caused me to become an original man. If he had agreed to guide me probably I would not have been an innovative man at all, I would have been another copy-print totally dependent on him. But luckily at that time I was very wild at my *Gurujī* that a man whom I considered as God should leave me on the ledge without guiding me along the way. Anyway this helped me to become strong both physically and mentally to continue my practice of what he taught and I began to build up brick by brick on that.

I came from a poor family and I had to find my own way to survive. For days and days I have lived only on water and practised yoga. That's why when people ask me, "What diet?", I do not comment because I have never had a good diet in my life. I have lived on tea and practised yoga, so naturally I don't speak on that subject. At the time there was nobody to cry if I died and nobody to be happy if I lived. And when I was on this precipice, this art – yoga – and people who came asking me to teach coincided in such a way that I said I would make or mar. So I came up!

Q.- Apart from the fact that your *Gurujī* didn't really help you actively, were there other things that came to influence you and inspire you once you had separated from him, perhaps the scriptures?

No, not at all, nothing of that kind. It was just a feeling of loneliness. When I was a boy of seventeen years, I was asked to teach. Then the real fight came from within. Should I read books and repeat like a parrot as others do, or should I work hard with attentiveness to give them something? This was the turning point of my life. I reasoned that there were hundreds of people available to teach through reading and studying the scriptures, but was there any single person available to teach who has done it practically himself? This made me penetrate the subject in depth.

Without food, without any financial, moral or intellectual support I used to practise ten, twelve hours each day, morning to night. People called me a lunatic. I wore only trunks and sat on the threshold of my door whenever I got tired. And after recovery I would go in and practise again. Whenever I failed I would come out and sit on the doorstep, then go in and try again. If I failed my mind was unhappy, and in success too my mind was unhappy, for I was questioning, "Is it a success?" Whatever *āsana* I tried, it ended in failure. It was this failure I faced that worked on my deeper consciousness to try again – try again! When I failed, it said try again. This way I went on for years. I am delighted to say now that, it is ending with fruitful results and from loneliness I have touched the fullness.

Q.- As you developed on the basis of your own practice only, did you find that the few things you read later confirmed your own practice?

Yes, yes that's how I came to know that I am on the right path. First I did not read any books at all. Even now I tell many people not to read in the beginning, because reading can create confusion. You read something, you experience something and they don't meet. But after experiencing, if you read about it, then you know the value of those statements. After many years of practice I started to let myself see what Patañjali said, what Svātmārāma said, what Gheraṇḍa said. I started reading the *Upaniṣads*. And some of the experiences that I had felt were there. At the start, while reading I thought: "Oh, everything I do is wrong, or what I read is wrong." Something would strike me, "This I have experienced", let me use that light as an indication that what I was doing is not on the wrong path.

Many a time when people read first before doing practice, their minds begin to dream. They remain in the spiritual dreamland which is a kind of a daydream of spirituality. One cannot dream of Self-realisation. It has to be factually experienced.

Thank God! The scriptures came to me afterwards. I never read the scriptures at first because if I had read the scriptures first I would have taken the experience from the scriptures. Because I first had the experience I could read the text to see whether I was going right or wrong. The real confirmed that I was in the right side.

Q.- In spite of the fact that I know that you stand, in the first instance at least, for a very practical, down-to-earth approach to the subject – there's no sort of extra-terrestrial nonsense about it – nevertheless yoga is definitely a subject with which there are unusual associations from historic writings and ancient writings, and it's not only in India, but I think throughout the Orient that there are things which to the western mind sound strange and even impossible. In your experience and in your practice, can you in any way throw a little light on what those things really mean and the way western people should try and understand them?

I know what you are referring to – it is the *Vibhūti Pāda,* supernatural powers. Each man has a different state of consciousness. Through the practice of yoga, when a person develops this high state of consciousness, it becomes so sharp, so subtle, so fine, that for an average intellectual it appears to be a supernatural power, but for the person concerned it's absolutely a natural development or you might call it an intellectual evolution.

Q.- Thank you, that explains it beautifully.

One must take it that the more you practise, the more it becomes a natural, not supernatural, process. That's why when you hear a person speaking of *kuṇḍalinī,* "My *kuṇḍalinī* is awakened", he has to prove that his *kūṇḍalinī* is awakened. If his *kuṇḍalinī* is awakened, he is a divine person living in the world, but is he divine in any way? If he smokes and drinks and so on, then his *kuṇḍalinī* is not awakened, it is all his imagination – your word. He has imagined but he has not experienced.

Q.- Can I say that I also think it's true that with the development of fineness you have also developed a good sense of humour?

(Laughing) Well, I am humorous in order to release myself. It is natural for me to become humorous because of the 'ferocity' that is sometimes created by these students. I can be in a pitch of anger, and as soon as you do very well you see my anger disappears in a split second. That means I can go up and down like a wave. You know my 'reputation' and without this balance I would have been a physical and mental wreck from the way I conduct classes. But my blood pressure has not gone up, mental disturbances have not taken place, I am not physically weak anywhere.

I have not lost that inner peace and stability. Take an actor who puts on different shows. The role changes but the person is the same, is he not? In the same way the yogi has to put on, as a teacher, several colours, in order to uplift the student. That's all I can say.

Q.- Do you find that as you've developed over the years, you have also gained an incredible memory?

See, it goes together. Without memory how do you know that you are progressing? But the trouble comes with yesterday's memory. As you practise yoga or whatever, when you practise you create an obstacle already, because you want to repeat the experience of yesterday. Yesterday I had it, why should I not have it today? You might have had less sleep or you might have overslept, your food might have changed, your way of thinking might have too. So what I say is question, how you develop on yesterday's experience. The memory is not required to repeat the experience but how to feel better than what you experienced yesterday. I keep a track with that memory on hand, and today, when I practise I practise with a fresh mind and fresh intelligence to see what new experiences arise – and I compare today's experience with those of yesterday.

Q.- Do you find that you are able to keep a completely fresh approach every day?

That is what made me continue, otherwise it would have been churned out as a monotonous subject and I would have left it. I have done forty-eight years and not once has it come into my head that it is boring. This shows that there is a tremendous freshness in it.

Q.- And you still practise as vigorously as ever? More I guess?

Yes, I have again doubled my own practices in the past year. I devote five or six hours to practice.

Q.- I don't mean this in any way to sound like a rude question, but a lot of time has passed since you began. You are definitely, if I may use the phrase, 'an older generation gentleman' now.

(Much laughter) Yes, I have to agree with that also.

Q.- Does it affect your practice?

If age affects my practice, that means I am degenerating, so if I completely degenerate, it is my bounden duty not to interfere in this subject or the art of teaching. That is my ethics. If I continue for another three or four,years and I am not successful, it would mean that I would have to accept that I have lost something, I have lost the fragrance and I should say "goodbye" to my pupils. But till then I will not say that. Naturally, at this age, one cannot expect the same energy to run, but with will power I am still persisting with my practice devotedly.

Q.- Do you feel that the subtleness of your practice is synonymous with energy?

Yes, that is what I feel and want to say, "Yes. They are synonymous terms." They go together, the moment you lose the subtleness, the energy also drips backwards – it does not go forward. So that is how I have learned that the energy and consciousness go together. So in order to maintain the quietness of energy you have to maintain the quietness of consciousness. Secondly, in order to maintain the quietness of consciousness you have to see that energy is not depleted or inflated, and that depletion and inflation of energy does not disturb your consciousness or subtlety. But it is bound to have an effect because I know that the energy is depleting so it has to affect me, and for that reason I am practising so that the flow of energy remains alive in my body, mind and self.

Q.- Can you see any end to this practice, or will it continue?

The end cannot come at all. Just as you are advancing in your music, so I am advancing in my yoga. Will you be, any day, satisfied that you have reached the peak? It's the same in yoga. Due to the constant destroying and regenerating of cells, every day life is not the same as yesterday. As the life in the cells is new, so the thinking process and the action has to be new so the practice cannot be stopped. Experiences also become fresh and new. So there is no end.

But the infinite can be experienced. It comes in glimpses. It cannot be maintained. Even men like Ramana Maharshi were not in an infinite state throughout. Ramakrishna Paramahamsa was not in the infinite state throughout, otherwise he wouldn't have talked to people, and he wouldn't have guided the people.

They experience the infinite and, having experienced that state, they again come to the natural level so that they can help those who come to them. So being in the infinite state is not a continual experience, and the moment you find that you are in the infinite state, you are 'dead' because you are one with infinity, and that's all I can tell you!

THE BODY MY TEMPLE*

"My father, Bellur Krishnamachar, came from a poor family in a village called Bellur, in Kolar district, now part of the Karnataka State." So begins the autobiography of B.K.S. Iyengar, with the stark simplicity of a person who has made of his life what he had wanted to make of it, and has no need either to offer apologies for anything in his life or for any reference other than his own achievements to give it value.

*For years, life was very hard for Iyengar. He was frail and unhealthy, his formal education was negligible, and he was wretchedly poor. His self-transformation into what he is today was an act of will and devotion though he was lucky to have in his brother-in-law a distinguished yoga teacher, patronised by the Mahar*ā*ja of Mysore as a guru. While still in his teens Iyengar himself set out as a yoga teacher, sometimes walking (because he could not afford the bus fare) as much as eighteen miles daily to teach a single student for a fee of nothing more than one meal at the student's house. In 1937, Iyengar, then aged nineteen, moved to Pune. "All my worldly goods were a pair of shirts and dhotis and bedding", he writes. "I used one dhoti as a towel. I had no soap. I had no money even for a shave. I bought a razor blade for one* paisa *and with that naked blade shaved twice without soap during the month."*

Today, Iyengar runs a highly successful yoga school at Pune and he can count among his pupils some very distinguished persons, including J. Krishnamurthi and Jayaprakash Narayan. Iyengar is one of the greatest yoga instructors of our times, authoritative and exacting, yet open and innovative. In the clinical applications of yoga, his work has been outstanding. Short statured, wiry and beetle-browed, with a hawkish demeanour, Iyengar is an activist. There is a suggestion of impatience about him, as was evident during his yoga demonstration at the Bharatiya Vidya Bhavan Hall in Madras recently. But then, Iyengar does not claim to be a Bhagavan *or a* Maharishi *or a* sannyāsi*; he is simply and superbly a yoga researcher and instructor. During his recent visit to Madras, ASIDE interviewed him.*

---

* Published by *Aside*, Chennai, vol. 8, August 1980.

Q.- Traditionally the purpose of yoga was not the attainment of physical health or even mental equipoise, but something beyond that. But today the emphasis is on the clinical aspects. Can you comment on it?

Yes, yoga has now become a clinical practice, like naturopathy, allopathy or homeopathy, though it is not a "pathy" at all. It is a way of life which shows the path towards the Ultimate.

The world has become so small because of the communicating network that the speed, the strain and the stress on each individual has increased enormously. Naturally all these 's' sap the energy of people so much that they almost become physical and mental wrecks. Yoga, from that angle, is a panacea. But beyond improving the physical health of human beings, yoga also has the power to improve discrimination and effectiveness in decision-making. It gives strength like a tonic for emotional stability and intellectual clarity. From that angle too, yoga has tremendous clinical value.

Physical and mental health for better living has become as essential as food, water, air and shelter. And without having these minimum essential requirements one cannot think of higher aspects which are beyond one's grasp/understanding.

Again, if the emphasis is on clinical aspects, Patañjali has already said that disease is an obstacle in the path of yoga and practice of yoga alone can remove this obstacle. He even recommends prevention saying that the sorrows that have not yet come but are in waiting can be avoided. So what else would we want?

Q.- Doesn't this place yoga on the same plane as any other system of physical conditioning?

No! Yoga is not like any other system - it is not just a physical exercise, it is more an organic exercise, though it helps to realign the musculo-skeletal body. The technique of performing the *āsana* is such that each cell, each area, each organ, each system of the body is dealt with advertent attention and awareness in providing the oxygenated blood supply in the cells for the body to get united, energised energy - *prāṇa śakti,* awareness in mind and invigorated consciousness - *prajñā,* which is definitely not possible with other types of exercises. In other exercises one can develop one's thighs or one's biceps or triceps, but how can one develop one's heart or liver or intestines or spleen? From the organic standpoint of view, I don't think there is any exercise which ever can come closer to yogic *āsana.* So, I would not call it a physical exercise but a physiological or organic exercise.

Q.- This is to say that, while other exercises may develop certain anatomical parts, yoga can strengthen all parts and organs of the body. But, does it take you beyond that?

It does! It does! Let me tell you this. Among the more than two hundred- thousand people that I have taught yoga, not one of them had come to me saying that he or she had only a philosophical interest in learning yoga. They have come in the beginning with complaints of physical, physiological or mental problems, unhappiness or other reasons. So, we have to train them through certain *āsana* to keep the brain quiet, their emotional centres calm. In every individual there is a conflict between their intellectual calibre and the emotional standard. Yoga brings unity between the two, clarity in the brain and stability in the mind, so that the practitioner can withstand any stress.

Q.- None of these takes you beyond temporal compulsions, as yoga is supposed to...

That is what I am coming to. The mind is the instrument that unites the body and the soul. The character of senses of perception – the *jñānendriya* – is to perceive and put the imprint of what they perceive on the mind. The mind plays the dual role of pleasing the senses and pleasing the self. Practice of yoga makes the body look after itself. Yoga brings the health to the body not only making it disease-free but attachment-free also. Obviously the senses get drawn in. The mind is cut off from the senses, and since it has nothing else to do, it turns inwards to trace its source. So, until the time the body can look after itself, and forces the mind to look towards the self, yoga is not a spiritual pursuit, but when each organ looks after itself and the mind is free to turn inwards, it becomes a spiritual pursuit.

Q.- But such an exploration of the self, as you call it, does it not involve certain taboos of food, rituals, etc.?

No, it does not. Each cell, I tell you, has an individuality of its own, an intelligence of its own, and by the practice of yoga, each cell tells you if the diet you are taking is congenial or not. There are drunkards and smokers who have come to me; I have not told any of them to leave off smoking or drinking. Yet, they tell me that after four or five months, a transformation has taken place in them to stop such habits themselves. Because the stimulation which nicotine or alcohol provides is now provided naturally by the body itself. They don't require any external stimuli.

Q.- But this was not the traditional attitude of yoga, was it? Traditionally certain austerities were required of the novice before he began the yoga practice, isn't it?

Yes, the system was different in olden days, the social set-up and circumstances were different... If we insist on such austerities today, then people will never turn up to learn yoga. As teacher, I make them stay in an *āsana* for a certain period of time focusing their attention on certain parts of the body as needed in each *āsana*, which automatically diverts their minds to the movements of breath and an active attention on the required parts of the body.

Q.- So, you believe in adapting yoga to suit the contemporary social culture?

Yes! Yes! Why not? If the traditional yoga has proved its value, is it not our duty to see how it can be adapted to free oneself from contemporary social problems? We are living in this modern age and not in the *vedic* era. We need to bring about a transformation.

Q.- The contemporary emphasis is on *haṭha yoga* and physical exercises, but aren't we supposed to proceed from *haṭha yoga* to *rāja yoga*, which in turn leads to spiritual emancipation?

It is true. *Haṭhaṁ vinā rāja yogaḥ, rāja yogaṁ vinā haṭhaḥ* (*H.Y.P.,* II.76) meaning, one cannot obtain perfection in *rāja yoga* without *haṭha yoga* and vice versa. They cannot be separated. With due respect to Swami Vivekananda, who was a great intellectual, it was he who was responsible for the bifurcation of yoga. Since then the notion has spread that *haṭha yoga* is purely a physical discipline while *pātañjala yoga* is a mental discipline. But the texts do not say so. *Haṭha Yoga* starts with the body and ends with the soul, while *pātañjala yoga* starts with the self and comes back to the body. Of all the reasons for ill health, Patañjali gives only two physical causes, *vyādhi* or disease and *ālasya* or laziness, the rest are all on the mental plane. We do not know where the body ends and the mind begins or where the mind ends and the self begins. As I said, the mind plays a dual role, serving both body and soul. When the body is independent and takes care of itself, the mind says, "Well, you are fine, so let me turn towards the self." If there is a pressure on the body, it will affect the mind and vice versa, because they are interrelated.

Q.- Would you say that *rāja yoga* is one of the final avenues – like *karma yoga, jñāna yoga* or *bhakti yoga* – which man has to take for the attainment of Self, while *haṭha yoga* is the preliminary broad avenue from which you can branch into any of the particular paths to Self-realisation?

No! I do not agree with your statement. First of all yoga is one. Yoga is inclusive of *karma, jñāna, bhakti, rāja* and *haṭha*. They are not separate. If one is explicit, the others are hidden. All these are encompassed in yoga. Let this be clear to you. Yoga itself is a final avenue.

The journey of the practice of yoga is from body to soul, from health to Self-realisation. It is not that you take or choose only *karma, jñāna* and *bhakti* for the attainment of the Self. The words such as *karma yoga, jñāna yoga, bhakti yoga* came into existence recently. Otherwise yoga was all-inclusive. So yoga is the path of Self-realisation.

The fact is that in order to have Self-realisation one needs health. Body aches, pains, diseases distract one from the inner journey. One needs first to eradicate these distractions.

Now another ignorance about *haṭha yoga* is that it is to do with physical body in order to eradicate diseases. That is false knowledge. *Ha* stands for sun – the soul, *ṭha* stands for moon – the consciousness. When consciousness – *citta* – becomes as pure as soul, it is equal to soul. Yoga is practised to bring this purity equal to that of the soul.

Now look at J. Krishnamurti, the finest intellectual in the world today, a *jñāni*, but why should he do yoga for three hours every day? Does he not practise yoga every day? How many people are not able to serve the world because of ill health? If there is no good health, you cannot do good *karma* They are interrelated. If I am perfectly healthy, and a good thinker, the action is good. When Ramana Maharshi got cancer, he offered his hand to be amputated. Why? The hand started giving trouble. He asked the surgeon to cut it off if he wanted. Study his tranquil state of mind when he was afflicted with cancer of the hand. When Vivekananda suffered from tuberculosis, he said that he did *prāṇāyāma* and used to feel well, but due to reasons known to him, he gave up the practice. Yoga gives the strength to bear the sufferings in life.

Q.- You are a major factor in popularising yoga around the world. But in universalising yoga, are you not diluting the Hindu metaphysical concepts which are basic to yoga?

No, not at all. Even Patañjali, who lived between 500 and 200 BC, never said, think of a particular god only. Whatever you like, you accept. Yoga is a universal culture. It is not confined to any particular place, time or culture. Patañjali did not propound yoga as a Hindu religion but as a Universal Religion.

Now, where is the question of dilution of metaphysics? It is your misunderstanding if you think that I am teaching yoga to Westerners by diluting the metaphysics of yoga. All the practitioners, to whichever country or religion they belong, have to cleanse and purify their body, organs of action, senses of perception, mind, intelligence, consciousness and conscience. Is this not a process dealing with metaphysical concepts?

Q.- May I approach this problem from another angle – how does the concept of *karma* relate to yoga?

Yes, yoga and *karma* have a connection. We believe in continuous refinement. The present life leads to and determines the next life. The last and profound thought in our mind is the seed for the next life. Yoga teaches us to burn out our last thought, to burn away the impurities, so that we attain *mukti*. Yoga does not allow *karma* to accumulate.

Q.- That is to say, yoga is a means of escaping from the consequences of *karma*?

Not escaping. Facing, cleansing and getting rid of. Positively. There is no running away.

Q.- How is it that, though traditionally they are closely related, there is not much of a link between *āyurveda* and yoga in modern times?

Āyurveda and yoga are both *mukti śāstra* or *mokṣa śāstra*. *Āyurveda* means *veda* or knowledge of *āyu* or life. There is a similarity between *āyurveda* and yoga throughout: they help each other. While yoga talks of *triguṇa* – the three qualities, namely, *sattva, rajas* and *tamas*, *āyurveda* talks of *tridoṣa* – the three humours (*vāta, pitta* and *śleṣma*, i.e., bile, phlegm and wind) of the body. But while in yoga we believe in our own inner energy to match the *tāmasic guṇa* of the body and the *rājasic guṇa* of the mind to the *sāttvic guṇa* of the soul, *āyurveda* believes in the use of certain external medicines to harmonise the three humours so that they can build up subjectively the harmonious health through yoga. That is the only dissimilarity.

Q.- Let's move on to another area. One problem, which so many people who want to learn yoga say is that the system is enormously complicated – would you comment?

It is all in the fixed and rigid frame of mind. Let me give you an example. In deep sleep, one can experience serenity in the body and the mind, but is it not difficult to experience that state of serenity in awareness which one experiences in sleep? In sleep you don't say you are serene. You wake up and say, "What a sound sleep I had." But who is the witness to that serenity? The soul witnesses the serenity, therefore when you wake up you say you were serene. Now the question is, how to maintain the serenity of deep sleep in a wakeful state? In order to experience this serenity in the waking state, one must assume that state of being actively, and not negatively as in sleep. And this is the process of *dhyāna*. You are awake but imitating the action of sleep thoughtfully and without wavering. That requires special effort and guidance. To imbibe this state one has to practise all the aspects of yoga, including clinical yoga. Otherwise your attention remains all the time with the diseased body. Hence, it is not a complicated subject but an advertant system.

Q.- What about the time frame? How much time can a person devote to yoga in the midst of a busy, active life?

Here, you are coming back to your earlier question. If one has to have spiritual emancipation, can one frame yoga in the frame of time? Again, you say that with a busy and active life you cannot afford to give more time.

So I frame the programme according to the requirements of the practitioner which you brand as physical yoga, clinical yoga, *haṭha yoga* and what not.

Knowing very well these problems, I have to give some solutions.

Suppose you come to me for guidance, then I can lead you to the solution of your problem easily. One reads so many advertisements of medicines but one needs a doctor to guide one. I prescribe a few *āsana* straightaway and it makes it so easy to follow. Then the complicated art becomes a simple art.

Q.- So, you prescribe only a few specific *āsana* and never the full course?

Do not read me incorrectly. Go back to your questions so that my answers are interpreted in the right perspective. Know that it is certainly not possible to give a full course to everybody in that short period when people cannot afford to give time. Only a few *āsana* are prescribed. For example, if you are a high-strung person, then brain stimulating *āsana* should not be done by you. The brain must be quietened and the emotional areas should be expanded. For hypertension, the horizontal place of the intellect should be expanded when you get fully absorbed into the subject, naturally you would yourself like to go in for the full course.

Q.- How important is the role of the *guru* in learning yoga? Can't one learn the *āsana* by oneself, from the books?

It is possible to learn yoga without a teacher, but it is desirable to have a teacher. The *āsana* should be done perfectly and with full knowledge of what they mean; otherwise they may injure the body as well as the mind. But of course a good book is better than a bad teacher!

THE GURU WHO IS JUST A FAMILY MAN*

B.K.S. Iyengar is quite unlike the accepted western idea of a guru. To find him you do not have to trek to a remote Indian countryside or seek entrance into an āśram. *He is a family man who lives a normal family life in Pune, 170 kilometres from Mumbai.*

He has a simple house where he lives with his children and grandchildren. In front of the house stands the Institute which has been built by grateful students so that he might pass on what he has spent years studying – the art of yoga.

Rare among yogis, he demonstrates by his simple, unpretentious life that liberation from physical, mental and emotional slavery can be achieved by all who sincerely and regularly practise yoga, whether they be male or female, Eastern or Western, young or old. He also holds daily classes at the Institute in Pune that is dedicated to his late wife and called the Ramāmaṇi Iyengar Memorial Yoga Institute. These are attended by Indians and Westerners alike.

From time to time he holds intensive courses for overseas students who have only limited time to spend in Pune. It was during one of these courses that I spoke to him about various aspects of yoga, and his teaching and practice of the art.

The philosophy of yoga was first systematised by Patañjali around 300 BC. This yoga is usually referred to as rāja yoga. *A subsequent work by Svātmārāma is considered to be the basis of* haṭha yoga *which is widely practised in the West.*

Q.- What is the difference between *haṭha yoga* and *rāja yoga?*

Just as the Mother Earth is supported by the Universal God, so is *haṭha yoga* a support to *rāja yoga.*

There is no difference between Patañjali's *rāja yoga* and Svātmārāma's *haṭha yoga. Haṭhayoga Pradīpikā* starts with the body and ends with the soul and Patañjali starts with the soul and comes to the body. In the very first chapter Patañjali mentions the various obstacles

---

* Interview by Pauline Dowling. Published by *Here's Health,* November 1981, vol. 26, no. 301, pp. 132-134.

such as dullness and disease, which distract the mind. Aren't these obstacles creating impediments for the body? Once you have conquered these, then you are in a state of freedom.

So, *haṭha yoga* starts from the body and takes us to the pinnacle of life – freedom. *Rāja yoga* starts by explaining what freedom is, then explains the obstacles which come in the way while achieving this freedom. Ultimately, you need to overcome these obstacles and you are free. So there is no difference at all. One starts from the base, the other starts from the top but both reach the same point. *Haṭha yoga* is like a turtle shell for all branches of yoga. It is not fair to differentiate between the body and the self, even though the body is a cover. As the skin of the fruit is a part of the fruit, similarly *haṭha vidyā* is a part of yoga. *Haṭha yoga* makes the cover of the self to be kept intact so that the self moves freely in the entire system of the *sādhaka*. Your self cannot jump here and there but is full within yourself, as a single unit. When the mind is completely merged in the self, differentiation between the body and the mind disappears, only then one remains as the Self. Experiencing this state of being is called *rāja yoga*. *Rāja yoga, samādhi, unmanī,* oneness as a *manonmanī, śūnyāśūnya, laya, amanaskatva,* etc.,[1] convey the same meaning without any difference. So the end of yoga is known as *rāja yoga* because you are one with the Universal Soul. It is said that *haṭha yoga* acts as ladder to reach *rāja yoga*, which has several connotations. Yoga begins from the body and ends with the soul.[2] If *haṭha yoga* is the beginning, then *rāja yoga* is the ending.

By the by, let me remind you that Patañjali nowhere called yoga *rāja yoga*. He has not given a special name for his treatise. In fact, it is Svātmārāma who gives the name *haṭha yoga* for his treatise and declares that it leads towards *rāja yoga*. The commentator of the *Haṭhayoga Pradīpikā* explains the *rājayoga* as *pātañjala yoga*. Therefore neither Patañjali nor Svātmārāma are demarcating or confusing us. It is the practitioners who are confused.

Q.- Is it necessary to devote yourself entirely to yoga in order to reach this state?

Yes! If you are a genuine *sādhaka,* you need to devote yourself totally until you reach the goal. For instance, as a teacher I have to devote my entire time to this subject. Preachers are different from teachers. A preacher may not be a practitioner with religiosity. He only throws knowledge and goes away. But when I'm teaching it means I have taken the complete responsibility of guiding day in and day out on myself. The pupils have transferred their problems to me and hence I have to work on them in order to make them free from problems.

---

1 *Rāja yoga* (the royal yoga), *samādhi* (total absorption), *unmanī* (beyond mind), *manonmanī* (extinction of mind), *amaratva* (immortality), *laya* (absorption), *tattva* (truth), *śūnyāśūnya* (void and yet no-void), *paramapada* (the supreme state), *amanaska* (transcending the mind), *advaita* (non-duality), *nirālamba* (without support), *nirañjana* (pure), *jīvanmukti* (liberation while in the body), *sahaja* (natural state), *turīyā* (the fourth state) (*H.Y.P.,* IV.3-4).

2 *Tapas svādhyāya īśvarapraṇidhānāni kriyāyogaḥ* (*Y.S.,* II.1).

Q.- Even for teachers in the West with complex lives?

It's a must. Otherwise the fineness of the art will never come to them. As teachers they have to communicate this fineness. They have to illumine their pupils.

Q.- So if they have diverse interests, is this not possible?

Not to the highest extent. Can a musician with diverse attention become a genius?

Q.- Does it depend on what his other interests are? If he's interested in going to the theatre, reading, wandering in the countryside, then these can assist.

If those are akin to the subject and not diverse, then I say yes, they help. Anything which is akin to the subject is worth pursuing. Patañjali also says that if your thought is fixed throughout on the subject whatever it may be, as long as it is in line with your way of thinking, then it is not a diversion of the mind. This is the state of the mind one requires to become a genius. Any interest which is akin to the subject will be wonderful. It will add to your own experience. All your experiences become finer and finer as you continue practice with oneness in *sādhanā*. But if you pick up something else and divert your attention from yoga, it will not help at all. On the contrary, the downfall will begin.

Note that there are two types of yoga practitioners. One type can practise just to be balanced, healthy and peaceful. This practice is meant for just the well-being of oneself which is fine in one way. Most of them belong to this category. Obviously the practitioners of this category will not study the subject in-depth.

There is also a second type of practitioner which is rarely found. A person like me who is totally devoted and dedicated does not even think of anything other than yoga. The complex life is not only in the West but in the East too. In fact, life itself is complex. Yoga is meant to solve this complexity of the mind and unknot it. The self has to become one with the Universal Soul. This type of *sādhaka* prefers to practise for the ultimate end, ultimate freedom. Such people do not have diverse interests at all. I too may enjoy music or reading but it will not be for my sensual or mental amusement. Basically the mind and the consciousness have to gravitate towards the core.

Q.- There is plenty of evidence that the *āsana* can improve physical health. Can you explain how they do the same for mental health?

No man is separate from soma and psyche. Can somatic body function without psyche's influence? He is connected to both. Yoga as a subject definitely deals with the mind more than the body. The body cannot move independently of the mind. It is wrong to differentiate the body and mind as separate entities. The moment we differentiate between them we are already ill as the body is the gross form of the mind and the mind is the gross form of the self. As such there is no difference between body and mind. If your body is pricked, it affects the mind. Suppose you are in sorrow, misery, unhappiness, is not the body affected by these? So it is inter-related. Therefore, it is wrong to say that physical diseases are different from psychological diseases. Any psychological fault, pressure, depends upon the physical non-well-being. If there is a physical upset, it affects the mind and the mind broods on it. We may then call it a psychological disease, but the foundation of the psychological pressure is the disease of the physical body. It is the vital body or the physiological organs like the liver, spleen, pancreas, intestines, heart, lungs that get affected. So, when you speak of the physical body you have to always correlate the physical and physiological bodies. When there is some upset in the physical or physiological body, it has a bearing on the mind. You cannot control with the mind an organ that is not well. But you can work on the affected organ through the physical and physiological body.

Why were the varieties of *āsana* and *prāṇāyāma* given? They were given so that you concentrate on the physical and physiological bodies and make yourself free from their shackles. What role does yoga play? The mind is normally attached all the time to the body. From the practice of *āsana* and *prāṇāyāma* we learn to make the mind free from the contact of the body. The moment the mind is free from the contact of the body, it no longer wants to run after the exhibitive nature saying, "Let me enjoy this, let me enjoy that". When you have this peace of mind, free from the contact of attachments and allurements, your existence becomes spiritual. The mind turns inwards to go beyond this poise and peace, to trace the eternal core which has no sorrow and no pleasure. This is how the signs of spiritual progress in yoga take place.

Q.- The majority of people do yoga on a "once a week" basis. What would you say is the value of yoga done this way?

Something is better than nothing. Today people cannot find sufficient time to practise. Under the guidance of a teacher, if they work once a week, the right thought will be imprinted on their minds and it will have a good effect. And this effect will last for about two or three days on the entire human system. Then it starts deteriorating. If people go to a teacher once a week to learn correct presentations and practise at home twice or thrice a week, retardation will not take place. The functioning of the human system and the clarity in the brain and maintenance of equilibrium in body and mind will increase if one practises daily.

I have already said that you will find many people who want to do yoga for health and peace attending once or twice a week. Though it is fine in one way, they cannot grumble if they don't reach the unbiased freedom which is the aim of yoga.

Q.- How can students recognise a good teacher?

First of all, if yoga is taken from the commercial point of view it is definitely unfair. A good teacher shall be truthful to yoga and the sign of a good yoga teacher is in practice and presentation of the art. This demands intense discipline and sincerity of purpose behind each individual's practices and as long as the teacher does not practise, the pupils who go to him should be a little bit guarded. They should ask the teachers every now and then to present what they are saying and not just to accept their words. Teaching without showing what is the right practice is cheating the public.

Q.- For many students practising alone is difficult, so they attend many classes a week instead. Is this advisable?

There is a very peculiar feeling in western minds as well as eastern, that by going to different teachers they are able to accumulate knowledge. Knowledge can be acquired – it cannot be accumulated, except where it is accumulated by one's own experience and practice. Objective view of knowledge comes through the study of books, but subjective knowledge cannot come from study of books or through a teacher but comes only through one's own practical experience. Just as a farmer cultivates and looks after the plant, you have to work yourself in order to grow within yourself. For this reason when students think that they can accumulate a little from here, a little from there, the confusion comes. Suppose I am confused. If I go to another teacher, I am going to be more confused because I am already confused. Suppose I continue with one teacher and absorb whatever he says, then there is a little bit of understanding in me to discriminate with my experience when I study with another teacher. But going from one teacher to the other is not going to bring maturity of knowledge at all.

Even if you go to one teacher and attend the classes everyday, you need to study and do it by yourself to understand your capacity, your standard, your weakness, your faults or your achievements. You can judge your will power and may throw a great challenge on yourself.

Q.- Does a serious study of yoga also presuppose a belief in reincarnation?

It will not occur to a yogi at all. A true yogi will never think of an incarnation. That's the beauty of perfect practice. As his practice and ways of giving make him purer and purer, the idea never strikes him. There are three types of actions. We call it *kriyamāṇa* - present actions, *sañcita* - accumulated actions, and *prārabdha* - the effect of those accumulated actions.

In the practice of yoga - it's the same whether for *āsana* or *prāṇāyāma* - suppose you are stretching your right leg and do nothing with your left leg, you have left room for a reaction. Suppose you react on the left leg when you are acting on the right leg. Reaction and action meet together and hence, there is no room for further action. In the same way your reincarnations shorten because you have created in this very life actions without leaving room for reactions. As a writer, don't you like to improve the presentation of your words - don't you want to become finer and finer and more sensitive in intelligence? Is not this a sign of reincarnation of intelligence in you?

- *Yes. All the time.* -

All the time. Indians call it reincarnation. Westerners say, "I want to become better and better, finer and finer. I want to become the finest in the art."

I can give you another example regarding divinity and precision in instruments. Technologists today say that they have got precise instruments conveying from every angle that their products are perfect. And in ancient times they did not use the word 'perfection' but they used the word 'divinity'. What difference does this make in words? Perfection is purity and purity is divinity. Perfection is pure. So perfection is divine. Is it not?

When there is a will or wish to get better, to improve and become perfect, it obviously means reincarnation or rebirth. Life is a continuous process. Death is a part of life and not the end of life. As the wrong or bad actions get accumulated in the form of fate or destiny, similarly good thoughts, good aims which may remain unfulfilled in this life, the next life alone is the answer for rebirth which you term as reincarnation.

Q.- But unfortunately words like divine and spiritual today have lost their currency. They are used exclusively in orthodox, organised religion.

That is what I'm saying. So the technical words for divinity today are precision and perfection. Your instrument, the body, the mind, the intelligence should be very precise and perfect. When the body is perfect, the mind gets non-attached to the body and moves towards religious thought of righteousness and virtue. This, I say is the sign of perfectness in yoga.

All religions talk of perfection which is fullness – *pūrṇam*.

Q.- There are many therapies on offer in the West today which promise instant enlightenment. Can these therapies achieve for people the liberation they gain from yoga?

Tell me, is there anything in the world which is instant?

– *Apart from coffee, food.* –

No, not even if there is instant coffee. You have to boil water and have milk to add to the so called instant coffee powder. Is it not?

It is the same with instant therapy. It is like the petals of a flower, which blossom and then drop off. Like a leaf or like the petal of a flower, these instant therapies drop. Then you don't pay any respect to it. Whereas in yoga the petals are kept as fresh as ever, forever. That is the difference. In yoga there is a discipline involved. If a farmer does not look after the land, if he does not remove the weeds, can he grow anything?

May be accidentally something can be grown. But how many centuries it may take, nobody knows. But suppose the farmer tends to his land, is he not sure about the crops? It is the same with yoga. This instant effect is accidental but not permanent.

Q.- You have been described by many people in many different ways – dynamic, mercurial, creative. Thousands of students all over the world have studied with you – each one sees you differently. How would you describe yourself and your teaching?

I am made of many different facets. I'm not a single faceted man, a mono-type. I can face anything at any time, according to the situation. I am a man of principle, and a man of principle will not have two minds.

When I'm teaching I'm creative. But I do not change my base. From that base I am cultivating lots of things, because I have got the maturity and hence grip of the subject. In my teaching, I'm trying my best to make each individual an original person. Only while teaching I am a tiger. You can call me a lion, you can call me a tiger. There I'm a dictator. But afterwards I'm very soft. And even though I am strong while teaching, my heart melts if I see people suffering, going wrong and committing mistakes. So I go out of my way to help them – to relieve them. Because I am so mobile inside I change the entire system for that person who is wrong. In that mobility I am unpredictable. My teaching is never the same – ABCD. I can teach ABCD, CBDA or I can teach DCBA.

Q.- Would you say that, as a result of your years of study, you and yoga are the same thing?

We are almost one. We are what you call synonymous, Iyengar and yoga – yoga and Iyengar. In my subject I can tell you that in whatever I have done up to now or what I am doing, I am 100 percent clear and sure about it. I do not even touch a person on an *āsana* or on a teaching point which I have not experienced.

Q.- India today has become a spiritual haven for thousands of Westerners searching for the missing dimension in their lives, what they call spirituality. How would you say that you as a yogi, as a teacher, differ from all the other *gurus?*

I am a non-attached person. Because I am non-attached, if the people come, it's for them. I've not invited anyone to come. That's one difference. Others advertise that they will do this or do that. I don't say that. That is why I say that I am still innocent of the worldly life. I'm just like an ordinary man. When I go out on to the street, nobody can recognise me as a yogi. When the *gurus* walk on the street you see the crowd of pupils around them. Unlike others, I don't ask my followers to come with me. This is the difference between me and others which anybody can see.

I have faith in what I practise. This does not mean that I want people to follow me blindly. I want them to do with open eyes and mind to trace their mistakes and get rectified. I do not claim that by my blessings they reach the goal. I might have been a guide to them but the fruit they derive is from their own right *sādhanā*. It is one hundred percent their efforts and their achievements.

My way of living is quite different. I live like an ordinary innocent man. I'm not an ideal to anybody. I'm a family man. You ask my children, they will say, "Our father does not care for us". Why should they say that when I'm a family man, when I am their father? It does not mean that I do not care for them. It means that I am non-attached even to my children. I have no desires in life. The desires have all gone. My desire is only to practise and to teach those who come to me.

Q.- And if nobody came?

That is still fine. I will say that it is the blessings of God for me to use my time for more practice or from that day on I may go into a voluntary retirement. Though I have stamina, strength, confidence and clarity, I may withdraw voluntarily from teaching. But I will never stop my practice. I will be at the Institute going nowhere. But I will be practising myself so that pupils build up courage to continue practice like me. I will not stop my practice, this is certain, and note that I shall practise in real peace.

Q.- But people don't want to know that. They don't want to take responsibility for themselves.

In the practice of yoga, it will clearly come to the person that peace is within himself and he need not depend on anyone. He need not run after anyone. Peace is not an outer search, it is an inner state of being.

THE SEARCH IN ALIGNEMENT LED ME TO EXPERIENCE THE INNER MIND*

In November of 1981 I returned to India to participate in my second intensive course with B.K.S. Iyengar. I found him in a remarkably different mood than on my first trip: friendlier and more approachable, almost gentle. There were several days in class when I felt my eyes filling with tears of simple affection for this unique person.

Just following the last āsana *class of the intensive on December 11, 1981, I spent about an hour and a half with Mr. Iyengar recording the following interview. We were in the library in the basement of the Institute. It was my first opportunity (or should I say, the first opportunity I took) to get to know B.K.S. Iyengar as a person outside the classroom. Accustomed as I was to watching him perform fantastic things with his body or storm around class, it was a different experience to see him sitting in a chair, wrapped in a grey wool sweater on a chilly day, sipping coffee. Still, one could never mistake him for an average man on the street; his dancing eyes and those fantastically expressive eyebrows gave a clue to the agility of the mind inside.*

As we talked, I realised I had found Mr. Iyengar in a very open mood. I felt a tremendous connection with him, and he was willing to answer any questions I asked. Perhaps he has reached a point in his life where he can relax some of his driving force and put his life in perspective – as people do only after they have lived a long time. I hope this interview will deepen your understanding of B.K.S. Iyengar as a person and a teacher, just as it deepened mine.

Q.- How did your teaching method evolve?

Circumstances made me a yoga practitioner, rather than my own zeal. I started doing *yogāsana* in 1934 for my health. In 1936 I was asked by my *guru* to teach in the northern part of Karnataka. I felt a great responsibility: if I was going to teach, I felt I should know something about yoga. Just doing a few *āsana* for my health would not give me a grip on the art of teaching. The challenge

* Interview by Carol Cavanaugh. First published by *The I.Y.T.E. Review,* vol. 2, no. 3, January 1982. Published by *Yoga Journal,* July/August 1982, pp. 30-37.

at that age was beyond my physical and mental limitations. I said, "Let me take a chance." When I started teaching, I asked myself what is the use in reading books and following those methods, when we do not even understand ourselves. I continued for about a year with half-hearted effort, then I was called to Pune in 1937.

I saw lots of youngsters from college who had enrolled for yoga classes but I was the youngest. It was very difficult for me, for I was immature both in yoga and in knowing the ways of conducting the classes or understanding the meaning of life. I knew I would have to devote all my time and that I should show something more about yoga than what they could grasp. I knew I should present yoga in such a way that even people who had done it before would know they were hearing something new for the first time. That made me revolutionise the subject. The idea struck me in 1937, but did not fructify for several years.

In 1944 I began getting clues from my hard work, realising the normal way *āsana* should be done this way rather than that way. I started realising the importance of linking the external actions with the inner-body, the mercurial mind and the sharp intelligence. My inward journey began there. Then I tried to find the correct way to work in each and every *āsana*. Between 1937 and 1944, my teaching was completely immature. The advantage was that I was young. Vanity was in the pupils and in me. If I had to prove my superiority, naturally I had to express my vanity more. The only way I could do this was through my practice of yoga. I could see that my own pupils were doing better than me, and that gave me a clue that if they could do well, I should do better. I was always thinking ahead of them, looking for clues from the best of the class. I used to look at each limb separately. I first used a prop in 1948 when I was not getting *Baddha Koṇāsana* at all. I started using bricks, the heavy stones which were available in the street. But the idea to use props on a large scale and a systematic way really struck me in 1975, when the Institute came into existence, and I was planning what to put into it.

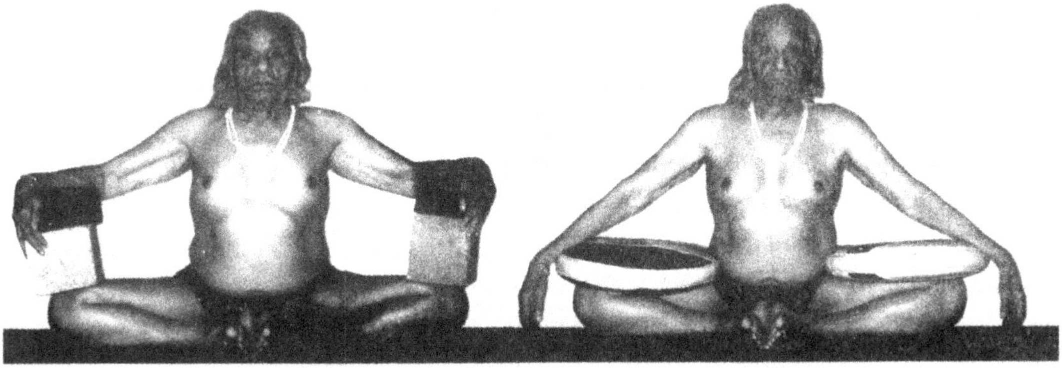

Plate n. 3 – The first props were with bricks and stones, now weights are used

It wasn't until then that the idea struck me that alignment is the most important thing. Yoga is alignment. This word was there theoretically, but no one explained what it meant. Almost all were saying that *āsana* are only physical and have nothing to do with the spiritual. That criticism was also in my head and meant to guide me. I had to accept all kinds of stupid and wise statements given to me by people, then sit at home and toss them over. I asked myself what is right, what is wrong; should I take this one's word or that one's word? I began to look at photographs of people, drawing lines between their way and my way of doing it, chest to chest, hand to hand, elbow to elbow. The *āsana* were performed, but the position of the body was not aligned. In head balance, the head was in one place and one leg was straight and the other leg was turning. I wondered why there was this difference. Where was that alignment that yoga talks about when it says one has to be balanced? Where was the equilibrium or balance – *samatvam?*

In order to know what alignment is, it is important to realise that the central portion of the body is the median plane in each and every part. If you take your finger and divide it down the middle, you get the median plane. When we stretch, are we in the median plane on either side, or are we overstretching from the median plane on one side and understretching on the other side? If there is overstretch somewhere, there must be understretch elsewhere. The median plane is the god: it is what brings you to the art of precision. From the outer part, inner part, front part and back part – you always have to measure how much you are extending from the median plane. There is no overstretch; you are balanced exactly in the middle.

Later, with this alignment of the skeleto-muscular body, I began to align my mind, intelligence and consciousness, which made me look within. This new frame of study and observation made me engulf all the instruments of the self and made the very self occupy the body – its frontiers – as *citta prasādana* and *ātma prasādana.*

Q.- Could you talk about why the skin is so important?

When I did yoga in the early days, I perspired profusely because of the diseases I had. To buy medicines was beyond our financial situation. The smell of my perspiration was unbearable to my relatives and colleagues. In my heart of hearts I knew that I was definitely unhealthy, otherwise, why would it smell? I didn't follow the old theories; I felt that if I am sweating I should sweat but without smell. When I noted the density of perspiration gradually changing, my attention went to the skin. I asked myself: what is the skin's duty while performing *āsana*; is it just an anatomical cover of the body, or is it an organ of perception? The skin had to be expressing something within; how should it alone produce this smell? I started thinking about the skin. I would feel that while doing an *āsana*, there was no response, no action. I wondered why. Is my skin connected to my body, or is it outside of my body? If it is connected, then it should move also. So, let me learn with skin movement. When I started moving the skin, I realised the truth of ancient peoples' word that the skin is an organ of perception. I would feel thick patches of skin at some places and thin at some places. This made me think and then I started working on the skin. As it became thinner I soon noticed that the smell began to disappear, I decided that the quality of the skin will tell the quality of the organs inside. That is why, even today, my emphasis is on the skin.

The skin has a sensitivity of touch. When the skin comes into contact with the object outside it gives us the message. But with the practice, when I began to feel the thinness of skin, the sensitivity of touch began to come from within. This sensitivity from inside brought a great change not only in the practice of *āsana* but also in *prāṇāyāma, dhāraṇā* and *dhyāna*.

Q.- You said in class that the flesh is anatomical and the skin is an organ of intelligence.

Yes. According to *sāṁkhya* philosophy, the five senses of perception, and five organs of action, are connected to the elements – earth, water, fire, air and ether, and their qualities, smell, taste, shape, touch and sound. The five senses are meant to feel the body temperature, the reactions to the *āsana*, where heat is created, where it is not, where the coolness is felt and where not. I started understanding through observation and developed the sense of creating space in each joint while doing *āsana* or in walking. I used all these qualities of the elements as a source of understanding when I was doing *āsana*. That developed me to understand the *āsana* more and more.

The *Bhagavad Gītā* says that the body is the field, the self is the fielder. The agriculturist acts as a fielder and produces something by cultivating the field. I use the body as a field and the inner intelligence as the fielder, to find out the quality of the field and how the fielder has to work so that both the body and the intelligence work out and meet together. I started balancing the awareness in awareness of the intelligence as the anatomical body has sensitivity of its own. Flesh is an anatomical conative system: the skin is an organ of perception. It is cognitive and sensitive, unlike the muscles. The muscles act but they are not sensitive. They don't convey the message. The skin and the nerves convey the message. If there is a formation of pus or something, it tells on the skin. Otherwise disease remains hidden.

While practising I observe the flow of energy in the nerves and the skin, which gives the feeling of alignment, sensitivity and intelligence. Muscles may get aligned but they don't convey it to the self.

Q.- One of my favourite things that you say is that the diaphragm is the mediator between the physical body and the spiritual self. How?

The diaphragm balances our physical and mental bodies. When people suffer from a catastrophe, depression, sorrows and miseries, they say their solar plexus – the navel region, is tight and cramped. Why? What is the medium for our existence? It is the diaphragm. If the diaphragm is cut, can a man survive? Although it is a physical organ, you can see that it has tremendous bearing on the mental state. It is the only muscle which makes you draw the vital energy. If the diaphragm loses its freedom, the navel gets cramps. When there is fear or sorrow, the breathing is heavy because the diaphragm does not take an aligned movement upon inhaling or exhaling. We pant and wheeze. Everything affects the diaphragm first.

Suppose someone comes up to you and screams, "I will stab you!" You hold and contract the diaphragm. On the other hand, when you see the setting sun, or an old friend whom you have not seen for years, think of how you stretch the diaphragm and how the diaphragm opens. In yoga we learn to develop the elasticity of the diaphragm. *Prāṇāyāma* plays a very important role, as does *āsana*. In olden days people suffered from mental diseases; today there are stress diseases. They suffer the same. Why? Because there is no elasticity in the diaphragm. Tension and pressure make the diaphragm harder. "I ought to be like that." "I have to be competitive in life." "Come what may, I want to take that challenge." Although they take the challenge from the head, where does it grip? It starts from the diaphragm. The diaphragm is the window of the self. The more tension you have, the more the window of the diaphragm gets closed. If the diaphragm is spread, it takes any load, whether intellectual, emotional or physical. If you shorten it, or harden it, it has no room.

Q.- You are always getting after us of doing postures with our mind rather than with our body. Why?

In Western countries they have still not found the spiritual seat of the mind. The mind exists everywhere; the intellect exists only in the head. Emotional intelligence exists in the heart. The intelligence is of two types, namely emotional and intellectual. Now man has reached the moon. It is a vertical growth, a technological growth, an intellectual development. But today the mind is so small; everyone is only an individual. We think only of the head, whereas in the olden days, they were thinking of the heart, the seat of the sun giving room, inviting people and mixing with them.

The other day a doctor asked me if I could tell him where the mind is. I said I could give him a clue. If a married man is unfaithful with another woman, when he comes in and looks at his wife, where is the guilt felt? Is it in the brain or some other part? It's the heart. Actually, according to medical science, you would have to say it's the diaphragm that constricts: that's the seat of the intelligence of the heart. In yoga we try to open the emotional centre more and more, so that the broad-thinking comes and one appreciates what compassion and friendliness are. From your head you cannot understand what compassion is, what sympathy is, what friendliness is. Friendliness and compassion belong to the seat of the heart, the emotional centre. When there is harmony between the head and the heart, one is a saint. Otherwise, one is only an intellectual person. How many of us say, "He has an intellectual mind, but he is a stupid or egoistic fellow; he cannot understand how to live with his neighbours." That means that his mind is not cultivated, only his head has grown. Conscience is the seat of the mind. The head is an object, like another limb.

Q.- Could you talk about discipline and freedom?

Without discipline you cannot succeed in action. For example, if you walk zigzag in the street and a car hits you, this freedom may cause an accident. Discipline is a safety measure. It appears in the beginning as regimentation, but the moment you labour with love, discipline disappears and passion for the ultimate aim sets in. Until then, one thinks of it as discipline. But for us, we discipline ourselves to reach that passion of the ultimate goal. When transformation takes place, discipline suddenly vanishes and you become part and parcel of that object for which you and I are struggling.

I was struggling and nothing was coming. So I had to discipline tremendously and follow rigidly, to reach that state. For me there were only two ways on the precipice – either I have to fall in or I have to fall out, to accept or say good-bye. I couldn't play the middle. The moment I crossed the precipice, it no longer was a discipline – it became a passion, an urge to pursue. That was the change. Then I experienced freedom. Freedom comes when the discipline revolutionises the discipline as a passion for the art.

Q.- I would like to ask you a few questions about the medical aspects of yoga. If you have an injured part of the body, most medical people will say to avoid using that part. Your approach is make a point of working that area.

This is true. Suppose you have an injury to your heel. In yoga there are two methods – a recuperative method and an irritative method. Other systems of exercise have no recuperative or stimulative method to rest the injured part. If a runner has torn a muscle, he cannot run. If he does, he ends up in the hospital. With yoga, there are movements which revitalise and stimulate the injured part, so it heals. There is a healing touch in yoga. We say to go ahead because *āsana* supplies blood to those areas, helping them heal faster. Western doctors use ultraviolet rays to improve circulation. Yoga does the same. The *āsana* bring blood to an area by stretching and blocking other areas. For example, you do *Utthita Trikoṇāsana*. If on the right side the extension is good, the blood moves and flows well, and on the left side contraction takes place and the blood flow is blocked. Similarly, when you do it on the other side, the left side draws in blood and the right side does not (see Vol 3, Pl. n. 25). That is why we emphasise, "Do this, do that". A weight-lifter develops his biceps, triceps and looks muscular. How many people ask him how to develop the liver or the spleen? He may develop muscles, but how does he get his liver in good shape? Here yoga has an answer. *Yogāsana* are gravitational movements, which flush out the impure blood and bring in oxygenated blood to the area, making it healthier. Gravitational forces have a tremendous effect. Whenever I teach, I bring attention to maximising blood circulation, because unless and until the circulation improves, the organ will not be healthy. This is the supplying of the energy through the blood current to various areas, so the cells may become healthier.

The *āsana* teach you how to deal with the injured part. While doing the *āsana,* the injured area is not dealt with directly. If the knee or ankle is injured, the *āsana* are done in such a way that the weight of the body is not put directly. So the anti-gravitational *āsana* are introduced. The inverted *āsana* help to return the venous blood.

If the back is hurt, the lateral twistings are introduced in such a way that muscles do not get squeezed and the spine does not get compressed. Such actions in *āsana* will be stimulative, passive and curative whereas sometimes we give active movements when the joints are calcified due to injury. These active actions may seem irritative or painful at that moment, but they break the calcified particles and remove stiffness.

How can an untouched or unused part heal the injured area if not attended to with carefulness and discretion? Yoga basically gives the discriminative sensitivity to reach the injured area.

Q.- Are there any physical conditions that yoga cannot cure?

How can I say that? An effort should be made. Even if there is five percent progress, I say it is a success for yoga. You have seen how I work with children who have genetic defects. Even if their progress is one percent, I should consider it a great success. Yoga, being the art of action, has to bring an effect. It may or may not bring the maximum effect. Sometimes the seed may take two days to sprout; sometimes it may take one or two years. Perseverance is the key. Hence, it is not the physical condition that is involved but advertent attention in practice which is needed.

The question is not about the cure but it is a way of living one has to understand. Hence, I am sure that yogic practice shows the way to better living.

I repeat here what I answered in the previous question. There are innumerable *āsana*. We have innumerable methods with which to work in the affected areas. It is not just the accomplishment; it helps to see the placement of the different areas, various cells of the body in a healthy way in each *āsana*. It is a great science that teaches how to use one's body, how to energise the different areas of the body and how to bring the mind and will to that area where attention is needed.

"Yoga is meant for one and all, be they young, old, diseased, physically or mentally challenged, provided one has a will to do." If there is a will, there is a way, says *Haṭhayoga Pradīpikā*.[1]

Q.- We often hear people in yoga talk about strengthening the nerves, a concept not often discussed in Western medicine. I wonder if you could talk about that?

No, it is not strengthening the nerves. It is the culture of endurance and optimum level of the flow of energy in the nerves. The power of endurance depends on nerve cells. Nerves carry what is called bio-energy, supplied by the current of blood, like electricity. If there is a storehouse of this bio-energy in the nerve cells, then a person has tremendous patience to take any amount of load and stress with comfort. If there is stress and strain, the person's energy becomes a spent-force like a man who has an account with no bank balance. The bio-energy is consumed a lot due to intellectual thinking and emotional brooding. Some waste energy through unwanted movements of limbs and gestures, and often we see them collapsing. The *yogāsana*, by various right-extensions, movements and stability, help the blood current to flow to each and every part

---

1 *Yuvā vṛddho'tivṛddho vyādhito durbalo'pi vā /*
abhyāsāt siddhimāpnoti sarvayogeṣvatandritaḥ //
(*H.Y.P.*, I.64)

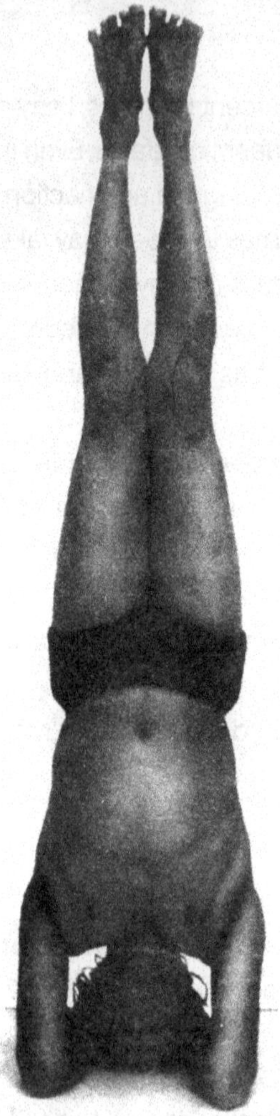

Plate n. 4 – ***Sālamba Śīrṣāsana***

of the body and supply the needed energy through the blood currents. That is why *prāṇāyāma* is also essential. Without the healthy functioning of the respiratory system, pure blood is not supplied to the system.

Yoga does not eat away energy; it supplies. That's the beauty of it. When you do *Sālamba Śīrṣāsana*, the blood is circulated in the head. When you come down, you feel completely refreshed. When you do *Setu bandha Sarvāṅgāsana* on the bench, the blood is supplied to the chest. Naturally, when you come down, you feel as if your chest has been renewed and is in a state of peace and poise.

Q.- Do you think people can reach a balanced mental state without yoga?

It may be possible for a very few gifted ones. But know that people like Ramakrishna Paramahamsa or Ramana Maharshi may seem to us that they did not do *yoga-sādhanā*, but you cannot forget that they did some *sādhanā* and yoga was there in their previous life's *sādhanā*. The *sādhanā* was refined as it was already flowing in their blood. An average man cannot compare himself with them. An average man thinks that he has a balanced mental state but the disturbances at the physical and mental levels afflict him immediately and he loses the balance easily.

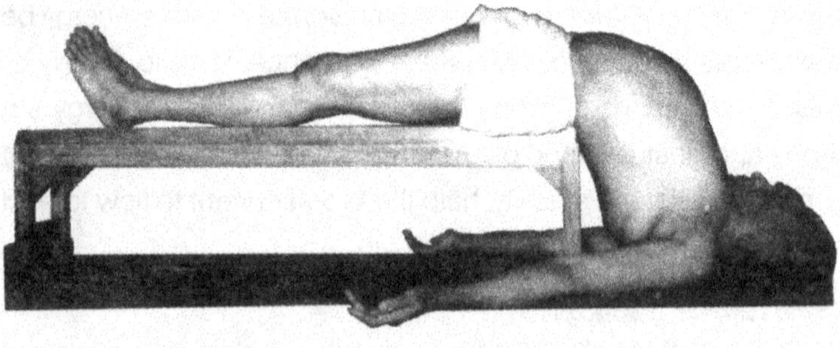

Plate n. 5 – ***Setu bandha Sarvāṅgāsana* on a bench**

If our brain and mind are the conscious intelligence, the nerves are the unconscious mind. When this conscious intelligence of brain and mind are weak, psychiatrists can guide a person. When the nerves collapse, or when there is a breakdown in the nervous system, then he or she may collapse and a psychiatrist cannot supply the needed energy or strength in the mind. He advises shock treatment or sedatives. In yoga, there is tremendous feeding of the nerves to store energy in the nervous system. Then there is no possibility of the mind breaking.

I have seen and met people who practised meditation without developing stability and lost balance both in body and mind. When people are not of a stable body and mind, they are advised medication or meditation. Meditation is an introverting art. It takes one inwards. When such unstable and unbalanced people become introverted, they become negative. So we have to make them extroverted so that they pay attention to the body and become positive. They need the practice of *āsana* and *prāṇāyāma*, which make one come out of the depression or the dreamy illusions they have created around themselves. These aspects build up the strength in the nerves, senses and mind to be positive. If an introverted person goes into meditation, he becomes diseased; that is why they face failure and dejection. Yoga says an extrovert should become an introvert and an introvert should become an extrovert. The first five aspects of yoga bring a proper balance between these two tendencies, namely, extroversion and introversion. Then a person can travel out or travel in with ease. When a person knows what extroversion and introversion are, he is complete in the sense that he does not get disturbed or perturbed. His body, mind, senses, nerves, brain and intelligence co-operate and co-ordinate properly. To a negative person, meditation is a negative approach and by doing that he gets shaky and confused. That is why the earlier, outer parts of yoga, namely *yama, niyama, āsana* and *prāṇāyāma,* are taught to make the practitioner strong in body and mind before one moves into the inner layers of yoga, namely, *pratyāhāra, dhāraṇā* and *dhyāna.*

Wrong practice of yoga can disturb the balance of the elements in the body and bring diseases leading to complications.

Q.- We know that incorrect practice of yoga can cause physical problems. Could it also cause difficulties in the psychological state?

Yes, yes. That is what I am explaining. The first ill-effect of a wrong practice is irritability. People read books and think that they have improved in yoga. They begin to believe that since they do not care for worldly matters, they are "irritable". The sign of irritability should not be mistaken for renunciation. Practice of yoga needs self-study and examination of oneself. One needs to learn to know one's own mistakes and weaknesses and learn to rectify them first.

I ask myself why, if I was not irritable yesterday, why am I today? How can this happen? Something must have gone wrong in my practice, this is why my nerves are disturbed. As my nerves are disturbed, they become shaky inside, creating irritability. So I work; I say, "Let me see tomorrow. Let me see how I did it yesterday. Can I repeat that?" If I again feel the irritability, that means I have done wrong practice. Just as you have to climb steps one after another, in yoga you have to climb according to your capacity. You have to see how much clarity and how much confusion you have. If there is confusion, how can you move ahead? You have to go slowly to get confidence. You have to think and recollect your practice, where you went wrong as well as to see where the unrhythmic non-sequential methods set in for irritability, mental disturbances and all these. Then, yoga is a friend; otherwise, it is a foe.

The psychological disturbance is possible if practice is wrong or overdone or underdone. So it is safe to build up the body's intelligence through *āsana*, and its energy through *prāṇāyāma* before jumping to the other subtle aspects of yoga.

Q.- How has yoga changed your psychological state?

I had tremendous power to endure pain as well as pleasure. I used to go to the depths of pain when I was doing the *āsana*. I had to struggle. But in that struggle I found out the range of pain which came to me, and I absorbed all those things. After absorbing, only I knew what is right practice and what is wrong practice. If I had a little pain, I would ask, why did that pain come? Is there pain on the other side also? If the pain is not on the other side, why is it paining on the first side? My logic commences at that moment. This way I understood myself. This helped me to know what happens to others. If someone says, "I am getting this pricking pain", I am quick to say, "Your hand is placed wrongly". I correct the problem immediately. If I had not suffered, how would I know? Due to the pains and suffering I underwent in my early days ~~and~~ determination in pursuit of the subject, steady psychological growth took place in me. Secondly, the will to know the mistakes made me re-think. This acted as a stepping stone for evolution in my mental make-up.

The accurate sequencing of *āsana*, balancing rhythmically the various diverse parts of the body to bring unity was learnt by adoption and adaptation and made my mind steady for further study.[1]

---

[1] *Kramānyatvam pariṇāmānyatve hetuḥ* (*Y.S.*, III.15). Order of successive sequencing the *āsana* practice brings not only different feelings of transformation but later leads to a right distinct thought wave.

Q.- Where are you in your own practice?

While I am teaching intensely my mind is diverted into an external approach and in my own practice I move inwards to act from the core of the being. Who knows, a new light may come to me. That is why I go within. Now, I am teaching in such a way to convert *bahiraṅga* into *antaraṅga sādhanā* in *āsana* and *prāṇāyāma*. I have lived a rigid life from childhood. Soon I may convert my profession into a hobby. A hobby doesn't mean doing yoga casually or changing the subject matter. Let me go in my practice to integrate and unite body with senses, senses with mind, mind with energy to understand the flow of energy, connecting energy with intelligence and intelligence with the self. Actually it is hard for me to talk about my going inwards. Factually I lose my individuality and feel the cosmic sense or the sense of non-division in the *sādhanā*.

Q.- How do you see your role as a teacher? What are you aiming at when you walk in the classroom and see a group of students in front of you?

One good thing is that I don't aim at all. But when I start working, I ask if it is possible to bring these people to my level in a shorter period than I took, that is the only reason why I am strong in class which appears as aggressive. Why should you waste your time as I did in my earlier days – not knowing what alignment is, what rhythm is? My brain was thinking and my body forgetting, or the body remembering and the head thinking something else. All these things I had to face in my early days. Is it essential for everyone to go through that? Why not show a direct path and proceed? So I look at my students, keenly observe their response which nourishes me with the feedback to work with renewed ideas on the subject and keep their minds away from the time factor. This freedom from the time factor helps me with what to teach and how much to teach and when to stop so that they are not bored.

Q.- When do you think a student of yoga can start to teach? Are there certain characteristics that need to develop before a person can begin?

We need to differentiate between teaching yoga and teaching *āsana*. Confidence, clarity and compassion – these three are sufficient to teach *āsana*. Clarity, because if you have to teach, you should be clear in what you know. For instance, if I know only ten *āsana*, I should be clear in those ten *āsana*, so I can say, "I know these ten". If somebody can teach you better than me, I should admit that. If something is new, I will not try it on another person, I will try it on me. I take risks on myself and not on others.

This is how my approach was. That's why now I talk confidently and create confidence in all of you. I know to what degree a raw body can provoke the teacher to handle that body and mind. In this manner, I think and work out a strategy for the student. My body is so sensitive, so mobile and so elastic, I stretch to experience the feelings of my students by imitating their ways of presentation. I struggle more than them to penetrate their psyche in order to learn what is needed for them to progress. I get clarity, then I teach and see how they bring progress in their practice.

Also, if one has to teach yoga, then one needs a thorough knowledge of it. One has to be very disciplined, honest, practical and devoted to the *sādhanā*.

Q.- Do you teach Westerners differently from Easterners?

No, not at all. That is a misunderstanding. I have the power to bear emotional upheavals with patience. I tap that intelligence to use it in the emotional area. We are lethargic. I have to behave like a slave driver. If I were lazy, I would probably not have come to this level. Having worked hard, I know how much effort it requires to experience this. Though Easterners go on saying, "I have a pain here, I have a pain there", they will not cry like the Westerners. They only complain. Western people want to solve everything intellectually, even the *āsana* or the pains. An emotional disease has to be worked on emotionally. So one has to think what one could give to this person. I cannot think only intellectually. I have to weigh the intellectual and emotional capabilities before handling the student.

One has to think of what area affects them. What is the feeling? How do their minds behave? Observing all this one has to feed those areas.

Yoga is a universal subject. As the physics and chemistry cannot change for Westerners or Easterners so also yoga cannot be changed. All the rules, regulations, principles remain the same for both. Still it is a subject to be dealt with individually according to their capacity of physical, mental, emotional, psychological, intellectual levels. Therefore, it may strike one that the system may be different for Westerners.

The weather in India is different from the weather in your countries. People in my country get exhausted quickly due to the heat. Therefore they need *sādhanā* that is adapted to sustain their energy in a slightly different way.

In case the pollution level is high it affects not only the body but the mind also. Therefore, the approach may differ but the teaching does not differ.

Ultimately, it depends upon the practitioner, whether he or she is a Westerner or an Easterner, to grasp and absorb the subject.

Q.- You explained in class one day why it is that you slap people in class, and how that brings awareness. Could you repeat that?

Actually, the word is not "slapping". Because often slapping means on the face.

The dull part is very, very insensitive. With all the power of their intelligence, students may still not observe the dullness of the particular part. At that moment, I go and hit precisely that part where one is dull so that their attention is brought to that needed part. My hit not only brings about awareness but adjusts the part at par with the other. I go and teach a certain movement according to the demands of the skin, ribs or muscles. If it is too dull, too broad, my instinctive fingers adjust and spread at once to cover the area to bring sensations in that part. By the correct touch or hit I create action, and they get the *āsana* and feel happy.

Also why don't you appreciate the other side of it. You say that I slap, but when you do *Sālamba Śīrṣāsana* and do not get the balance, I use my knee on the dorsal back to get the balance. Then do you call it a slap? Why don't you call it "skill"? Can anyone else give such exactness or balance? My body has learnt that. My touch or hit too will be only that much, a measured hit so that it works.

– *Yes, I've had direct experience of your method. (Both laugh!)* –

One may be very intelligent, but would that intelligence be of any use if it does not discriminate and work on the dull area? We have developed our intelligence to work in the outer world; but that same intelligence of ours does not work to feel the inner world in us. Why waste forty or fifty years? Learn quickly to observe these things and live a harmonious life in body, mind and self.

If I am soft, it may take a long time for you to progress. Now I create intelligence and sensitivity at once while in the earlier days I was not that quick in creating that intelligence on my pupils. I was making them act mechanically. It means repetition of the same for days and days. As constructive change took place in me, my teaching method changed. I try to create that intelligence and sensitivity so the students learn and become original in their practice and teaching.

I am giving links of the chain of each *āsana*, making each one to understand that the knowledge grows up subjectively. I am making each and everyone become more and more subjective and sensitive rather than just objective. As a teacher, I make everyone experience subjectively rather than know the subject objectively.

Previously I had to work like a donkey to create interest in each and everyone. Today, the interest is there. Now my job is not necessarily to create further interest but to ignite the fire in my students by making them understand themselves. Previously, I used to present each aspect of what I do and how you all do. Now, my students who are in touch with me become aware with just my touch and adjust the inner body and respond well.

Q.- Do you have anything more to say?

Yoga is a light which once lit can never fade out. The more you do, the brighter the flame burns in you. Yoga is a fountain for all things in the world. It has been given to us, but we do not know how to make use of it. When we rightly understand and adopt it in the right way, the whole world will be revolutionised.

"TUNE YOURSELF TO THE MUSIC OF YOGA"*

Q.- What made you follow the path of yoga?

It is rather hard for me to recollect the situation which is fifty years old. You see, I have come from a very poor orthodox family of Karnataka. My father then was a primary school teacher. My parents had thirteen children. I was the eleventh child. Fortunately or unfortunately I was born at a time when the whole world was engulfed with the epidemic disease of influenza in 1918. My mother was affected by this fever, yet, providence saved both of us to survive but it left an impact on my state of health, with thin legs and arms, protruded abdomen and drooping head. Soon, we lost our father which added to our difficulties.

It was common in those days to undergo a medical check up once in six months in schools. While I was studying in the middle school, the doctor suspected that I had contracted tuberculosis. There were no antibiotic drugs and I had to leave my future to destiny. At that time, my brother-in-law – my elder sister's husband – an adept in yoga, asked me why I should not do yoga to gain health. He introduced me to a few yogic *āsana*, which slowly and surely became a turning point in my life. My nagging negative life was turned to hope and confidence thereafter.

Q.- What was the driving force behind your career as a yoga teacher and what was it that inspired you to continue?

In 1936, the late Mahārāja of Mysore sent my *gurujī* to propagate yoga in Mumbai and parts of Northern Karnataka, then in the Bombay Presidency. My *gurujī* asked me to follow him along with his senior students. Our yogic presentation attracted interest in the public and many desired my *gurujī* to conduct classes. He readily agreed. There were many women in the group who were keen to learn but were reluctant to learn from the elderly persons. In those days women were very shy even to stand in front of men. So my *gurujī* asked them whether they had any

* Interview by Burjor Taraporewala and Sam Motivala for *Eve's Weekly*, September, 4-10, 1982.

objections to learn from me. As I was the youngest in the group, they readily agreed, but I was nervous. I knew very little of yoga but the responsibility was great. First I almost became hysterical. Knowing that I was just a novice in yoga, I was placed in a very sensitive situation and yet within myself I thought that I should prove my worth and agreed to teach them. This way the inspiration to teach yoga was planted in me by the lady members of Dharwar.

In the thirties and forties, yoga was unknown even to Indians. Very few were interested. People were under the impression that those who had quarrelled at home, dejected in life or mentally unsound were turning towards yoga. So I made up my mind to work more on the practical aspects than on the philosophical aspects to remove these misapprehensions. This idea of practical presentation started igniting interest in people rather than just curiosity. This probably was the driving force to build up my career as a yoga teacher. New challenges from human personalities inspired me to find a solution through yogic practices.

Q.- What according to you are the special qualities required to make a good yoga student? At what age should one start?

There are no special qualities required to be a student of yoga but certain characteristics are a must. Of course, these characteristics need to be cultivated to acquire or to stick in the chosen path without deviation of thought. One must have courage to face failures that come in the way and to persistently persevere with faith and vigour in the turmoils of ups and downs in one's efforts and develop sharp memory so that one can compare and watch the progress within oneself. One must develop one's awareness with attention by acquainting intelligence with each and every fibre and cell of the body. Lastly one has to labour with love. These are the qualities required from a student not only in yoga but in all forms of art. These qualities are a must to master any art and yoga is no exception.

Remember that yoga is the basic art of all arts. In yoga one has to depend upon the inner resources of energy and strength and use the body, mind and will as instruments to tune oneself to live fully to the music of life, whereas in other arts like music, dance, painting, architecture or sculpture, one has to depend on external resources to express one's spiritual light.

Yoga can be taught from the age of six or seven. Children should be taught in such a way so that they imbibe an interest in it as conative exercises. Then at adolescence, yoga can be taught on a physiological level as organic exercises to be performed with grace, and from the age of twenty-five onwards as mental culture, so that when fully matured, it can be practised as a spiritual pursuit towards Self-realisation.

Q.- In your opinion, are women more attracted to yoga discipline than men? If so, why?

It is a fact that women take to yoga more than men. Being a man myself, it is not easy for me to find the reasons for it. But as far as I study, man thinks vertically and so acts from his head. Women's intelligence is ruled by the heart. They think and act according to the heart, so they have a broad mind. Man is content with his success, selfish in his outlook and heedless towards his health. Hope men forgive me for my remarks!

Women are more prone towards compassion and go out to console and help others. A woman tries to keep everyone pleased, happy and contented. By nature she is a self sacrificing person. She conceals all her sufferings. Knowing that she cannot conceal for long, she looks for avenues to gain health, mental poise and strength so that she has the power to endure and keep harmony at home. She turns towards yoga which helps both body and mind to gain emotional peace and poise. I think she is more enlightened than man to take to yoga for keeping fit in body and clear in mental balance.

Secondly, yogic exercises are not violent movements. So it befits her. Yoga being a non-competitive exercise, man shows less inclination.

Yet, man too now realises the importance of yoga as a remedy for stress and strain and now a good number of men too are taking to yoga.

Q.- What in your opinion are the similarities and dissimilarities in yoga discipline amongst your pupils in affluent and non-affluent countries?

Affluent countries have everything in abundance. They have plenty of resources to develop their physical, mental, intellectual and financial potencies. So chances of abuse are also more. They analyse factual problems like love, sex, compassion and friendliness from the intellectual calibre rather than from the seat of the heart. Their study is more objective than subjective. They do everything by sheer intellectual will power and cannot take pains and failures with patience and tolerance.

In non-affluent countries, people have to struggle for existence. As such their minds have a limited approach. Not that they have no intellectual potency. They have a great deal of knowledge acquired through experience. So the knowledge is subjective. As avenues to acquire the knowledge are not there due to economic wants, they bear all sufferings and face life magnanimously. In affluent countries people do everything in excess. In the non-affluent countries it is a problem to balance the body mechanism without proper nourishment. Hence, the ultimate end is the same. The affluent lose health by overindulgence and non-affluent people lose health due to wants. Hence, yoga is taught to the affluent to remove the toxins created by over-nourishment and for the non-affluent it is taught to assimilate the body they take and make them feed from within by proper energy circulation to balance the hormones. While teaching the affluent, we work from the intellect towards emotion whereas for the non-affluent, we build them from the emotional seat of the heart towards the intellectual clarity of the head.

Q.- You have taught yoga in different continents for over 40 years and are considered as one of the best yoga teachers throughout the world. Why is it that you are more famous outside your country?

It is a fact all over the world outstanding people are kept out-standing! But in India it is more visible that outstanding people are kept out. There is an adage that "no prophet is respected in his own country". I think our government is the last to open its eyes to recognise the potentialities of our own men. Only when other parts of the world recognise the achievements of our artists and scientists does our government begin to scrutinise whether such a person exists in India or not.

It was in the year 1952, when Pandit Nehru invited the world famous violinist Mr. Yehudi Menuhin to India, this great artist recognised my talent in yoga. He improved on his violin through my teaching and called me, "my best violin teacher". He transmitted all my techniques to his violin playing and found them very useful. He invited me to the West and presented me to the people of the West. Again it is through him that my method of teaching was adopted in the educational institutions of England. America. Africa and Japan too invited me and there too it spread. Students came from Pakistan, Europe, New Zealand and Australia and spread my art in their respective countries. I think the success of my work may be attributed to my strict discipline, sincerity, honesty of purpose and compassion to all though I appear harsh and rough from outside.

When Mr. Menuhin introduced me to the late Prime Minister, Shri Jawaharlal Nehru, in 1954 and asked him to show his practice to me, he declined saying that he did not want to show his weakness to one who was not half his age. In India, there is the feeling that yoga is to be adopted in old age. The teacher should be aged, it is as though youngsters cannot take to it. According to Indian thought yoga is meant for *aśramaits* like *vānaprasthi* and *sannyāsi,* and not for *brahmacāri* and *gṛhasthi.* Again, there is a misunderstanding that yoga means to sit and meditate and move away from the activities of the world. If I am not famous in India it does not matter to me since yoga is not practised to gain popularity. I feel only sorry that such a great science and way of leading one's life which has been shown by our ancestors, is not only being neglected but even criticised by us. I am doing my best for people to recognise its value sooner or later.

Q.- Does yoga discipline help to change the mental outlook of the individual?

In the beginning, the immediate effect is the feeling of well-being. This alone is the key to persevere, though the progress is agonisingly slow and takes years for changes to appear. By persistent yogic practice, intelligence becomes mobile and extends and expands in each of the *āsana*-practice, and is made to interpenetrate from the skin towards the self and outerpenetrate from the self towards the skin. This brings the flow of alertness in intelligence and creates awareness in the cells making the *sādhaka* live totally as a single unit from the cells of the skin to the self. This is the beginning of knowing thyself. From then on mental attitude makes a return journey towards its source. This is the turning point in yoga.

This way change in mental outlook dawns as one perseveres in practice.

Q.- Can you give some idea of your experiences with drug addicts and prisoners?

Addicts are primarily empty and absent-minded. While accepting them, I have to think what *āsana* would help to remove the vacuum in them. As they go silent, empty and dull within, I have to be with them moment to moment to fill the awareness and attention in their way of living while practising. I have to make them work on *āsana* to live in the present that creates exhilaration. I have to show them that nature abounds with exhilarating principles through which yogic *āsana* tickle and trigger their nerves. This sensation in them has made many to be free from smoking, alcoholic and drug addictions and transforms them for better living and high thinking.

Regarding prisoners, they are aggressive and destructive, yet soft in their hearts. Their intelligence is limited in understanding moral behaviour. In prison they do repent for their crimes and like to find solace. Mild practice does not convince them. They love the speedy sequences of doing *āsana,* which exhilarate the brain, and difficult *āsana,* which attract them. So we teach what they ask and slowly change them for the better. At San Francisco, seeing a few hard core prisoners was a delight for me. They all embraced me and kissed me when I talked to them and showed what they can do in their cells to keep lively. They liked it and are as humane as we are, but circumstances make them choose that path. With compassion, firmness and a friendly approach in *āsana,* they come to smile.

The sequences of *āsana* for the mental state of addicts and prisoners differ. I feel the disappointments, sorrow, negative attitude, too much money or poverty, dissatisfaction of family life, broken families, cause them to take to addiction and crime.

Yet, we need to discuss with them first their basic requirements so that we plan the *āsana* or *prāṇāyāma* which are beneficial to them. A friendly approach is needed to make them develop constructive ideas so that they become aware of their weaknesses and get uplifted from their present mind-pit.

For the addicts, as I told you, I choose the *āsana* and *prāṇāyāma* which remove the emptiness, defeat and dejection in them. The standing *āsana,* inversions and backward extensions are very effective. Relaxing *āsana* like forward extensions do not help them much as their minds go towards depression. Therefore they need to be kept active.

Sometimes I make them do the standing *āsana* and backward extensions very fast to refresh their minds. *Āsana* such as *Ūrdhva Dhanurāsana, Viparīta Daṇḍāsana, Viparīta Chakrāsana* (see plate n. 29), or *Adho Mukha Vṛkṣāsana, Pinca Mayurāsana,* exhilarate and bring cheerfulness in them. *Āsana* like *Sālamba Śīrṣāsana, Sālamba* and *Sarvāṅgāsana* sharpen their brain. Doing *Halāsana* and *Paścimottanāsana* repeatedly in quick succession acts like a bath as brainwashing which soon stimulates and freshens for better living and higher thinking. The *āsana* brings chemical changes. The smoker begins to enjoy the fresh air, the addict no more likes the dullness or dope. The stomach and liver, and finally the entire body system reject alcohol.

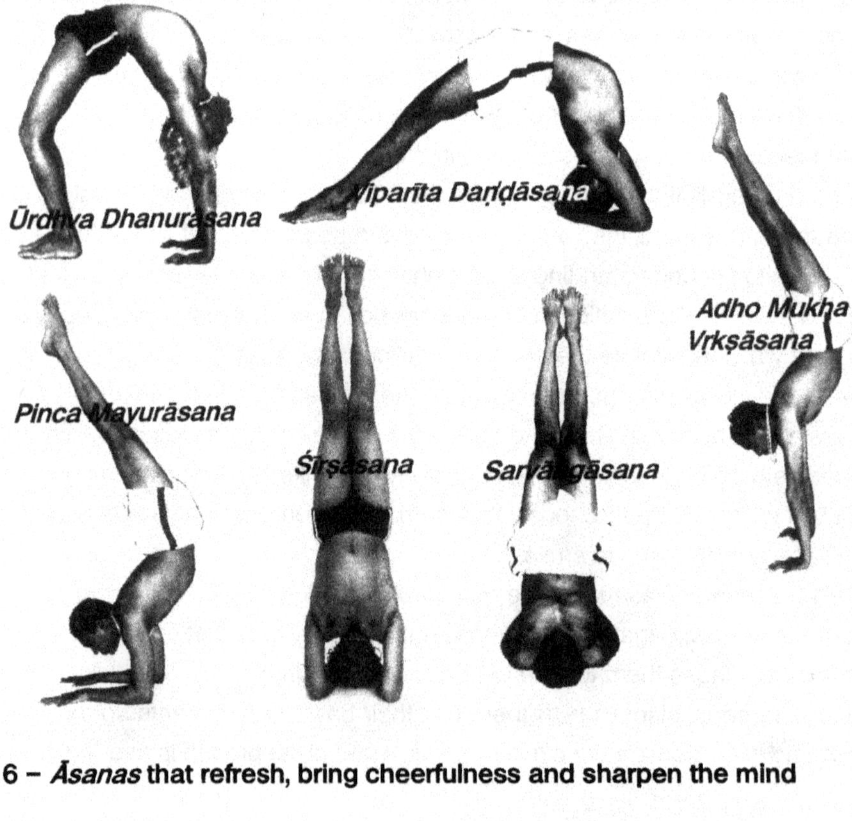

Plate n. 6 – *Āsanas* that refresh, bring cheerfulness and sharpen the mind

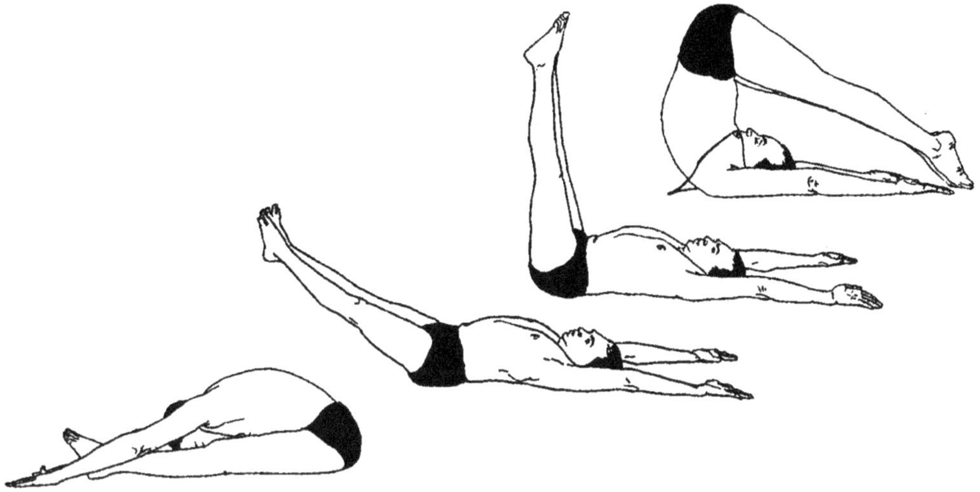

Plate n. 7 – *Halāsana* and *Paścimottanāsana* repeatedly in quick succession

Q.- What impelled you to write your two books *Light on Yoga* and *Light on Prāṇāyāma*?

I must have been born to become a teacher and not an author. No doubt, by the grace of God I transformed the natural ability that I had into talent which was acquired through strong will and efforts in the art of teaching yoga. Not once did the thought come to my mind to take to writing. Mr. Jal Taraporewala of Taraporewala Publishers called me to his office in 1959 to consult regarding publication of a yoga book. He had many photos of various yoga masters and asked me to bring my photos. He compared each one and asked why should I not write a book with such good photographs. I said, I would consider and slept on it for months.

Then my pupils encouraged me and insisted that I should make an attempt and they would help me later. As they coaxed me, I hesitantly started to make a beginning. Meanwhile Taraporewala intimated to me that he was not interested in my book with so many illustrations. As I had started it, I made up my mind to finish it with the help of my pupils. I also informed my pupils in London that I was working on a book on yoga. A pupil of mine, Mrs. Beatrice Harthan asked me to bring the script and photos with me as I was visiting London. I took the script and photos. She was a friend of Mr. Gerald Yorke, the literary adviser of George Allen & Unwin Ltd. He carefully went through the script, showed me guidelines on how to write a book and promised to edit the entire work. Thus the credit and merit of these two monumental manuals go to him as they are considered classics. Believe me, *Light on Yoga* took me five years to complete while *Light on Prāṇāyāma* took eight years.

Never in my life did I think that I would be an author. The word 'yoga' was never in my heart. When friends and circumstances forced me, I began writing and tearing the papers and re-writing dozens of times for *Light on Yoga.* This work on *Light on Yoga* gave me hope and confidence to touch the other aspects of yoga.

Q.- Can you mention one or two unforgettable moments in your life?

There are many such instances in my life. But the most unforgettable ones are: when I and my wife dreamt a good omen the same night in 1946. Lord of the Seven Hills, Bālājī came in my dream, gave me a few grains of rice from one hand[1] and told me that from then on I need not worry about day to day survival for existence, and with the other hand, blessed me to carry on with my practice. As soon as I got up, I narrated this dream to my wife, who in turn surprised me with her dream. She saw Goddess Lakṣmi who placed a small silver coin in her palm saying that she owed that to me and disappeared. Since that day we were not in want. Slowly people started asking for yoga tuitions and certainly, my teaching grew from individuals towards institutions. Until 1981, I never realised that the dream would have a complete cycle. I started with *āsana* and *prāṇāyāma* and I never knew that they would terminate in the form of two classics. So I went to Tirupati and offered as an oblation my *Light on Yoga* and *Light on Prāṇāyāma*[2] in March '81. I did not offer the first book when released, as my work was half done.

The second incident was my lecture/demonstration at the Central Hall, Westminster, in London in 1972. It was a big hall which accommodates 2,350 people. The stakes were high, the rent of the hall was too much. I was nervous to give a demonstration in such a big hall with a few hundred people. I was worried whether they would meet the expenses at all. My pupils were encouraging me not to bother. They were more optimistic than me. As they expected more members, they wanted me to guide them to raise a high platform. So I went to the auditorium in the morning to guide and arrange seats and so on. While helping I got a severe catch in my back which made it difficult to stand or turn. I was annoyed with the catch and disgusted with myself. I took leave of my pupils to go home as the soreness increased. I went home, rested the back to relieve the spasms; prayed to God to help me out that night. With a heavy heart I reached the hall half an hour before time. I was to encounter for the first time such a huge audience coming from all parts of England. After speaking on the philosophy of yoga I showed the art of *prāṇāyāma* and

---

1 See *Aṣṭadaḷa Yogamālā,* vol. 1.

2 Published by Harper Collins, London.

its effects. To my surprise, after I finished my *prāṇāyāma*, I felt relief in my back and from then on I gave one of my finest presentations of *āsana* demonstrations, which lasted more than two hours. After these hours of trials and tribulations it all ended in triumph.

Q.- Does incorrect practice of yoga cause physical problems and difficulties in one's mental condition?

The practitioner of yoga can invite physical and mental problems, if the practice is incorrect. Wrong practice can cause uneasiness, irritation, aches and pains and may invite some diseases too such as indigestion, constipation, anaemia and so on. As far as the mental condition of the practitioner is concerned, not only wrong practice but faulty notions about yogic methodology can also cause problems. First of all, while practising *āsana, prāṇāyāma* or *dhyāna*, the nervous system plays a major role. Nerves are the bridge between the body and mind. If the nerves are disturbed, then both the body and the mind are disturbed which may cause the above mentioned problems on a physical level and bring shakiness of nerves, fear, anxiety, depression, aggressiveness or even laziness, inertia, dullness and so on.

Again, there is a wrong notion about yoga. Yoga is undoubtedly a path of renunciation - *vairāgya*. But it does not begin with renunciation. It begins with practice - *abhyāsa*, and one sees the renunciation as effect or fruit of practice. However, some people reverse the process and begin with so-called renunciation. They think that they have to become detached from everything. Therefore, they suddenly change their daily routine, their attitude and their interaction with others overnight. Such undue imposed discipline on oneself without any proper background or previous practice or any understanding of the concept of renunciation is wrong, causing tremendous disturbance in the nerves. It disturbs the mind too. People jump on the practice of meditation, retention of breath - *kuṁbhaka* -, forceful breathing techniques without having a proper hold on the body, nerves, breath or mind. Such practice can derange the nerves, which can cause emotional and mental imbalance.

Therefore, while practising yoga one should climb the ladder step by step. One has to have a retrospection after the practice on one's physical, mental and intellectual aspects. Body ache, disturbance in the mental state, sudden energy-fall, lethargic approach, undue disinterest towards family and society, heedlessness to one's responsibilities, sudden increase or decrease of desires, emotional upheaval or emotional dryness and emptiness, intellectual arrogance, tendency towards dry, non-fruitful and non-conclusive faulty arguments, non-coherent talking, all these indicate the wrong practice of yoga.

Careless practice of yoga is like walking inattentively on the street, and ending with an accident. One has to learn to climb the ladder of yoga according to one's capacity, constitution, strength and pliability. So watch carefully the reactions of a healthy growth and practice.

One need not get alarmed, but by knowing the other side of the effects, one should learn to be on the right path.

Q.- How has yoga changed your own mental make-up since you began practising?

My practice not only evolved but revolutionised me. Transformation in body and sharpness in mind were visible. To see good and weak points dispassionately in me and others developed. I developed a tremendous power of enduring pain as though it is a pleasure and a joy. I could go to the depths of pain and absorb them and at the same time work to find out the causes and the way of remedies by repeated performances. If one side was paining and not the other side, logically I was having a dialogue with the other side while doing, i.e. finding ways by adjusting and remodelling the *āsana*. Tolerating all these deliberate as well as natural pains, I understood inside and outside of me. New things began to strike me in a flash which became intuition. It taught me when to be tolerant, steadfast, patient, when to use the will power or to surrender it, and how to work to overcome limitations.

Q.- The Ramāmaṇi Iyengar Memorial Yoga Institute built in memory of your wife is considered unique in its field. Could you enlighten us what makes it so?

Are you asking me about the uniqueness of the building or my method of yoga? First of all this Institute is a gift from friends and lovers of yoga who 'adored' my wife's way of life. It is no doubt a unique structure in Asia wherein the concepts of yoga are expressed. Yoga's eight aspects are represented by the eight columns; the centre beam represents the healthy spine, with white paint on the ceiling for clarity in brain; three storeys represent body, mind and soul. The God Hanumān on the top of the building and the buttresses on the roof represent the merging of individual paths as well as the individuals with God. In this way, the building is unique.

Regarding my practice and teaching methods, I worked with sincerity in purpose to go beyond my mental capacity and actually took on myself the load of everyone's suffering and prayed Lord Hanumān to bring happiness to those who came to me to learn yoga. Similarly, the

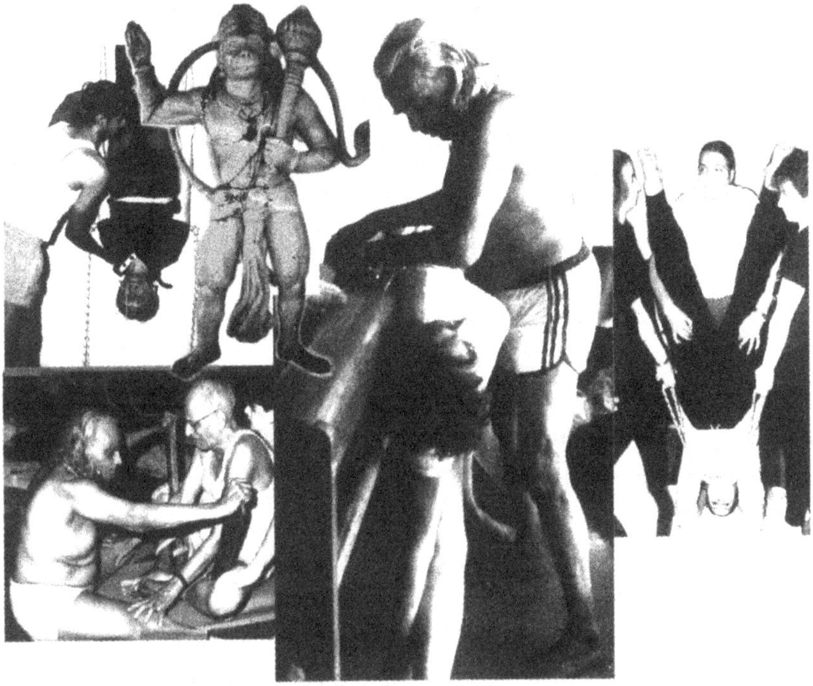

Plate n. 8 – The character of helping

teachers who help pick up this character of mine by which I serve the students has led people to consider the Institute to be unique. The motto is to help each and everyone towards perfection and precision as precision is the only way to understand truth. Mahatma Gandhi said truth is God; here each one is made to see God through perfection.

Q.- Have you any special message to give to the readers of *Eve's Weekly?*

Yoga is a light which once lit can never fade out. The more you do, the brighter the flame burns. It is a fountain for knowledge of the material world as well as the spiritual world. The sages of yore gave us this discipline, but we have to learn to make use of it as it brings physical and mental health. By this physical health and mental poise a new world will be built if we all practise it. For years the seed of yoga never sprouted.

With the blessings of God, thousands of teachers trained by me have taken the responsibility of teaching yoga. I am sure now that yoga has germinated well and is spreading all over the globe. Their responsibilities are going to increase as days go by and I have faith in them carrying out this art with attention, absorption, dedication and devotion for the people in the world to drink the nectar of health, peace and prosperity.

PATHS ARE MANY, BUT THE GOAL IS ONE AND THE SAME*

Q.- During the intensive you have emphasised the unity of all yoga practices and it has only been in recent times that they have been separated into categories of yoga practice. Please comment on this.

There is a tremendous historical background for the break of the continuity of our Indian traditions in art, science and philosophy. Once upon a time our country was completely free. People used to move without any hindrances or fear complexes. Our country was attacked from the north-west. The country was plundered, the people were massacred and its wealth was looted and carried away. This created fear complexes in the people.

Their religious traditions were forced on us. This had a tremendous bearing on the loss of our great ancient art. The Indian people had to live guarding their women in order to see that they maintained their purity. So each one was suspicious of the others, and they formed small groups and protected themselves. Due to this break-up a communication gap set in. Due to this communication gap as well as the destruction of our many sacred books, knowledge and understanding were lost and yoga and other allied subjects kept as secret subjects. Therefore it could not spread. Yoga was the way of life before the invasion of India from outside and was known to each and everyone. This invasion created turmoil in people who left for remote places where various subcastes and sects developed in the Hindu family.

Groups of people carried away whatever manuscripts they had to remote places and saved them for posterity. Today we are all depending on those manuscripts to work and build-up the knowledge again. Luckily, the human chain of civilisation did not break. The methodology had to be rebuilt connecting the possible links in order to reach that goal of realisation. This is how the traditions deviated. Even today one can see the impact of that deviation as several groups of individuals began practising their innovations in our Indian art and tradition. On account of these interruptions the real essence of that flow of intelligence is lost, therefore someone had

---

* This interview was taken 1st December 1982, by Norman Mackenzie. Published in two parts in *Yoga Center of Victoria Newsletter,* March and April, 1983.

to find out where the old knowledge and present time understanding could meet and how it could be integrated. On that basis I am working on my pet art, yoga, and trying my best to bring the various aspects of yoga together. When I say this, please, know that my practice of yoga, as far as I am concerned, is a total and complete path which is inclusive of *jñāna, karma* and *bhakti*.

Q.- In the West it seems misunderstanding has lead to divisions of yoga, such as *bhakti yoga, jñāna yoga* and so on. Can you discuss this?

The division appears to have arisen with intellectuals. Yoga is union, hence it is one but the paths – *mārga* – are many. They are *jñāna mārga, karma mārga, bhakti mārga* and *yoga mārga*. All these four paths are meant to reach the same destination, i.e., Self-realisation. These paths were given to us to take initiative according to one's tendencies or inclinations. Later on those who were explicit in one path, though the others are implicit in it, began naming the paths as yoga, as *karma yoga, jñāna yoga, rāja yoga, bhakti yoga* and *haṭha yoga* and so forth. For example *karma mārga* is not possible unless there is *bhakti mārga* and *jñāna mārga*. If action in *karma yoga* is predominant, it is termed as *karma mārga*. The same vocabulary follows with *jñāna* and *bhakti yoga*. Know also that yoga similarly covers all paths.

If one who is interested in gaining knowledge analytically and predominantly acts as a thinker, naturally he is called a *jñāna yogi*. Such people pride themselves as *jñāna yogi*. If one follows *bhakti yoga* then *jñāna, karma* and *yoga* get submerged and the *bhakti* takes the lead. If one is more emotional, then the devotional aspects are emphasised and expressed more than *jñāna, karma* or *yoga*. As far as my understanding goes, none can differentiate these four paths except on the part which may predominate in the *sādhaka*. So these paths cannot be divided. It is just weakness of the aspirants to miss the potential of the other paths as the seeds of *yoga, jñāna, karma* and *bhakti* are interwoven within one another. Please note that one path is not complete without the intermingling of the other paths.

If I am devoting my time to practise *āsana, prāṇāyāma* or *dhyāna*, they become my key to *sādhanā*. From that practice I have to develop my root of knowledge into a trunk and a tree, in building up the intelligence and cultivating understanding. So the *sādhaka* in day to day life practises following the facets of the various paths after viewing them through study. Without this study, or without knowing the reason or the purpose, one cannot proceed towards *sādhanā*. This study is *jñāna*. Again, without zeal, passion and love on the subject one cannot proceed. If devotion is *bhakti*, action becomes *karma*. You may have tremendous knowledge – *jñāna* –, but if you have no compassion – *bhakti* –, and concern for being good – *karma* – to your neighbour, society, fellow beings, then what is the use of that *jñāna*? If you have tremendous desire to help and do not know the way to help, then what is the use of that *bhakti?* All these are interconnected. Is it correct for any person, or any aspirant to say, "I am this and I am not that", or "I am a *jñāna* yogi," or "a *bhakti* yogi"?

Patañjali explains these paths beautifully as *kriyā yoga*, connecting all the four *mārga*. *Tapaḥ svādhyāya Īśvarapraṇidhānāni kriyāyogaḥ* (*Y.S.*, II.1).[1] In this *sūtra* he describes *kriyā yoga* as all paths intermingled and interwoven. Some like Swami Yogananda and others have said, "We teach *kriyā yoga* as a new method." It is not at all a new method as Patañjali had already described it in his aphorism. The proper definition has not been given in any of their books which I have read. They speak only of *prāṇāyāma* as *kriyā yoga*. For them the *antara* and *bāhya kuṁbhaka*, which the *Bhagavad Gītā*[2] says is a *yajña* or surrendering or offering of breath as an oblation to the soul in the fire of our body, is considered as *kriyā yoga*. From Patañjali's point of view it is *tapas*.

Tapas means tremendous discipline, tremendous cleanliness, to purge the weaknesses in every human being. Burning desire, burning passion, the love to purge these weaknesses, is the meaning of *tapas*. *Tapas* indicates fire or heat. Our transitory desires must be burnt to ashes from moment to moment. To burn these sensual desires, what do we do? We act. This is a part of *kriyā yoga* as *karma mārga*.

Then, Patañjali speaks of *svādhyāya*. After disciplining ourselves by certain actions to get ourselves purified, he makes us understand ourselves from body to the self as self-study. He leads us to know ourselves through our behaviour with neighbours. By this we understand the moods and modes of our mind. We are made to study what is the right mind and what is the wrong mind. Hence, *svādhyāya* is a process of re-discovering ourselves. At some places and times *svādhyāya* is translated as studying of books in order to understand the character and quality of ourselves and the Self. Actually, we have to work on our own to understand ourselves, though the sacred books are our guides.

Studying ourselves and the ways and movements of body and mind would form a book. How am I behaving with my neighbour? How is my neighbour behaving with me? Should I react? What is the way to come together in a communion? This way of study in one's own nature and one's own behaviour, one's own actions and interactions is *svādhyāya* or self study. As *svādhyāya* means self-study, one needs *jñāna*, knowledge and understanding. So if *svādhyāya* is *jñāna mārga*, *tapas* stands for *karma mārga*.

---

[1] Burning zeal in practice, self-study and study of scriptures, and surrender to God are the acts of yoga. See the author's *Light on the Yoga Sūtras of Patañjali*, pp. 102-104.

[2] *Āpane juhvati prāṇaṁ prāṇe'pānaṁ tathā'pare /*
prāṇāpānagatī ruddhvā prāṇāyāmaparāyaṇāḥ // (*B.G.*, IV.29)
Still some others who are inclined to breath control, having restrained the paths of outgoing breath *(prāṇa)* and ingoing breath *(apāna)* pour as sacrifice *prāṇa* into *apāna* and *apāna* into *prāṇa*.

Lastly he speaks of *Īśvara praṇidhāna*. *Īśvara* means God. *Praṇidhāna* means devotion to God with single pointed attention. After acquiring the inner and outer cleanliness that are needed, after acquiring the tremendous amount of awareness of one's own mind, one is lead towards the path of surrender to God which is *bhakti mārga*.

This way Patañjali has made us imbibe the path of the eight petals of yoga to absorb and to receive the essence of the other paths.

Please know that Patañjali has not used the word *rāja-yoga* in his entire works. He only uses the word *kriyā-yoga* in one aphorism, covering all paths – *mārga* – as *kriyā yoga*.

Kriyā means *sādhanā* or practice. Patañjali explains what this *sādhanā* means, which covers *karma mārga*, *jñāna mārga* and *bhakti mārga* and the ways of using the eight aspects of yoga, namely, *yama*, *niyama*, *āsana*, *prāṇāyāma*, *pratyāhāra*, *dhāraṇā*, *dhyāna* and *samādhi* for the paths of *karma*, *jñāna* and *bhakti*. Careful study of the *Yoga Sūtra* reveals that *karma mārga* is involved from *yama* to *prāṇāyāma* of the *Sādhana Pāda*.

Please look at the *Sādhana Pāda* wherein you find *samādhisiddhiḥ Īśvara praṇidhānāt* (*Y.S.*, II.45).[1] There, he says that *samādhi* is reached only by *bhakti*, devotion or surrendering to the Lord. Is this not *bhakti mārga*?

Again he says, *yogāṅgānuṣṭhānāt aśuddhikṣaye jñānadīptiḥ āvivekakhyāteḥ* (*Y.S.*, II.28).[2] By the regular practice of yoga what do the *sādhaka* develop? The ignorance in the *sādhaka* gets destroyed and knowledge dawns. Does it not convey the path of *jñāna mārga?* I feel that the *aṣṭadaḷa* of the flower of yoga pivot around these paths of *karma*, *jñāna* and *bhakti*. They cannot be separated from each other. Those who call this *aṣṭadaḷa yoga* as *rāja yoga* want to exhibit as though they are teaching something special or extraordinary. The word *rāja* has come, not in Patañjali's *Yoga Sūtra*, but only in *Haṭhayoga Pradīpikā* of Svātmārāma.

Haṭhayoga Pradīpikā (IV.29) creates questions and answers concerning mind. It asks who is the king of the senses and answers that mind is the king of the senses; then proceeds further telling that the king of the mind is the breath. Questioning who the king of the breath is, it says that the nerves are the controller and soother of the breath. There the text uses the word *laya*. *Laya* means absorption. For the average practitioner of yoga, the experience of absorption comes only through the nerves when they are controlled and soothed. When the breath is going rhythmically, the nerves too recede. *Laya* also means rhythm. If the energy in the nerves moves unrhythmically or zigzag, it disturbs the breath and the mind as well as the senses. If the nerves are rhythmic, the breathing goes rhythmically, if the breath is rhythmic, the mind is under control. If the mind is under control, senses are also under control. Or, if the senses are controlled, then

---

1 Surrender to God brings perfection in *samādhi*. See the author's *Light on the Yoga Sūtras of Patañjali*, pp. 148-149.

2 By dedicated practice of various aspects of yoga, impurities are destroyed: the crown of wisdom radiates in glory. See the author's *Light on the Yoga Sūtras of Patañjali*, pp. 132-134.

mind is under control. If the mind is wandering, the breath has to be regulated. The regulation and control of the breath depend upon the strength and endurance of the nerves. Therefore, the nerves have to have the rhythmic flow of energy. The absorption is experienced when the energy in the nerves and in the breath flow with soft, smooth and serene rhythm, so that the mind and the senses reverse their flow towards the soul. This is *nāda*, the inner sound.

Patañjali says, *yogaḥ cittavṛtti nirodhaḥ* (*Y.S.*, I.2), *citta* – consciousness – is the interior expression of the mind and the mind is the outer expression of the intelligence and consciousness. Those who call *pātañjala yoga* as *rāja yoga* have taken the term "mind" from the *haṭha yoga* texts. I have said in earlier volumes that *cittavṛtti* describes the *rājasic* nature of the outer mind. Mind, which is closer to the senses, wanders with the senses in various directions. How can you bring it to a *sāttvic* nature, when the mind is *tāmasic* or *rājasic?* Yoga helps to sublimate these lower natures of the mind to bring the light of *sattvic* nature which is illumination. The *Yoga Sūtra* of Patañjali describes the word *nirodha* for the sublimation of the wandering *rājasic* nature of the mind for *citta* to experience the *sāttvic* state.

When the *rājasic* nature comes to the uppermost and controls this vibrant flow of the mind, then one reaches the state of being which is equal to benign *sattvic* state. Because of the misinterpretation of *citta* as mind – *manas* –, neo-translators have called *Patañjali's Yoga Sūtra* as *rāja yoga* or mental yoga. It is true that *citta* and *manas* are two different aspects, whereas for a common man, the mind or *manas* and *citta* seems to be one and the same. The *Haṭhayoga Pradīpikā* uses the word mind for *citta*[1] in this gross sense for a common man who understands the mind but not the consciousness – *citta*. Hence, *Haṭhayoga Pradīpikā* explains the control over the mind as *rāja yoga*, for the simple reason that mind is the king of the senses. Therefore the text says that without *haṭha yoga*, *rāja yoga* is impossible.

The traditional way of expression is *jñāna mārga, bhakti mārga* and *karma mārga* and not *jñāna yoga, bhakti yoga* and *karma yoga*. However, Patañjali includes all three in one word, *kriyā yoga*. *Karma* means action, *kriyā* also means action. If *karma* is a noun, then *kriyā* is a verb. *Karma* is just objectively taken, whereas *kriyā* is to do the *karma* functionally. So *karma* is objective and *kriyā* is subjective.

When Patañjali speaks of *kriyā yoga*, it means that one has to do it, and cannot get out of it. Yoga has to begin with actions. That is why I say the word *kriyā-yoga* is used whether one does *tapas, svādhyāya* or *Īśvara praṇidhāna*. One has to understand why Patañjali used the word *kriyā* for *karma*. So, *karma* is *kriyā*, *jñāna* is *kriyā*, and *bhakti* too is *kriyā*. Discipline is also *kriyā*, so *anuśāsana* is also *kriyā*. *Kriyā* only indicates the practicality of yoga and not merely a theoretical explanation. This practicality includes *karma, jñāna* and *bhakti* in *yoga*.

---

[1] It uses the term *citta* only once (IV.22) and in a different sense than *Yoga Sūtras* of Patañjali.

Q.- Is yoga, according to you, meant for all? How do we understand the path one has to choose?

It is not the question of choosing the path. Any path you accept, you have to stick to it. You have to make up your mind, your tendencies and your intentions to stick to the path.

For example, if you want to be good to others and if your mind is unhealthy, how can you help? There are savants in the West and the East with unhealthy bodies who have done a lot of work. But they are rare.

For example if you want to follow *karma mārga,* you may have to go with compassion to help those who are physically challenged with an unhealthy body, you may go out to help afflicted and unhealthy people. Suppose you are mentally disturbed or impulsive, are you in a position to help others in that condition? Is it not essential to have a healthy, calm and cool mind to help those who are mentally impaired? As such it is necessary to have a healthy body and a calm mind to help and guide others with compassion and friendliness. But do not take shelter under the guise of a few rare gifted persons as if you can also work and act like them. Why should we talk of such born saints when we are to a great extent selfish and self-centred? The question concerns 99.9% of the people whose ways of behaviour are important to be thought of and not the 0.1% of rare personalities. Here comes the importance of yoga for humanity as a whole.

In fact such rare persons come once in a hundred years, or maybe once in a thousand years. We have to take their ideals as examples for us to live a useful life. We have to live day to day, as we die, to be reborn. This being our nature and as we do not change, yoga helps us to build and develop a firm foundation for leading a good and useful life.

If we are healthy within and it rebounds outwards, then I am sure that in that healthy atmosphere we can serve our neighbours better. If one is unhealthy, tell me, in what way does one show compassion, when oneself seeks that compassion? When one is in agony and wants someone to help with compassion, how can one help others? Within a few years of agony, if one says, "I am collapsed" and hunts for something to recover from total collapse, I think from that point of view yoga comes to one's rescue. In order to pour out the energy, one needs to gain energy which through the practice of yoga helps one to live the rest of one's life in satisfaction and contentment.

Patañjali never overlooked helping even uneducated people. If a person has no knowledge, what can he do? If he has no understanding, what can he do? Modern saints say, "You should analyse". It is easy to say, "Analyse and find out". Even Ramaṇa Maharṣi said, "Find out. Know who I am." But how can a dull and uneducated man learn from this? So somebody has to show the way.

This is what Patañjali has done. He explains by dividing the mind into five categories, namely; *mūḍha* - dull, *kṣipta* - wandering, active, *vikṣipta* - oscillating (sometimes you have the power of concentration, sometimes you lose it and sometimes you have tremendous concentration), *ekāgra* - one-pointed and *niruddha* - restrained. Patañjali, with detailed explanations, devises the eight-fold aspects of yoga for persons, with five categories of the mind to progress from the dull state to a restrained state. If one is dull, one has to do certain things to get activated or stimulated. If one is slightly active and cheerful, one has to channel energy to do something concrete for stability. If one is extraordinarily intelligent, there are special instructions and practices in yoga that one can follow to channel intelligence for furthering the faculty of attention.

There lies the beauty of Patañjali's system wherein he has not left anyone out. I teach what Patañjali is asking us to do. He shows the path which is inclusive of all sorts of approaches and efforts required for the aspirants to go in a right direction. Therefore, I say that it is meant for all. As such I say that yoga presented by Patañjali is the foundation. After acquiring knowledge in this path, what impresses one according to one's intellectual capacity and growth has been covered by Patañjali in his treatise, which is known or recognised as *mārga* - the *karma*, the *yoga*, the *jñāna* and the *bhakti*.

In fact, we have to think and discriminate, whether in philosophy, art or science, how to help the majority of people. Today scientists are doing their research work on yogis who have supernatural powers. For example they do research work on yogis stopping their heart beats. How is this type of research going to help humanity at large? Is it going to help an ordinary man to lead a healthy life? The yoga researchers or scientists may do some research work on yoga and record it, but does it educate and ignite the ordinary people in the majority to take to yoga for health and happiness? A common man is keen to build-up health, happiness, peace of mind, discipline and control over himself, and have emotional stability.

I do feel that researchers of yoga do research to get credit for their research work. If it is not out of compassion, the research work in yoga is not done for the good of the people but for fame. In my case I have not done any scientific research but did work to attract hundreds and hundreds to yoga for health and happiness. This is what I have done. I wanted hundreds and hundreds to be available for scientific research on what yoga can do for humanity at large. Having suffered myself with ill health, I know what practical aspects of yoga are going to be good for people and I have worked from this practical point of view.

Q.- Was it out of that kind of thinking that the "non-traditional" *āsana* developed?

How can one produce anything from nothing? Without a traditional background discovery is not easy. Therefore, there is no non-traditional *āsana*, but one can add to the traditional *āsana*. To some extent, as I have said in the answer to the first question, these things were lost because people lost contact and the refined art disappeared. Now the *āsana* we see are a crude form. One does not see the flowing of vitality, superforce, superdynamism, superpresentations in the present yogis. What they say is all in the ancient texts and they are just repeating the same. If you question why, then you conclude that the refinement and precision have disappeared.

All *āsana* practices today are in a crude and superficial form. Someone had to struggle, strain and trace the missing links of refinement and precision. As I said, God graced me only to work and trace the subtle in the gross and crude presentations; he never allowed me to think of anything else in my life except *sādhanā* in this field. Of course, a good number of people tempted me to find the best in my *sādhanā*. "You have so much art, I will do this, I will do that, I will give you this, I will give you that." For example, nobody will believe that Swami Yogananda, in 1935 when he visited Mysore and our *yogaśālā*, as the guest of the Mahārāja of Mysore, offered to take me to America. He saw my demonstration and immediately said, "What a superb structural movement and control on the body you have got". "Come with me," he said, "I will give you all facilities." At that time I was just a raw yoga student and had no thoughts of my own. Still I told him, "As people have one father, one mother, one wife, one husband, so I have one *guru*. My *guru* is T. Krishnamacharya. I cannot have two *gurus*." I said, "I am sorry, I will not come and your offer does not tempt me at all".

I taught Krishnamurti for more than twenty years and lived in the same house with him, several times. I was not tempted to his teaching. Swami Sivananda once said, "I will give you *sannyāsa*. Why don't you come to Rishikesh?" Recently someone said, "For your art you should have orange robes". I said, "Why should I? I don't need any robes at all."

God graced me to stick to the subject of yoga, hence none could influence me to change my line. That grace of God and my determination and strength made me study each *āsana* in depth and I went on and on with them. By the grace of God I re-discovered something new and precise in each *āsana* which came to me and confirmed my practice though I have not broken the tradition.

---

[1] Swami Yogananda was the founder of Self-Realisation Society and the author of *Autobiography of a Yogi*, published by Self-Realisation Fellowship, Los Angeles, USA, 1959.

Q.- So you feel that at one time those *āsana* were, in fact, practised by the earlier yogis?

Otherwise how could the text proclaim eight hundred and eighty-four thousands of *āsana*? It is said that there are as many *āsana* as the species created by God. Yogis had the power of imagination. They had to think, they had to work out. For example, the other day I told you I had been to South Africa. I was taken to a zoo and saw the gorilla sitting in *Baddha Koṇāsana, Upaviṣtha Koṇāsana*, performing *Supta Pādānguṣṭhāsana* so perfectly. Unbelievable! I said, "We struggle and for these gorillas they appear as natural poses." *(Laughter).* You have not seen them doing such *āsana* at all? Please go and see how the gorillas sit. You will be surprised. To some extent I see this and learn.

Perhaps you have not but I have seen the Ellora caves where yogic postures are carved.[1] Or the old temples where the *āsana* are carved on pillars. I saw a *Kaṇḍāsana* statue in a temple in the old Alwar State.

Some years ago I was asked whether I could give a demonstration for the members of the United Nations. My demonstration was for one and a half hours. I finished everything and one intelligent man stood up on the platform and said, "You have shown so many things. You haven't shown the *āsana* called *Bhujaṅgāsana*". I had shown the scorpion pose and all. The man should be ashamed to ask this when thousands of people were watching me. He said, "You have not shown this at all and it's a major pose." You will be surprised to know what I told him.

I asked him, "Have you seen a cobra?" He said he had. "Do you know *Bhujaṅgāsana*?" He said, "Yes". "How do you do it?" He said "We press our hands and we lift up". I said, "You press your hands? Have you seen a cobra with hands?" *(Laughter).* In front of so many people he thought he was putting a very intelligent question. I made him a completely stupid person on the platform.

Then I showed him my *Bhujaṅgāsana*, how I use my hands on the knees. I said, "That is *Bhujaṅgāsana*. Have I taken any support on my trunk?" He said, "No." Then I said, "Now can you do it?" He said, "No." Then I said, "Don't ask such questions next time when you see others demonstrating in a given time. In a presentation of hundreds of *āsana*, if one misses one, one should not complain. When one presents better *āsana*, you should never question them for overlooking a gross, simple *āsana*. Sir, probably you may not know that as an artist I cover the simple *āsana* in the advanced *āsana*.

---

[1] The Ellora and Ajanta caves are situated in Maharashtra State, India.

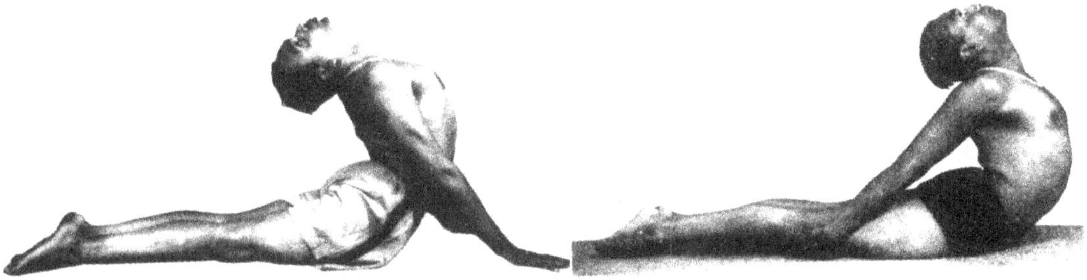

Plate n. 9 – *Bhujaṅgāsana* I & II for comparative study

Now, *Bhujaṅgāsana* I is a traditional *āsana,* but *Bhujaṅgāsana* II which is seen very rarely may seem to be non-traditional. But it was existing originally and that is how my *guru* taught me. I am performing, and my pupils are also doing the same. So *āsana* are there from time immemorial. It was all in vogue but we lost them due to historical reasons and time factors.[1] That is why this friend of mine questioned about *Bhujaṅgāsana* I and I showed him the real *Bhujaṅga* – serpent – without the hands.

Q.- You've talked quite a bit from time to time during the session of the art of teaching. It was mentioned that someone has requested you to write a book.

The art of teaching is a practical subject, not a theoretical subject. How could the art of teaching be written? It is direct perception. The direct perception has to be explained, observed and made to be handled. A book cannot be written on the art of teaching except the basics. But I have been asked by my publisher to write on the art of yoga, which I am doing. I think they want to boost some of my final poses of *Light on Yoga* as they saw the laminated photographs which were exhibited in London in 1984. He said, "We want a book, *Light on the Art of Yoga.*" So it is the latest.[2]

They were only asking about teaching but I said, "No, how can I teach the art of teaching? It can't be written in books; it is hand to hand." A doctor can become a doctor, but as soon as he gets the degree he has to work under the experienced doctor. Even an experienced doctor cannot teach him through a book. The neophyte doctor has to undergo training with the

[1] *Aṣṭadaḷa Yogamālā*, vol. 2, "From Moha to Mokṣa", p. 321.
[2] *Art of Yoga*, published by Harper Collins, London 1985.

experienced doctor. Yoga is a practical subject, so the teachers have to be trained, but not at all through books. Learning can be taught through books but teaching cannot be taught through books. Only certain guidelines and ideas can be given.[1]

Q.- Do you foresee any other publications?

I am translating *Yoga Sūtra* of Patañjali for the common man to understand. There are complicated translations done by lots of commentators, but I am trying to simplify it so that it is understood by an average person. Intellectuals are more academic than practical, they can grasp intellectually the subject with multiple interpretations; whereas I am trying to write this book so that a person with an average intellect can grasp this subject. I have drafted two chapters. Now I have been caught in writing this book and the *Art of Yoga* remains dormant. I don't know when I could complete both, but I am making a small contribution of my way of thinking in this book of Patañjali.[2]

It is going to be a long term project because there are so many controversies which are to be touched by me. I shall try to give new interpretations to some of the *sūtra*, which may cause conflicts. Either the critics will have to say that it is all out of the brain or they have to say let us rethink. It is easy to dismiss it. But if somebody tries to understand why I have written this way, probably they may re-think for some new light to dawn on them.

I am trying to be original in my thinking and writing but let me be clear with you that when the original works appear with the new way of thinking, some mistakes too may crop up. It may be true or it may be false. But my convictions have made me touch more new points, through my own filtered experiences of the practice of *āsana, prāṇāyāma* and *dhyāna*, that fits into the exposition of *Yoga Sūtra*.

Many commentators on Patañjali's *Yoga Sūtra* have treated each *sūtra* as a chapter in itself. *Sūtra* means a linking, one *sūtra* linking to the other. As far as I have read, the commentators haven't linked the *sūtra* at all. That is why when one reads, one gets confused. Hence, I am trying to link the *sūtra* on similar topics from chapter to chapter and describe why certain words come before and some after.

---

[1] Recently *Gurujī* has brought out the book *Basic Guidelines for Teachers of Yoga*, B.K.S. and G.S. Iyengar, YOG Publication, Mumbai, 2002.

[2] *Light on the Yoga Sūtras of Patañjali*, Harper Collins, London, 1993, and *Light on Aṣṭāṅga Yoga*, YOG Publication, Mumbai, 2002.

Q.- So you look at it as a whole?

Yes. It's almost a new way of thinking. As I have done with *Light on Yoga* and *Light on Prāṇāyāma*, I should give a fresh touch to this book with my own interpretations.

- Light on Patañjali?

Light on the Yoga Sūtras of Patañjali, I would say.

Q.- Can you talk about the importance of ethics in terms of practice and relationship to yoga?

Ethics is a way of life. Moment to moment in each movement or action one has to observe the ethical pattern as ethics are the base for spiritual growth. As such, the ethical disciplines explained in the *Yoga Sūtra* of *yama* and *niyama* are the foundation to be followed. For example, while in *āsana*, if my one right toe is turning out and left toe is turning in, there are no ethics involved and it becomes an undisciplined practice. If it is incorrect on one side and right on the other side, readjustment of a wrong placing in the right direction is ethics.

As I said the other day when you were doing the *āsana*, if you are stretching more on the right side and less on the left you are doing *hiṁsā* to one part, *ahiṁsā* to the other. One part is moving in purity, the other part is moving in impurity. This is known as ethics.

If you remember, I told you today, when you were doing *Paśchimottānāsana*, if the right eye is moving forward and the left eye is not moving, one is in ethical discipline and the other is not. Ethics is not the way of just thinking but it is the way of doing with thinking. It is the process of re-alignment of body, senses, mind, intelligence and consciousness, which have to be put together.

You cannot separate ethics from physical or mental discipline. You cannot discipline physically without ethical means. Even the breath that you take has a certain regulated flow. That regulated flow is ethics. You sit for meditation and close your eyes; but how the eyes are to be closed is ethics. Ethics is not technical processes. So how can I say in a few words what ethics is when the whole life's moments and movements are involved?

Ethics and spiritual discipline are like two eyes of an individual. They cannot be separated. It is impossible for anyone to experience salvation or reach God without ethical discipline. Ethics is the starting point to reach spiritual *sādhanā*. If a man has no ethics, he can never be a spiritual man. They go together. So whoever practises spiritual practices has to have ethical discipline, and a man with ethical discipline is a spiritual man in his heart. Indiscipline and morality cannot go together.

Ethics and spirituality are like two sides of the same coin. The moment you say, "This is ethics", then regimentation comes. When you say, "This is not this" and "this is not that", then we lose advertent study.

If one is walking on the street without caring for the moving vehicles, then what happens? One gets hurt or injured. If a heedless way of walking makes you get hurt, you have broken the principles of walking on a busy road. So if you follow a certain discipline in your walking, it is called ethics.

Q.- Very practical : *(Laughter).* It's very important to remember that in Pune! We've seen you work on some of your senior teachers here. Can you describe what you feel are the important characteristics of a good teacher?

Clarity, confidence and to some extent even one should be very clever too, because clarity and cleverness are not the same. Cleverness is manipulation, clarity is purity. So sometimes with some students we have to be clever, but basically we should be clear. Tremendous confidence is required and, at the same time, compassion. So compassion, clarity, cleverness, confidence are essential to be a good teacher. You may know the art, but if you have no confidence, how can you teach? You may have clarity and the power of transmitting, but if you have no compassion, how can you give? In order to be compassionate you need to come to the level of the students, so you make them understand better. Never forget that compassion is not just softness. One has to be harsh too. If I have to do good to you, I cannot speak soft words only. If you have to improve fast, it is only through action, not mere words. Just patting a person on the back and saying, "I am sorry, my dear friend, for your suffering. I wish God bless you." This is not compassion. When you have a stressful period in suffering, there is no point in showing compassion through words. Rather I have to find means to bring the change in you through certain actions so that your suffering and stress are minimised or eradicated bringing this type of change in you. That is compassion. The teacher has to express his compassion.

In compassion, the teacher has to act, and that action appears harsh and cruel to the observer but maybe not so for the teacher or the participant. Understandably it is the observers who see, specially my teaching, and comment, "He's very cruel. He's very rough!"

Compassion is emotional, it is an emotional feel from the heart towards those who are suffering. The soothing words may bring solace for the time being, but not a solution. It needs a practical help to solve the problem. While teaching *āsana* as therapy, direct touch of the teacher is needed. The touch being a direct action demands stretching, extending, lengthening, bending, pressing, twisting and so forth in yoga. These adjustments are painful, but not cruel or rough. They are intense and strong. It is the intensive action to bring relief to the sufferers. When doctors do surgery they give you anaesthetics. Therefore you don't experience the pain. Later they give pain killers and healing drugs. My actions are like surgery but it is an intellectual surgery as I have to bring their *buddhi* and *citta* to act as surgical instruments to penetrate and this penetration irritates the areas, therefore they are painful. It pains, but then one is free from the original pain. Later, this new created pain too disappears.

Yesterday you saw the patients in the therapeutic class. How bad they were. You all saw a woman crying. I asked her, "Now when you are crying, why do you want to come to the class? What did she say? You heard. Ask Maureen Carruthers. She too knows what the lady patient said. She said, "No, I want to come because I am moving at least. It is painful. It is killing. But the after effect is very good for me."

– *That was the woman with arthritis.* –

Yes, you saw the man who comes on crutches. These people who are suffering tremendously are certainly agreeing that they are improving. You are witnessing their improvement. Such hopeless cases where nothing much can be expected are admitted though it is not a medical centre. In spite of knowing their limitations, we allow them to be in the class. When they admit they are improving, is this my cruelty or compassion? When I am teaching them or making them move their bodies, their joints, I make them do a little more than their limited capacities. This brings movement and they develop confidence. This confidence in them takes them to move beyond their capacities. I'm not playing with them, I am not experimenting with them, I don't say, "Try this."

I never use the word "try". If it appears possible, I make them do. If it's not possible, I work out and find some other means after observation. The other means seems to them hard but I have to get the right action in the affected areas. This compassion is very difficult for anyone to understand at a practical level.

If you go to a saint, he keeps his hand on your head and says, "I bless you" and you come out happily saying, "He blessed me!" Why? Because your mind was made receptive beforehand by your friends that you are going to meet so and so who has the power of healing. At that time there is a little bit of release in your nerves, which causes the effect. But you say that the blessing had an effect. It may be a momentary effect and as such those people also come for treatment to our institute.

When people come to me, they do not come with a relaxed body. They come with tensions assuming that Mr. Iyengar is harsh, hard, tough and cruel. *(Laughter).* Not that I do not know. That tension means they have created an obstruction in their system to follow me because they have heard people saying I am a tough teacher. So naturally I become tough because they are holding themselves. I have not only to break their physical problems but also their fears, prejudices and misunderstandings about me and yoga. Due to these emotional fears, morally they are not open to me as they show pettiness in their courage to face me. But when they go to a saint or a *sannyāsi*, they know that they are going with a passive reverent mind to have the blessings of a holy man and feel that being nice, soft and holy, he does not do any harm and feel the auto-effect before his blessings. If they come to Mr. Iyengar, they come with the fear that he may kick. *(Laughter)* This is how people read me. If I have to show compassion, I have to go out of my way to help a man. All my actions deal with the problem directly and in my techniques there are no "ifs and buts". Rumours spread that I am harsh and rough.

- *Compassion is the most direct route.* -

Ah! A direct route. *(Laughter).* So I can't help it otherwise. Otherwise I am cheating myself. Not only am I deceiving that person who has come for my help but I am also deceiving myself. If I don't act the way it has to be, knowing very well that unless I act in this way that man cannot improve at all, I would be a cheater. What do we do if there is some leakage in the house?

- *We try to fix it* -

What do you do before fixing it? You bring your hammers, hit more, create more space. Are you not injuring that wall?

- *Yes, we have to tear it apart to find the real source of the problem.* -

Similarly, we also tear apart their minds to find out the source. Nobody understands that. The engineer says, "It is leaking here, therefore it is probably coming from there." To get to that source of leakage in my system, I have to try from the periphery to find the source. Similarly, when I have to deal with the patients, I have to tap in so many directions to get into the cause of suffering. This tapping in various places seems to be cruel for you, because you think that when it is leaking at one place, why should I be cruel to the other areas? *(Laughter).* You want to do a patchwork and be satisfied. I am not satisfied with such work or a patchwork. When the pus is accumulated deep inside you cannot put a bandage outside. In order to repair one spot, you need to repair the surrounding parts too. For you it seems to be cruelty. For me it is a real compassion.

Yesterday you saw the man who could not walk? Did I not make him walk? When I said, "Ask your wife for help and take a few steps." Did you hear what he said? He said, "I can't trust my wife." I never said, "Have confidence in me." He has only come to me four or five times and he has lived with his wife for years. This is why the teacher should have tremendous confidence in himself in order to create confidence and hope in another person, even if it appears tough. That is the characteristic needed for a teacher.

I must know I can go to the maximum extent to make maximum use of this body without damaging it. It is not the maximum movement that I can think of in my body – my body may go beyond that range –, but what maximum movement can I take in that person who is affected? Secondly, as I know the range of movements, I take that maximum movement that is applicable and possible to the party to make him reach his maximum. It is my compassion which seems to appear harsh for an onlooker. If I give the minimum movement in that affected body, the effect is just like a scratch. It may appear soft. But for me it is cruel and heart burning.

If there is a wound and you go to the doctor and say, "I am scratching every day", the doctor says, "It has to be operated on. It's deep in." For example with a 'wet boil'. The boil which does not create pus for one to see but goes on growing. Doctors have to open it and convert it into a 'dry boil'.

Yoga is like that. All the diseases which come, we have to keep in mind about the boil which grows inside that has to be operated upon, again and again. We have to find out methods in yoga to see that it does not recur again, and therefore it has to be eradicated from the rest itself. This appears harsh on the surface but covers compassion inside.

Q.- Many teachers don't have the confidence to do that.

That's true. That is absolutely true. But I guide them in what way they should teach according to their knowledge and capacity to take the risk without damaging the patients. One has to study the patients' limitations and one should know how far they can rise to help.

In some cases I asked Dr. Bruce Carruthers and Dr. David Kell, "Can you treat this person if I give him to you?" They said, "Certainly not". Now see, what courage I must have to touch them?

- So the teachers must have not only confidence but also courage with knowledge and understanding.-

About me, I have courage. I have clarity; I am harsh and I have compassion; I've got five C's *(Laughs).* They are cruelty, compassion, courage, clarity, confidence, and I add cleverness. With some people I have to be dextrous – not with all. With 90% I can act with clarity; only with 10% I play with cleverness. When they are clever I also have to be clever.

- To match their cleverness! -

Yes, to match their cleverness. As I say in the class, if you show ego, I can also show ego. If you show vanity, I can also show vanity. If you show humility, I can also show humility. What is that? It is all hidden. It comes to the surface according to the behaviour of people or patients when they approach me. It depends on how they interact with me.

I have to be one inch above or one inch below. If I am one inch below, then I am not a teacher, because my pupil is one inch above in egoism. I have to prove by demonstration that I am one inch above the pupils. Today, I said in class, "You have all come for the intense course and you can't even do one *Uthitta Trikoṇāsana.* "You have seen me not just making a statement but I demonstrate with accuracy connecting hundreds of links of the body in a split moment.

This way I show how I am one inch above the pupils. This is all part of the great art of teaching. It is not that I am showing my vanity. It is to train my pupils to be careful, not to be egoistic without knowing it, to find the limitations and cross them.

If the pupil is humble and says, "Sir, I don't know", then my teaching will be quite different, filled with humility. I will go one inch below. I will have a friendly approach and say, "If you have not understood, why didn't you tell me before?" If one says, "I am dull", then I teach accordingly and bring him up. If you admit your ignorance, that is humility, humbleness; then I will also show humbleness. If you say, "I know it", and then I know that you do not know it, so naturally I jump into anger.

- Then you teach humility. (Laughter) -

Yes, you are right. My anger too is to make you humble.

Q.- You've accomplished a great deal in your life. That's evident here at the Institute and in the teachers you have trained. What remains for you, in terms of your goals?

Nothing in my life. What had to be done has been done. What had to be seen has been seen. What had to be achieved, has been achieved. What had to be felt has been felt. Nothing is left for me to do. What I am doing is to give other people the taste of the same nectar, the fragrance that I am experiencing. I have no aim in my life now, because what had to be fulfilled has been fulfilled.

The only ambition is, "Let me not lose what I have got." Then it is ethics, *(Laughs)* I don't say it is a spiritual thing. My principle is ethics. Who knows at what moment I may lose this fragrance if I neglect it. If it does not show me the further way, I will not be bothered. I don't mind if new ideas and things do not come, but let me not lose what has come to me with my labour. So let me maintain it.

The other thing is to give pupils a glimpse of that supreme feeling, which cannot be experienced by word; which is an experience instead. If they get it, then I am sure that I have done good work in this world. Otherwise, I will say I have not done anything.

For example, take Ramana Maharsi – a great man! Aurobindo – a great man! Mahatma Gandhi – a great man! There were three great men in the same century. Ramana Maharshi remained at one place and was open to all with advice for those who came to him. Aurobindo never mingled with the masses, but his works conveyed his knowledge and wisdom.

Ramana experienced the real directly but used very few words which have been expanded by the scholars who were following him.

Mahatma Gandhi, on the other hand, had qualities of Shri Ramana and Shri Aurobindo, and moved with the masses. It is he who uplifted the masses. His language was simple and expressions were straight forward. These three great men in the same century guided us in *jñāna, bhakti* and *karma mārga*. If *karma mārga* was predominant in Mahatma Gandhi, *jñāna* was predominant in Ramana and *bhakti* in Aurobindo. Hence, we were lucky to see those great men at one time.

Health is the foundation for anything. If the health is unsound, disease is waiting next to our skin. Just as two strong countries wait to win over the other, yet both are afraid and both are careful. Similarly, the disease is slightly outside the skin waiting for an opportunity to enter the body when the man is careless. Yoga is meant to keep the enemy – diseases – away. We practise yoga to keep the skin and disease away from coming in contact with each other. If my pupils carry this message of yoga, then I feel that I have done a good service.

I remember, and I think that you also have read the teachings of Lord Buddha. Lord Buddha said that if people give health, it is a great thing; if people give spiritual health, it is the greatest of all things. Today the world is topsy-turvy, so I say, if you give physical and mental health, you have done the greatest service to society, rather than saying you should give spiritual health.

Without this physical and mental health, spiritual health cannot come. The fruit cannot come without a tree. The tree is necessary in order to get the fruit. With these two things, physical and mental health, spiritual fruit will come on its own. If my pupils do that, they have served society and their lives are also meaningful and fulfilled.

Q.- You had many students from the West. You seem to have had a special role in bringing more awareness to people in the West. What are your observations of these people?

The cultures of the various places may be different, but the culture of yoga is meant for everyone. Yoga is a universal culture. It has nothing to do with any religion, neither is it without religion. Each human being, whether in the East or in the West, North or South, has the same problems.

The culture may be different, but the problems of emotional upheavals, intellectual cloudiness, whether it be the East or the West, is there any difference? That is why yoga is a universal culture; it is meant for humanity.

Culture, religion or civilisation do not interfere when every individual needs to have perfect physical health, stability in emotion and clarity in their heads.

Buddha was a single person. Christ was a single person. Krishna was a single person. Ramakrishna Paramahamsa was a single person. If you study them, one single person's culture became the civilisation of the world. If they had not been born, then what would the religion be?

One man's perfect culture is the civilisation of the world.

The culture and civilisation given by these great people have developed for the good of humanity. That's why they have survived. Their teachings survived, but they did not call their teachings as religion. Yoga has survived because it is for the good of humanity. Yoga is never associated with a particular sect. Patañjali does not call it religion.

Religion, if you ask me, is of two facets. One is man-made and the other is God-made. Religion is meant only to experience and realise a life free from emotional upheavals and intellectual disturbances. It is a process of learning how to use, day to day, our intelligence, activities, functioning and thoughts to reach God. Religion deals with ethics and morality so that the human being is transformed towards the spiritual.

There should be no quarrel from any angle, either of religion or of geographical region, as far as the realisation is concerned, to experience the unalloyed bliss and freedom. Christ said, "If you think of God you get dates." Why did he specify dates? Because dates were growing where he was preaching. Dates don't grow in India. Here you will get plenty of bananas and mangoes. It does not mean either that you worship God for dates and fruits. It indicates that human beings should preserve nature, environment, work and worship.

This is the way of leading people to change for good. All the old books speak of ethics more than the ways because they were inducing people to come to the right method. We cannot criticise them because the environments were like that in those days – they had to teach according to the environment also. The Westerners have one good thing – tremendous will power. The Easterners have tremendous tolerance, therefore they can bear any amount of pain. The West cannot tolerate pain. I am indicating some difference here and there.

Indians are a little bit slow to get stabilised. They are slow, but they will not stop. They have perseverance and so they continue, but slowly! Therefore, the establishment comes to them only after a gap of time. What you reach in ten days, it may take them years, but they still continue.

– *They have endurance.* –

Yes! They have tremendous emotional bearing. They cannot become instant victims of emotions. In the West, people become victims in a split second. See how Japanese women are – how quiet, how silent. How much they can bear the strain. These are 'geographical' and 'cultural' adjustments from their environments.

If this tolerance and emotional intelligence of the East can be combined with the will power and the vertical growth of intelligence of the West, then society will be tremendously unified. West moves through the head, East moves through the heart.

Some years ago while I was in England and America, many had approached me regarding their sex problems. Masculinity or virility is very personal and emotional. How can this emotional want be solved through the intellect of the head? Secretions of hormones play an important role in building up vigour. There are *āsana* that work on the hormonal development by developing the emotional seat. Divorce is very common in the West, because they want to settle everything through their heads, whereas this has to do with emotional build-up. So I ask the specialists in sexology, "How can you talk from your head regarding this emotional weakness or strength?" It has to do a lot with physiological and mental strength to develop.

We Indians try to solve emotional problems emotionally and intellectual problems intellectually. But in the West, people want to solve everything intellectually because for you science of the head is important and not the emotional intelligence of the heart. You can find out the facts through science, but you cannot find solutions for emotional wants. Here comes yoga as a science and art to help those who suffer from this weakness.

Sometimes it is unwanted, immoral, unethical sexual relationships that disturb the consciousness and conscience. Sex is not a sin. To have healthy sex, a healthy relationship between husband and wife is needed. In the East the couple gets attached to each other emotionally. Therefore, there is a mutual understanding between the wife and husband and they remain reposed and relaxed. Because of their mental state, health flows into the system both physically and mentally. Where there is absence of emotions, the confidence is lost. Therefore in the West they remain tense.

Emotional stability is repose. Without it the emotional side of disease goes on increasing. The nourishment from the emotional aspects comes through the practices in the art of yoga and improves the mental health. No other system opens the heart the way yoga does. It stretches like the trunk and branches of the tree in all directions, so it keeps the seat of the heart at rest and makes the intelligence of the head and the emotions of the heart extend and expand.

That's why when you practise yoga you develop more emotional stability. The moment emotional stability develops, clarity comes. When you want to solve such problems through your brain, you tense everything. You block the brain and nerves as you drain the circulatory system. The breathing becomes heavy and laboured. When breathing is laboured, how can one expect the *prāṇic* energy to flow? The faint flow of energy means the opening of the gates of disease. Due to the want of irrigation diseases go on increasing and they affect one giving worry and anxiety, which lead to mental stress and block the intellectual calibre also.

Yesterday you saw the diabetic patient. How was I explaining? Even in *Sālamba Sarvāṅgāsana* one has to find out how the liver and the pancreas work and how the bladder is gripped in the *āsana*.

You also saw me showing the four doctors who were present, the function of the pancreas in *Sālamba Sarvāṅgāsana*. I asked one of them to keep his fingers on the pancreas as I adjusted the person. They said, "Yes! We feel it, the spasms of its functioning appear." This is how *āsana* have to be adjusted for organic actions.

We are not saying that we are lessening the sugar level in diabetic patients, but we make them tone the liver, pancreas and kidneys. First the toning has to take place before thinking of whether *āsana* controls sugar or not. One cannot test immediately to find out whether the sugar was there or not before the toning of the organs. After toning takes place, the sugar level falls down.

I have explained how to teach *āsana* to help them to make the floor of the bladder strong to hold urine so that they may not pass urine so often. Therefore teaching involves both intellectual head and emotional heart.

If I say, "Take it and do it this way", without knowing what is happening, it is only intellectual thinking. I should also have an emotional mind to see and feel. Intellectually I have to think; emotionally I have to observe whether it is working or not. When the emotion and the intellect are blended together, they bring the harmonious growth and yoga acts as a key to bring this emotional intelligence and intellectual intelligence to balance evenly in all walks of life.

There is no other system to balance these two intelligences except yoga; yoga belongs to the heart, though you have to think through the brain. The practical side belongs to the heart, the thinking side belongs to the head. You have to use both. *(Laughter).*

I am explaining technologically. *Jñāna mārga* is from the head. *Karma mārga* is the work of the hands and legs. *Bhakti mārga* is nothing but dealing with emotions. Hence, a teacher should have all these three parts to work with understanding and in unison.

It is only the yoga of Patañjali which unifies these three as *kriyā yoga*. It blends the person and moulds him by regular practice to bring the body to co-operate with the mind, the mind with the self, and the self co-operating again with the mind and the body. That is the beauty of the union and the beauty of health, and this is what I make my pupils understand, the use of these three paths through yogic practice.

I have noticed that the senior students who practise regularly have definitely changed. Moulding in them is taking place, the behaviour of their heart is changing, and I am sure they are lighting the lamp of yoga more and more for many to enjoy harmony, health and a sound heart.

– *So you feel the West is learning slowly (Laughs).* –

Yes, not only the west but also the east are learning through yoga. Unfortunately, we have forgotten it but we have taken it. Now, the time has come to be taught and learn properly. Who knows, after fifty years the western practitioners may become the founders of yoga *(Laughs).* It was a forgotten, dead science, and I am happy that through my demonstrations as art and teaching, the subject is rejuvenating the people, so the revival has begun.

In my early days, everybody was saying that *haṭha yoga* was only physical, I was also under that impression. As I went on reading the text and continually practising it brought me much light. I realised its value, not only on the physical aspect, but also on the ethical, mental and intellectual levels. Today there are lots of yoga centres and advertisements everywhere which appear to be a good sign for yoga as thousands are available for scientific tests to find out the benefits of *āsana* and *prāṇāyāma*.

Whatever advertisement I see is an imitation of Iyengar's method. Any magazine you take, any advertisement of commercial concerns you find – yoga stretches better and for comfortable movements. In Indian papers, you can see some of my *āsana* like *Vīrabhadrāsana* I, *Ekapāda Śīrṣāsana* and *Hanumānāsana* and they say, their new designs stretch as the yogi stretches his body.

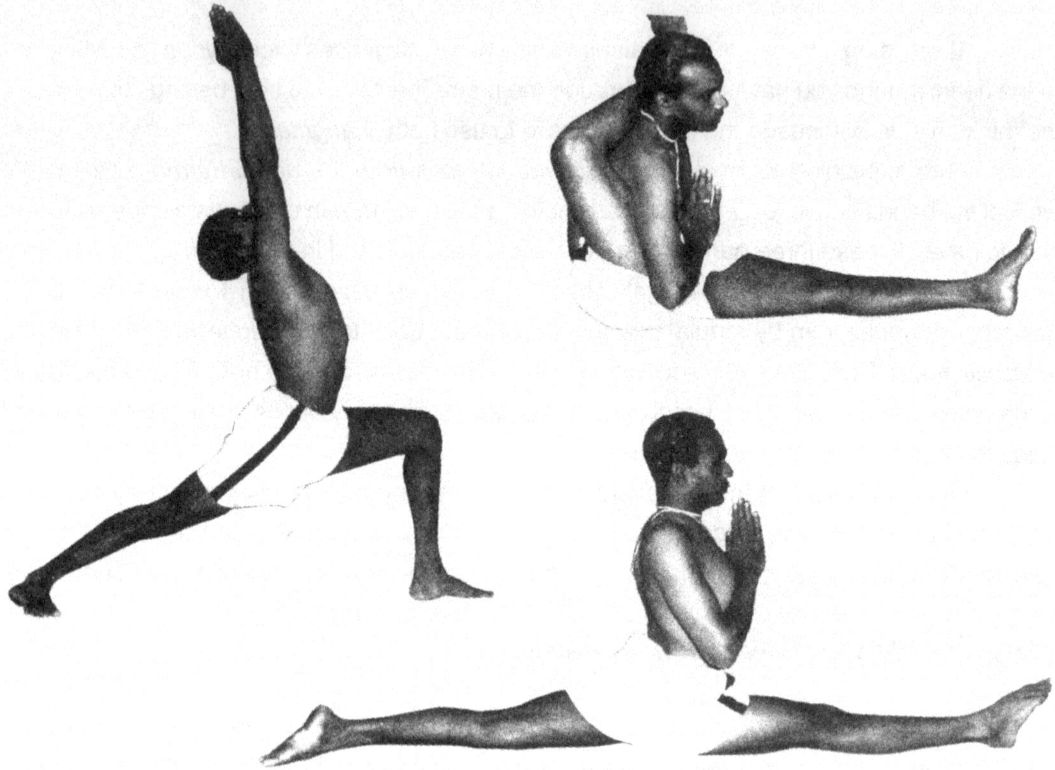

Plate n. 10 – *Vīrabhadrāsana* I, *Ekapāda Śīrṣāsana* and *Hanumānāsana*

I have been doing yoga since the 1930s. From that time I have meet *swami* after *swami* everywhere. They never took this art to the common man. They were only trying to get hold of the rich people or cream of the society so that they could become successful, and it was only I who went to the masses.

In India I was the first to introduce this art in schools and colleges. Now when educational institutions have accepted yoga and added it in their curriculum, everybody and every school of yoga is fighting for their method to be introduced and they have thrown me out. I was the first man to show how yoga could be done in the field without mats, without carpets. I adapted according to the conditions of the place. As the place was not congenial to head balance, they were not taught the head balance. Yogis criticised me for not teaching *Sālamba Śīrṣāsana*. I knew how to teach without any carpets and mats. So I took such challenges those days, to introduce yoga in schools and colleges. But I made enemies because I became popular with youngsters, which they could not. They, being older than me, began influencing the school authorities saying that "Yoga cannot be taught to the masses, but only on a one-to-one basis." This had the effect of closing my classes then, but now many are asking me for the authority to introduce yoga in their curriculum. As I did in India, to take yoga to educational institutions, I did this in England in 1972 and took yoga to schools and colleges; now you see yoga is spreading and people are attracted in large numbers to this art. In America community colleges have taken it up. This also I started in 1974. This way I planted a very good seed of yoga in these continents. Now it is the responsibility of pupils who must see that it does not fade.

– *There are many flowers.* –

So it will grow. I am happy about this work. I am only unhappy because intellectual pride is growing. What I am concerned with now is how to demolish this pride. Otherwise, if they just treat this yogic teaching as a service to God which we are doing, let us carry it to our utmost leaving pride behind. The utmost importance is honesty, sincerity and advertence.

Even if you know a minimum, even if in your minimum you do the utmost, you have done a good service to yourself, to society and to God. You need not even think of God. Once in London somebody asked me a very simple question: "Sir, have you to pray always to God?" Everybody was saying *bhakti mārga*, always think of God, think of God, think of God. I told them, "I don't think of God at all".

– *Very unfair as a yogi that you do not think of God.*–

Do you think of your father and mother all the twenty-four hours? Haven't you given your respect to your father and mother without thinking of them for all the twenty-four hours? So that's all. I have got respect for my God because I am paying my respects to Him already, through this art for man to become a better man. As we indirectly think of our parents, we think of God. "We think of God with each breath directly or indirectly, why is extra prayer required?", I said. *(Laughter).* Similarly, I accept God and think of him in my practice and before teaching, and pay my respects to him after the classes.

Sometimes of course I do laugh, when such questions come to me. It is a tricky question, you know. If I say, "Think of God", it is not possible to make someone do so. But, by my teaching yoga I have converted a person immediately to follow a right path. As I said already, though we don't think of our mother and father twenty-four hours a day it does not mean that we don't think of them at all but know our respect is not lost for them. It is the same with God. *(Laughter).*

"Why are you so egoistic?", some say. "Why are you so full of vanity when you are teaching?" I said, "Why should I not have the vanity when I have the clarity? You people have no clarity and you show vanity. But I have the clarity, so why should I not have the vanity?" As I said, I know also how to answer an egotist and also know how to behave with a humble man. That is why I say often, cleverness is also required for a teacher *(Laughter).*

God bless you all.

Thank you sir. –

Good work! Lucky that I was in a good mood! *(Laughter).*

B.K.S. IYENGAR TALKS ON YOGA*

Q.- Mr. Iyengar, you have worked with Westerners for over 30 years. In what way do you feel that the Western person needs yoga?

As yoga is a universal ethic and religion, health is also a universal ethic and religion. The need of yoga is found in everyone irrespective of caste, class, country, gender, in any part of the world. The western world embraced yoga for the simple reason that they developed their sense of comfort to such an extent that they were made to use their limbs less and less. Due to this lack of movements the joints and muscles started constricting. The muscles and the arteries get narrowed and the diseases began increasing. It is not only in the West, but it is also common in the East. At one time those from the East had to struggle very hard using their body movements. Though they were under-nourished, they were maintaining a certain amount of good health. As comforts started coming to them as well, their health also started taking its toll. So yoga really has become an essential part and parcel of our lives like food and rest, not just as an exercise but to keep man alive and healthy. Of course, yogic *āsana* are not exactly exercise, but are positions where each and every joint is thought of, made to feel and activated to function with sufficient supply of blood and energy.

In order to make a layman understand what yoga is, I say it is an all-round exercise. Here when I say all-round, I am not speaking from the physical level but on physiological, psychological, ethical, intellectual and mental levels also. Nothing can be forgotten in yoga, whereas in other types of exercises, emphasis is given to one part or the other. If you take yoga, you can really call it holistic because it works from the base – physical field up to the field of the spirit as a whole.

In the early stages of accepting yoga the need is limited to health and harmony. Now both the students and teachers of yoga have realised the effect of yoga is beyond health and harmony. They look with awareness about moral, ethical, mental, intellectual and spiritual health and well-being.

---

* Interview by Karin Stephan. Took place on January 1983, in Pune, India. Published in *Iyengar Yoga Institute Review*, San Francisco, vol. 5, no. 1, June, 1984. Reprinted in *Iyengar Yoga In Southern Africa*, vol. 2, Dec. 1985.

In this sense, yoga is an all-tonic exercise; nothing is neglected. Yoga is going to play a tremendous role as a living science since comforts of life increase and joints and muscles get rusted due to want of mobility.

Q.- Do you understand why you chose to take on the burden of other people to such and extent?

First of all I did not choose or take on myself the burden. The circumstances and environment forced me to accept this responsibility of releasing or minimising the burden of the people. This made me come out with all my affections as a way of compassion. If I have to bring my child up, I have to be strong; I have to find out whether the child is working or not, whether it is growing up or not. So all that we want in our own children, twenty-four hours a day, is their growth with health and happiness. In that case, parents sometimes use force to keep children in check. That force or admonition is filled only with love and affection. Is it not? For me, my pupils are like children. They come to me for solutions, they need my help. Obviously, I have to take the step as a philosopher, guide, father and friend as my duty to help them for which they come. It may be a physical problem from which they want to be relieved, or it may be to get some happiness or peace. It may be to get guidance in spiritual growth. They come with some anticipation of hope. If I give that hope by soft or hard means, then I not only feel that I have done my job well, but the grace of God too is there. And God exists everywhere, whether we see him or not, and every human being is a part of this divine force. So even if I lose my temper, which may seem to be a hard means, I am serving that God who is within the body of that student. And that is why I go out of my way to help my patients or students in order to make them reach beyond their mental capacities so that they feel the existence of God in their hearts one day or the other.

Q.- Yes, by demanding so much of us, you are challenging us to be our very best, which doesn't happen very often in one's lifetime.

Today, the broad emotional expansion of teachers has disappeared. They are very petty. They've got small eyes, small minds, but they expect big things. In order to do good you have to come out of your own self, do you not? Anyone who protects himself, how can he ever serve people? We have to give our life. We have to come out of our shells, in order to serve the God in those who come to us for help. If each and everyone thinks and works like this, then the society will be different; we will all be different. If we make up our minds to serve others well, this may happen in one's life time alone.

Secondly, you as pupils will be within your shells, and don't want to break the boundaries you try to put around yourselves. As a teacher it is my duty to break such limitations or the fencing which you build around you. My challenge is to bring the change, or rather the transformation in you in this very life.

Q.- So in a way what you're saying is that basically our sicknesses are first spiritual?

How can this be? There is no problem called a spiritual problem. There is no spiritual sickness. In fact all the problems belong to body, mind, intelligence, consciousness and conscience. These problems cover the soul. The soul has no problem. Therefore, when people say that they have different physical, physiological ailments and different psychological fear complexes, I have to start to work first with them on the body-level. I can't say, if one's mind is weak, to do certain things. The weakness of the mind reflects on the body too. When one has a certain psychological weakness which is taken by the heart as if it is going to burst, there must be some physical weakness somewhere for one to elaborate in depth on it mentally. So we say that there is a seed of that in physical form. Through yoga we work with physical weaknesses, by which the student develops confidence. This is what is known as a feedback system. The practice of *āsana* and *prāṇāyāma* play a great role here. Through practice we manufacture our own blood, our own vital energies, circulate them vigorously through the required parts of the body. If a patient is suffering from a liver problem, it is up to the yoga teacher to see that the patient works in such a way that he or she reaches that area and the liver directly receives circulation and energy. For this, the teacher has to think and act as to how to heal that part by blocking the circulation on the other area so that the blood supply increases on the afflicted part. This requires tremendous attention as well as affection from a teacher to go into that.

Q.- Do you feel that you pick up the physical problem in a person as soon as you see them?

Yes.

- Instantaneously? -

Yes.

- How? -

My years of practice have given me special eyes to see the weaknesses in others. It may seem to be intuition. Lord Krishna gave his devotee, Arjuna, divine eyes with which to see him.[1] In a way my practice of *āsana, prāṇāyāma* and *dhyāna* has given me these eyes to see, which you may not understand. The body, its structure, its positions and expressions convey the multiple hidden problems, diseases, as well as moods of their minds too. I not only perceive the physical problems but emotional and mental problems too. I build up the line of treatment with this intuition and perception of mine.

– *Yes! I can see that* –

Q.- One thing I've noticed is that you have more women coming to you from the West, but your students here seem to be predominantly male. Why do you think that is so?

You see, in India the traditional background is that men and women prefer to learn separately. I think in India my class is the only class where men and women are doing yoga together. And I have revolutionised it to such an extent that there are no fear complexes. Of course when the Indians come here they say, "We have the courage to come here and do it without fear". Women are usually shy here. It is a Herculean job to convince them to develop boldness and courage. That is the reason why you see more men here. In the West, the emotional understanding has slipped from the people due to the present technical and intellectual education. Women have to face emotional and family problems more than men. As yoga deals with the heart first and later with the head, women come to classes more in the West.

Q.- But you have also given women who come from the West a great deal of strength. We get so much even though we have had more chances to express ourselves.

Yes, because in the West background and culture are different though the psychology of man and woman is the same. Here, the cultural and traditional background is different. Here, there is no marriage within twenty-four hours and divorce within twenty-four hours. But in the West that freedom, that liberty has been used to such an extent that before people get married they act as if it were unbreakable, as if it were divine, and after a few more years, I hear that everything is quite different for them. How can such things happen? How can a good relationship overnight turn bad, I can't understand this type of talk. Is this judicious or is it libertinism? The man says, "If

---

[1] *Bhagavad Gītā,* XI.8.

this woman is not well, I will get another woman". The woman says, "If you go there, I'll get another man". This way of liberty is creating problems more than solutions. The fear of a split creates nervousness which constantly haunts you, due to the feel of insecurity in relationships. The trust gets broken as easily as a glass breaks. Can the emotional ties be broken by physical separation? In major parts of India these things are not there, which suggests that we are emotionally more stable. If there is a break in marriage here, society also has something to say about it, and people are afraid to go against social norms. At least they don't break the norms that easily. Whereas in the West one goes out of one's way to help society, in terms of his own life he says that it is a personal matter. You may have an association to heal the minds of divorcees, but you may not go to the root cause of problems to see why the divorce takes place at all. As we see the world, know that the world also sees our behaviour and selfish motives.

In India we cannot say it is our personal matter. We think of the responsibility towards society and try to live without double standards. In the marriage system, when we have committed ourselves to each other, we follow it. In India marriage is a norm meant for the good of society as well as individuals and we are made to take seven steps at the time of marriage promising that we are bound together and share together unhappiness and joy. But this depth of the meaning of marriage is not understood by the West. These days the contract or civil marriages have become so common that such marriages can be broken by breaking the contract easily.

Freedom of expression is good but it should not be at the individualistic level only. When one thinks of oneself as an individual, one has to respect the other person too as an individual. Even selfish motives must be within limits as society does not survive on selfish motives. Society survives on a give and take policy. Society is meant for the individual and the individual makes the society. There is an emotional tie between society and the individual.

Therefore, when I teach Westerners and give strength to them, I make them emotionally strong.

Q.- With your way in India, it would allow people to take their studies more seriously, to go more deeply into subjects because they're not so bothered by the multiple choices that exist.

Indians with a traditional background like to penetrate the philosophy of any art in depth. That is why the seriousness is there in imparting the subject.

Though multiple choices do exist here, they do not jump to varieties. They wait and stick to a line of thought persistently hoping that the result may dawn on them one day. It is this state of patience that pays dividends to them later in their efforts or *sādhanā*.

Q.- Do you feel that the Western students who come here are able to take yoga seriously?

To tell you the truth, the first time, they do not take it so seriously, but if they come for two or three times, there is a transformation in them. For example, when I went to London in 1954, I think I never had more than two students; when I came to America in 1956, I had only three or four people because nobody was interested in yoga in those days. I had to sow a good seed so that even if they didn't realise then, they did eventually. Even if there were only ten people, I gave them hope that they could know something about what this art is. It took a long time for the interest to grow in yoga. Now see the transformation everywhere. From two students in 1954, yoga has gone to hundreds of thousands now. They are continuing their studies, coming to India to further their knowledge on the nobility of life with total self-involvement.

Q.- How have you been able to manage your life as a spiritual teacher and yet have a large family?

My dear friend, if I had lived without being a family man, everybody would have said that this person has no responsibility in the world and what else has he except to talk on *adhyātmā vidyā*. Even though I am married and live in the external world, no one knows how I live within. I have all the contacts with the world and yet at the same time am unattached from everything. It appears I'm completely attached, but I'm not. That's why I could balance whether I'm with family or without family. Having lived as a family man, down to earth, I got the knowledge of the material world as well as the spiritual world. Besides these gains, my married life kept me away from sensual temptations of the west.

Q.- But in a way it has been a great inspiration for your students to know that you've been a family man and you have six children, so it makes those of us who have an ordinary life able to relate to yoga better.

This is true. If I had not lived the householder's life and practised yoga, people would have said, he's a celibate, what problems does he have? He has not faced life, he's living comfortably. Having married and living as a householder, I have faced turmoils in life. In turmoil I have practised, so that's why there is a beauty in my practices. This has taught me how to live in the world. I knew the problems of each and every one of you. Before a person told me what was wrong with him, I could catch it. I knew the causes of the sufferings. If I were a *sannyāsin*, I would have had to ask so many things. But having tasted the world, I have also undergone sufferings. These sufferings built in me compassion and affection besides love in yoga, and took yoga to people like you and proved the value of yoga.

Q.- Was there any one time when you felt that because of external circumstances, you couldn't teach, but you had to go on anyway?

Do you mean the external circumstances such as family, family life etc.? No! This never happened that I could not teach. In fact, yoga was my livelihood. I had to teach and earn. Yoga as a subject was forced on me. If I had chosen a path myself, I don't know in what direction I would have gone. I began to teach yoga due to the demands of the people though I felt within me that I was incapable of teaching, but I accepted the challenge. In the beginning there was tremendous fear inside, but outside, tremendous expression of confidence. This inside fear kept me within my limit to go with caution. This caution created boldness gradually to work out for the best in the art of practice and teaching.

Sometimes, there was confusion because of lack of understanding or want of knowledge. It was not certainly because of fear or any external circumstances. As I built up my practice, it built confidence and brought clarity. When clarity came, the confusion lessened and confidence occupied the place of confusion. This is how it happened to me.

Each person, each individual, whether married or celibate, wants to be healthy, strong, enduring – these are all by-products of yoga. The main product of yoga is Self-realisation. I learnt the needs of human beings from their elementary needs and began working on them so that one day they would also go towards the higher aspects of yoga.

Q.- You've worked with people with many different kinds of diseases. Do you feel that yoga can help overcome even the worst disease?

Friend, I don't go on that level saying that yoga is a panacea. I take it for granted that this person will never improve at all. But why not make an attempt? Who am I to decide whether or not the person can improve? Who am I to say I can't work on that person? So I make an attempt and while some ideas come into my head, I observe, I watch, I think, so my thinking and my acting go together; I see the reaction not only from the cells but from the eyes and the brain, how the person receives my instruction, and it works wonders on many cases and individuals.

Often, in certain diseases, one does not know how to make use of this instrument – the body, the organs, the limbs. One suffers with diseases and pains, the practice of yoga made me help those unfortunate ones, how to bear the suffering and tolerate it with ease. I worked on their cellular system, keeping in mind what they have come for and how they sustain recovery and maintain it through further adjustments for greater achievements.

Q.- You're not so concerned, then, in curing the disease?

It is not the question of concern. If one does the practice of yoga properly and judiciously, it has its effects on the body. It has to control or cure the disease. What one needs is how to make suffering people practise and how to gain the knowledge of yoga which includes body, mind and self.

Knowing what my job is, no matter what quality of blood the person has, what amount of energy one has. I begin to work on keeping the circulation of blood in good order, and it is through that alone that I help for their health and happiness. The windows of one's existence depend upon the circulatory and the respiratory systems, which ventilate the system for oxygenised circulation. If these windows are blocked, naturally, due to lack of ventilation, one suffocates. Similarly, if these two systems function well, then the rest of the systems sustain healthy and exhilarating functioning. Knowing that these two systems are the windows of the soul, I believe that there is no other way available to keep them working to the maximum except through yoga. We develop these systems with movement of vital energy into the blood system so that the blood irrigates all the areas of the body with various *āsana* to act in unison. Like a builder, after placing the bricks, sprays them with water so that the bricks may not break off, similarly yoga improves the blood circulation, supplying with sufficient energy to each and every cell in the body. You have to find out whether or not the blood is supplying the organs as it is only through the blood that we can nourish the body. Even if you eat food, the content has to be brought to the organs through the blood stream. So the yogi says, instead of storing, saturating that blood in one area, bring it to another area. That needs knowledge on the part of the teacher. Then the organ is supplied sufficiently and naturally with vital energy for its better functioning. Obviously, it has to improve. Improvement means a way towards a permanent cure.

The first attempt is to relieve the suffering, then building defensive strength, afterwards working for eradication of the disease.

Q.- Do you think we as your students can develop this same quality?

My dear friend, when one human being develops it, do you mean to say that another human being cannot? It is wrong to say that only one gets it. So I'm writing a new book[1] which says that I've developed the talent, but my talent appears to each and every one as if I were a genius. I'm not a genius, but I cultivated this art. But if you read the book on my life, you understand how much I struggled for growth in this art. If I had been a genius, then everything should have come to me easily. Is it not so?

After all, it is a science based on subjective practice. If all of you practise in the way I did and do with open and positive mind, with depth and penetration, you can develop the same qualities.

– *So you are giving an example. Rather you are a living example.* –

Yes, we can all reach. Patañjali, in the fourth chapter of the *Yoga Sūtra,* begins about the gifted accomplishments. The accomplishments may be attained through birth, by utilisation of the medicinal herbs, *mantra,* or by devotional practice as well as by profound meditation.[2] Perhaps what you see in me is the result of the last two.

Q.- If you had anything to impart to teachers, what would you say the most essential qualities would be? Or do these qualities develop from yoga?

Yes! These qualities develop through practice. But the teachers should be sincere, and should treat whomsoever they are teaching as if they were their own bodies. For example, a teacher might say, "Do it", even if the pupil cannot do it. This is wrong on the part of the teacher. Then, how can they help the pupil by ordering them? You need experience. In order to acquire experience, one has to go with the pupil and attend to his or her needs. If one has no experience, how does one know that what one says is correct? The oneness between the teacher and the taught comes with constructive suggestions and in understanding each other by mutual talk.

Suppose as a teacher you have a backache. What do you do? You will try all types of means to get relief as soon as possible. You have to go the same way with your pupils as if they are your kith and kin. It is called zealousness. In that zeal, though there is a separation between the teacher and the student, the mind enters into the other's body as if the teacher's mind is working in the pupil's body. This is love, affection and compassion. There has to be a mental

---

1 *The Art of Yoga,* Harper Collins, London, 1985.

2 *Janma auṣadhi mantra tapaḥ samādhijāḥ siddhayaḥ* (*Y.S.,* IV.1) See the author's *Light on the Yoga Sūtras of Patañjali,* pp. 230-231.

contact. These qualities attract the pupils towards the teacher. In order to grow as a teacher, one has to be strong. You try ways and means to help the pupil. Create artificial disparity between the teacher and the taught, but internally let love, compassion and affection flow in abundance. You have to struggle to see that each student of yours gets relief and poise as quickly as you worked on your own. Then the sparks of Divinity or the Grace of God will always protect you as a teacher. With this attitude, there is no self-interest as such in a teacher, and as the teacher helps others without having any selfish motivation, the conscience is clear and pure. When I am teaching or imparting knowledge, my pupils know that I am near, I am close to them. I am one with my pupils.

Q.- How long do you think it took for you to achieve that?

It is not a question of time. I was teaching and trying to help those who were aged, diseased and affected. As their lives were affected, I started teaching them to find some solace and freedom for them. Life for them became positive from a negative way of thinking. Through teaching them my observations sharpened. While practising, I used to imitate on my own body their ways of stiffness, weakness and presentation that occurred, and I began tracing ways to find relief for pains and guide them through their reactions. After twenty-five years or so I found the maturity setting in my practice, approach and knowledge. Now, I am exact, specific and quick.

Q.- So you think that a teacher is not mature before that?

Who knows, one may mature soon and one may not. No doubt it took me a long time to mature. Probably you do not know that I had no background nor any guidance. I had to start on my own from scratch. Luckily for you, the matured knowledge is ready-made and available. I had to experiment at every stage till the right idea and action struck, whereas now you have just to apply only. I have given you a sequential method whereas for me it was unknown. I had to work out myself with tremendous efforts to know, by changing sequences after sequences to strike the right sequence. Now, you have just to practise what has been made known to you.

As you keep on practising, the refinement comes. Refinement is a continuous process. If you want to be a precise teacher, you have to be a learner at the same time. When one teaches, one must always ask oneself how to impart ideas to the student and how to make them understand. If they cannot understand what I convey, then I have to think myself immediately, and work out ways so that I change my modes to fit into my students' way of thinking. Many in the West say, "Mr. Iyengar is an immature teacher because he changes all the time". They do not read that I'm mobile, my mind is flexible, my observation is quick and sharp. I go according to the students' mental standards and their way of working, which gives me time to change my explanations or adjustments if necessary. As a teacher, I watch many times their bodies faster than themselves and others, and in that observation of seeing, I adopt the right method to make them perform well in unison. This you may never know. In a split second my eyes move everywhere on all. If so-and-so is teaching, they may only see one person. When I'm touching one student, I see the members of the entire class and move fast and use words also faster. My touch tells me whether or not he or she is doing well or not. My intelligence goes out to see other presentations and give guidance.

There were many scientists who worked day and night to land on the moon. The success came after years. But the first scientist was a guide to the next. Similarly, I was the first to accept diseased people to work out with and experiment on the value of *āsana* courageously. As I have shown the way, now it is your duty to work to understand movements and ways of presentation. Observe the feelings from inside that help you to guide others confidently and fast. My study of the value of *āsana* and *prāṇāyāma* is purely a subjective experience and not based on reference or book knowledge.

Q.- Can you feel even from behind you?[1]

Yes, definitely. See, when the fire burns it has no limit. Is it not? So when I'm teaching, I'm nothing but fire. And the fire of yoga is to get rid of impurities. When I'm there my job is to see that the pupil is purified, so the fire in me burns. Others may not be having that fire to flame the light of knowledge in the pupil's body and mind. It is the fire that changes the pupil's body and mind.

- But this is an instinct that I think you have specially. -

You may call it instinct or intuition. I can see from the back because of the fire in me. The shadows of those doing wrong strike my brain. I receive the vibrations of wrong presentations as well as correct presentations. The wrong presentation disturbs me and I immediately go and correct. I get the indication at once even if someone is losing balance in *Sālamba Śīrṣāsana* behind me.

[1] This is a special but peculiar quality of *Gurujī*. He can make out the mistakes of a person even when he is not facing the person. For example, if he asks all to close the eyes and somebody behind him does not he can immediately detect.

Whether instinct or intuition, there is a source for it. You can call this source - God. It is not necessary that you have to give a name or form to God. As we say, "God helps those who help themselves." Similarly, I would say that my flawless *sādhanā,* devotion and adoration to this great art brought clarity and purity in me. Wherever there is purity, the spark of divinity shines. God says to Himself: "Let me be good". This divine grace of His pours in the form of energy or knowledge, since the Supreme is all pervading, omnipotent, omnipresent or omniscient. A new way of thinking, a new idea, if it strikes because of the purity within oneself, one should know that it comes from the unknown, the divine source.

Q.- Mr. Iyengar, could you say anything about how you see the next ten years of your life?

How can I see? It's ridiculous for a yogi to see the future. For me, second to second is a 'new' life. Why bother about it? You know, I'm not attached to my life to say what I will be in ten years. If God calls me, I should be prepared to go any moment. That is the beauty of my life. Natural plan. I did not plan to become a yoga teacher, so why should I bother now? It is He who makes me come to this level: it is for Him to make me do what I should do next. But one thing is, I shall maintain what has been given to me by this grace. That I will ensure. So if you ask me, I will say that I will not stop because after ten years, even if I am an invalid, whatever is possible in spite of that invalidity, I will do so much. According to my condition, I will say that is my maximum.

Q.- We just wanted to thank you for having remained faithful to us, no matter what limitations are.

You should always know that there are limitations. I'm not saying that the human soul cannot go beyond limitations. But see, if your limitations are up to a certain point, I see if I can take you to cross over that border line. Often the limitations are made by us – we don't want to see whether we can cross that borderline. So a little extra effort should be made. Maximum, only one knows, that is God. Between you and me, mine is the maximum compared to you, but if somebody is better than I am, then theirs become the maximum.

The evolution can be seen in someone. Everyone can progress, everyone can cross the border line of limitations. We limit ourselves. God has not limited us.

Q.- Everybody in the class seems to suffer for you, but I wonder when we are going to suffer for ourselves to go through what you went through in your personal suffering. How long did it take you and how can we learn that?

As long as God wants me to suffer, how can I know how long I've got to suffer? I have to suffer, is it not? I myself don't choose to suffer. It is He who gives me suffering and I have to face it.

What is suffering? Is it not *tapas?* Is it not a burning desire to reach perfection? You know that even the bread cannot be earned without taking pains. Here, do you not suffer for the sake of suffering? This is not the aim. I put all my efforts to see you learn self-discipline; you burn your impurities, you reach perfection. By putting my efforts I teach you how you have to be selfless. So, when I teach you, whether *āsana, prāṇāyāma* or *dhyāna*, I show the direction for you to put in your efforts. My keenness is not superficial. My keenness has its depth. Develop that intense keenness in yourself.

The time factor is not involved in it. The question is not of "how long". The question is of "how much".

The day you develop yourself in-depth, penetrate and burn all your physical, moral, mental impurities, then you are the master of yourself. I am not needed then.

Q.- But you do it and we don't. We don't go to that level in our own practice.

That's what I said. You require zeal, zest, a strong will power and discipline. Until that time I have to work for you. The teacher and taught should become one.

You are telling me that you work more for me than for yoga. But I don't believe it. You work more for yoga than for Iyengar because you have attachment to the art. Because you have taken it from me, there is a spark of attachment towards me, too. I'm not denying that. But at the same time it is not true that you are more concerned with me than with the art. Because how many are teaching? How can Iyengar come into the picture? Yoga comes into the picture. When you are teaching, Iyengar does not come, but the art comes first. You may teach what I teach, I am the instrument to convey the subject matter. You may teach the *āsana* I have taught you, with the methodology given by me. While teaching the *āsana*, the subject matter has to be at the forefront and not Mr Iyengar. Do not say in the class that you are teaching similar to what Mr Iyengar has taught. Then in that case the subject matter goes to the background and personality comes to the foreground. Undoubtedly, I have given you a method and undoubtedly you have to follow the method. But as a teacher things have to come from the heart. If you teach, saying that Mr Iyengar has taught me and this is the way to do it, then it does not come from your heart. It comes from your head. Then no more is it art. The art comes from the heart, though the science and methodology comes from the head. Art is first. Methodology is later. I too developed first as art, then I gave the methodology which was the outcome of art.

- *The art comes first.* -

Yes! So you're not working for Iyengar, are you? I am there, as a background; you cannot help but be aware of it. It's an established fact because you have learned from me. But when you are teaching, you cannot say you're working for me. You are working for the good of the person who is in front of you. After you have finished, you can say, "Thank God, Mr. Iyengar has taught me." Only because my guidance is there, it acts as a background. In music, you know, there is that background music. Because you have experienced a certain refinement in the method, naturally there is background. In that case you are not safeguarding Mr. Iyengar; you are safeguarding the art. The subject is important, though the subject is purified and sanctified by the *guru*, because of their *sādhanā*, their *tapas*, their sacrifice and their devotion.

IYENGAR TALKS ABOUT THE *SŪTRAS**

B.K.S. Iyengar fascinated me when I first met him at a yoga intensive in 1977. Arguing and hitting his students one moment, then joking and laughing the next, he reminded me of a lion strutting in his territory, proud and vibrant, daring to be himself.

Over the past fifty years, Iyengar, now sixty-five, has developed an innovative approach to haṭha yoga *that is noted for its thoroughness, precision and therapeutic effectiveness. Author of two classics in the field –* Light on Yoga *and* Light on Prāṇāyāma *– he has taught thousands of Westerners at his Ramāmaṇi Iyengar Memorial Yoga Institute in Pune, India, and his senior students now teach in a score of countries world-wide.*

Iyengar seems such a physical person – yet I sensed great depth as well. Learning that he was writing a book on Patañjali's Yoga Sūtra, *I decided that an interview on the subject would bring out other aspects of the man that I felt had not yet been properly exposed to the world. And I was not disappointed. Beneath the intense, imperious façade, I found a man of genuine compassion and love, using screams and slaps to move students beyond their limitations.*

The following interview was conducted in Pune in July 1983 with the assistance of Manouso Manos, a senior Iyengar teacher from San Francisco and chairman of the First International B.K.S. Iyengar Yoga Convention.

Q.- What inspired you to write a book on Patañjali's *Yoga Sūtra?*

I did not undertake to write for my satisfaction. I am writing because everybody insisted that I should write. The purpose of writing on the *Yoga Sūtra* of Patañjali is quite different. I said to myself, "Do the *Yoga Sūtra* coincide with my own practices? Can I present them with my teachings? I am a practical man; probably my book will not be interesting to the academic, because I give practical meanings. The theoretical explanations are found in many other published books written by so many authors. I am interested to present that each *sūtra* has a bearing with one's own

* Interview by Elise Miller in Pune in July 1983, Published by *Yoga Journal*, July/August 1984, pp. 29-31 and 66-67.

practical experience that reveals the meeting point if they practise on this point. I want to bring out the practical aspects with a subjective touch.

For example, Patañjali composed a series of aphorisms - *sūtra* -, which means pearls of wisdom woven into a thread. However, each *sūtra* is a book in itself. Very often, one does not find a connection of one *sūtra* with the next one, so the reader can get lost. That's why many consider it confusing. I'm trying my best to find out the connections from the start to the finish. Is there any connecting link between the aphorisms on the whole that may clear up the unnecessary confusion? As I find a great deal of logical connecting links between all the four chapters,[1] I have undertaken this task of presenting the homogeneity of the entire presentation of Patañjali.

Q.- Have you always been interested in the *Yoga Sūtras*, or is your interest more recent?

When I was a young boy and had practised yoga for several years, I found Patañjali very difficult to understand. Like many of you, I said, "I am not fit for this. Let me close this book". Then, as I started developing my practice, the hidden meaning of the *sūtra* began to emerge because it was already in my blood. So I said, "Something here connects with my practice. Let me learn more". Naturally I started reading randomly where I could relate it to my experiences, and for the past three years I have been discovering where and how it can lead one, and whether even the common person can understand Patañjali's teachings.

Q.- Are you concentrating on any particular area in the *Yoga Sūtras?*

How can you say "any area"? There are 196 *sūtra*. The key for me is only my own practice of *āsana* and *prāṇāyāma* and *dhyāna*. That is where I would like to penetrate.

Q.- In teaching the *āsana*, you refer regularly to Patañjali, urging us to go deeper than just the body to deal with the mind, to probe why we are doing yoga. Obviously, you see the *āsana* as more than just physical movements.

You're right. You have to know how to penetrate inside the skin. Everything is dark inside. Neither can one see or feel. So we have to develop that mental intelligence that can understand and cope

---

[1] See *Aṣṭadaḷa Yogamālā* vol.1, section III - "The Yoga Sūtra codified According to the Themes for Ready Reference". Also see *Light on the Yoga Sūtras of Patañjali*, appendices I and II.

with the intelligence of the body, which has its own intelligence. The advertent practice of each *āsana* develops a different sensitivity to see and feel in balancing the intelligence of the intellect and the intelligence of the body. Due to ignorance, people have equated *āsana* with the physical movements and the physical movements in *āsana* as *haṭha yoga*. So they insist on the idea that the aspect of *āsana* mentioned by Patañjali is not the same as that mentioned by Svātmārāma. The practitioners of yoga should remember and realise the fact that *āsana* has a great role to play in the entire yogic *sādhanā*. Actually practice of *āsana* brings new awareness and makes us shake hands not only with the body but with the organs of action, senses of perception, mind, energy, intelligence, I-ness and consciousness. Besides these transformations, a day may come when one has to realise the seer. Actually, the seen used as instrument is nothing but the seer himself. Though the seer and the seen are the same, the seer as seen is used as an instrument and when the seen merges in the seer, the seen loses its identity and presents itself as the seer. (See *Y.S.*, I.41).[1]

Patañjali has not divided yoga into *yama, niyama, āsana* and so forth. These are the limbs, or aspects, or petals of yoga which have to be concurrently followed. It cannot be divided or separated. They are interconnected. However, at one place, between *āsana* and *prāṇāyāma,* he has given a stage but not at all on the other aspects of yoga which have to be followed concurrently: while between *āsana* and *prāṇāyāma,* he wants one to first master the *āsana* before taking the *prāṇāyāma* course.

Patañjali at this place only says that after gaining perfection in *āsana* one should take up *prāṇāyāma*. He does not mean, as some people interpret, that you can sit in any comfortable position and do *prāṇāyāma*. The *āsana* are given in order to ensure that the *prāṇic* energy that has been drawn in is made to flow and is absorbed into the system without any interruption. This requires cleanliness and tenderness inside the body. Hence the *āsana* are done to keep the inner fibres completely clean. Water spreads evenly even if the level is uneven. Similarly, the energy spreads by itself in the body evenly through practice of various *āsana*. As soon as the breath is taken in, the energy and consciousness are both sensitised, which is witnessed when the breath is spread all over the body evenly. The very breath also is vitalised and charged. If there are obstacles or hindrances in the body, how can you make use of this energy hidden in the gross breath? The energy does not reach the inner body and therefore it cannot penetrate at all. As this is the actual condition, how can one say that you are getting the benefit of *prāṇāyāma?* It has to be felt. That is why I think Patañjali has not advised any comfortable posture, but rather the perfection of the *āsana* for cleanliness within, so that obstacles are eradicated for the smooth

---

[1] *Kṣīṇavṛtteḥ abhijātasya iva maṇeḥ grahītṛ grahaṇa grāhyeṣu tatstha tadañjanatā samāpattiḥ* (*Y.S.*, I.41). The yogi knows that the knower, the instrument of knowing and the known are one, himself, the seer. Like a pure transparent jewel, he reflects an unsullied purity.

flow of energy. In this sense, the *āsana* are not physical postures or exercises, as they make our intelligence and consciousness through *prāṇa* to go within to come in contact with our inner being.

- I think that is an important distinction. -

Yes, the effort has to cease. When the effort ceases, the *āsana* becomes perfect and comfortable. But you have to make an effort to become perfect. The *sūtra* II.47[1] that deals about the cessation of effort by concentrating on *Ananta* – the Infinite – has a double meaning. You cannot perfect *Bhujaṅgāsana* – cobra pose or *Anantāsana* – the *āsana* that resembles Lord Vishnu's sleeping position as well as indicating the couch – simply by thinking of the thousand-headed cobra. The *Ananta* stands for the king of the cobras, it also means infinite. You have to concentrate on the *āsana* first; then, if you think of *Ananta*, you forget the effort. Like people who lift weights – they make sounds, don't they? In that sound, they forget the effort they are exerting. Similarly, Patañjali has said that while you are making an effort, have the name of God in your mind so that when your effort is at an optimum level you would not feel the exertion even though it may be there. The real point is that when your body is totally making a full effort and when the mind does not feel that effort, it is considered effortless, and this effortless state in mind makes your body become one by uniting with the Infinite – i.e., the self and through self towards the Universal Self.

Q.- *How to Know God* – a translation of Patañjali's *sūtras* by *Swami* Prabhavananda and Christopher Isherwood – mentions *karma yoga* and *bhakti yoga* as well as other types of yoga. Isherwood, in his translation, states that certain yogis have more of a tendency toward one type of yoga than toward another. Do you feel that his translation is accurate, and do you consider yourself a *haṭha yogi?*

It is none of my business to comment on your first query regarding the translations of any author. Everyone has the freedom of expression. I am not here to check whether somebody is accurate or not. Your question which is directly pointed at me is whether I am a *haṭha yogi* since you conceive the idea that there are different types of yoga. Perhaps you want to categorise yoga and put me in one of the categories. Let me answer that point.

---

1 *Prayatna śaithilya ananta samāpattibhyām* (*Y.S.*, II.47). Perfection in an *āsana* is achieved when the effort to perform it becomes effortless and the infinite being within is reached.

First of all, yoga is one and there are no different types of yoga. Even if, for the time being, you call each path a different type of yoga, one type cannot be separated from the other, although no doubt one path may be predominant. A human being is made up of three inseparable parts – hand, head and heart. Hands and legs are meant for action, head is meant for thinking and heart is meant for loving. People distinguish between a *haṭha yogi*, a *karma yogi*, a *jñāna yogi* and a *bhakti yogi*, but Patañjali does not separate them. This division came later, when individuals started writing books about yoga. Patañjali does speak about the types of yoga, but he does not say that his is *rāja yoga* or any particular yoga. Svātmārāma names *samādhi* as *rājayoga*, since it is the ultimate state. This state does not differ from what Patañjali mentions. However, Patañjali mentions *kriyā yoga*. See *sūtra* II.1, *tapaḥ svādhyāya Īśvarapraṇidhānāni kriyāyogaḥ*.[1] Here he speaks of *tapas* for keeping the hands clean – path of *karma*; *svādhyāya* or knowledge for keeping the head clear – path of *jñāna;* and *Īśvara praṇidhāna* for keeping the heart humble in order to be free from the ego – path of *bhakti*. So Patañjali's yoga is inclusive of all. When he explains a part explicitly, the others are implicit. According to Patañjali, as I understand him, I feel that all the different yoga, I prefer to call them paths, have to be followed at the same time as they are all interwoven between hands, head and heart.

For your information, first of all there are no different types of yoga. Yoga is one. The path which unites us to the Supreme is yoga. One creates the path according to one's capacity, understanding and inclination. So yoga is one but one may emphasise on particular *sādhanā* in order to reach the Supreme.

Patañjali used the word *kriyā yoga* for the very methodology of yoga which includes *tapas*, *svādhyāya* and *Īśvara praṇidhāna* and *aṣṭāṅga,* eight aspects or petals of yoga. *Kriyā* literally means work or with intense activity. Whether it is *karma* – action –, *bhakti* – love, – or *jñāna* – knowledge –, intense activity is involved in all aspects of yoga. Even thinking is action. To surrender to God is an action. To discipline yourself is an action. To do *japa* is an action. Without action, you cannot make progress in any field, let alone the branches or petals of yoga. Action is the practical part of *sādhanā*. So to brand me indirectly as a physical yogi or a *haṭha yogi* has no meaning. To see *haṭha yoga* as just physical is limiting of one's intelligence or it may be a perversion of intelligence – *viparyaya*. *Haṭha* means will. In learning yoga, first of all one needs discipline of will. How can one discipline oneself without will?[2]

In addition, we have to remember that mind is like a mirror that reflects. If the mind cannot reflect my actions, then what is the use of that mind, the mirror, in my practice of yoga? Each and every thing has to make an imprint on one's mind, on one's intelligence and on one's consciousness. Then one will know where one is wrong and where one is right. This much is

---

1 Burning zeal in practice, self-study and study of scriptures, and surrender to God are the acts of yoga.

2 For details see *Aṣṭadaḷa Yogamālā* vol. 2 – section II – *Haṭha Yoga*.

enough for one to say that much more is involved than the physical aspect in *haṭha yoga*. How can I just be in my arms and in my legs without my head and my heart?

Therefore, let me conclude the fact that *haṭha yoga* is not a physical yoga. There are no different types of yoga. The path of yoga shown by Patañjali and Svātmārāma is inclusive of *jñāna*, *karma* and *bhakti* though he does not mention them by name. I am simply a *sādhaka*, a devotee of yoga. I practise humbly what Patañjali has said.

Q.- In the third chapter, Patañjali speaks on *saṁyama*, in which concentration, meditation and absorption come to bear on one subject. He speaks of making *saṁyama* on the back of the head, on the navel, on the hollow of the throat, on the heart. Isn't this what you're doing through the teaching of the *āsana* and *prāṇāyāma* – giving your students the experience of *saṁyama* and therefore making it a meditation?

Instead of speaking of concentration or meditation, let us come to the level of the intelligence of an ordinary person. For him the body is the gross self, the mind is the subtle self and the soul is the subtlest. Then *saṁyama* here means the integration of these three: body, mind and soul. In the beginning certain projections have to be given to focus the attention. Everyone is not highly intelligent to go inwards to the Self at once and one cannot become an expert without refining one's repeated experiences. When one has reached maturity in all the areas of attention, and no area is left out, it is *saṁyama*. If all the areas of the body are made into a single unit in your practice, whether in *āsana* or *prāṇāyāma*, you will find out that you are one with each part at the same time. Patañjali very clearly says that one-pointedness should remain as all-pointedness forever. If you are one-pointed, this one-pointedness is a part of a compartment or a part of the brain. Yet with this growth are we not disturbed and waver again and again? There are many stages or levels of one-pointedness. The highest level is said to be "seedless", where one-pointedness transforms into all-pointedness. This state of all-pointedness is very difficult to maintain because attention is like electrical voltage, which drops down or goes up. Similarly, our attention suddenly becomes very brilliant and then fades away. Therefore, we must cultivate that power in us through yogic discipline so that the voltage of intellectual attention and observation may not wax or wane.

Q.- And this is why you keep going back over the details of the *āsana* instructions.

Aah! Now you understand why we say, "Do this, don't do that" – so that you develop the power of attention by using your own body, your own mind, your own intelligence and your own consciousness.

Q.- Would that mean that the common person has some experience in the lower states of *samādhi*, hitting that level of consciousness for a short period of time?

Common person does experience the characteristics of *samādhi* when he lives in intellectual and mental state of silence and serenity.

Yes. Experiences do come to each and every one of us in a split second like a flash. Those who are intelligent can catch it, and pursue it. Those who are not intelligent cannot. So they have to wait patiently without loosening their efforts.

Q.- Patañjali talks about the *siddhis*, or powers, that one obtains by making *saṁyama*. I'm sure that you have attained some of these powers in your practices. How do you deal with these powers, and how do you advise your students to deal with them?

First of all, you have to be very careful about *siddhi*. Patañjali gives thirty-four fruits[1] that one can achieve from the practice of yoga. If you experience one of these, it's a sign that you are on the right path and your *sādhanā* is right. These powers, or sensitivities, as they are called, should not be considered as supernatural or supernormal powers. They are superlative sensitivities, which come in various forms and indicate that you are on the right path. But you should not hold on to them as if these were your own.

The powers do come as the effects or fruits of the *sādhanā* but one should not be caught in these but pursue the *sādhanā* as if one is innocent of *siddhi*. Therefore, Patañjali advises us not to abandon the base. Not to give up *kriyā yoga*. *Siddhi* should not interfere in the memory of *sādhanā*.

[1] See the author's *Light on the Yoga Sūtras of Patañjali*, pp. 33-34.

Q.- Doesn't Patañjali tell us to avoid them?

No, he doesn't tell us to avoid but cautions that though these sensations or sensibilities are great achievements, yet they are obstacles to *samādhi*. These are actually impediments for further development. That is why he has added the fourth chapter, entitled "Liberation". He could have closed the subject after describing how to master yoga in the first or second chapter. In the third chapter, *Vibhūti Pāda,* he explains what one gets once one has mastered it. Here, he explains the good and the bad effects of yoga, and then goes to the fourth chapter, *Kaivalya Pāda*. The *siddhi* or the powers are the result of conquest of *prakṛti*. In a way it is the total, complete evolution of *prakṛti*. But that is not the end. Now Patañjali wants the *sādhaka* to know how to go for the involution of *prakṛti*. Therefore, he shows the ways of how to live with all these powers, by developing an "exalted" intelligence, which has two facets – attention and awareness. The first is uninterrupted intelligence of attention, and the second is intelligence of awareness that has reached the pinnacle where there is absolutely no movement or fluctuation, waning or waxing. The first is vibrant. The second is luminous. This is *vivekaja jñānam* or exalted intelligence.

In order to learn, you have to be *rājasic*, or vibrant. That is why you are advised to manage with uninterrupted attention and awareness to stop the fluctuations or impediments that come in the way. When you have reached this pinnacle of yoga, your intelligence and consciousness are balanced and brought to the level of the purity of the self; then there is no difference between the two. That is exalted intelligence. The discriminative intelligence – *viveka khyāti* – has to lead towards exalted intelligence – *vivekaja jñānam*. This has to be utilised for the process of involution which leads towards *kaivalya,* the crowning glory of the yoga *sādhanā*.

Q.- You have used the word *rājasic*. Could you talk about the three *guṇa* – *sattva, rajas* and *tamas* – which Patañjali describes in the first chapter?

Let me talk more on the *rājasic* force. Concentration, or meditation, is vibrant. Is it not? That is why it is *rājasic* in nature. As I said earlier, the moment you move away from vibrancy the *āsana* become perfect and the effort ceases. As the effort of vibrancy ceases, one becomes luminous; one just shines. As we do not know when the cloud will cover the sun, similarly, we may not know at what time the clouds of doubt, want of attention, loss of observing awareness, may cover our exalted illumination. Hence, vibrant practice is needed in order to make sure that the cloud of attachment does not come and cover our luminous intelligence.

All humans are endowed with the three types of *guṇa: sattva*, meaning luminous; *rajas*, meaning vibrant, and *tamas*, meaning inert. These three fundamental ingredients of *prakṛti* form a kind of wheel that just rolls on and on. One of the three becomes predominant and dominates the other two. It revolves in turns. Therefore sometimes one experiences that one is inert, sometimes vibrant and sometimes luminous. We experience all these three, day in and day out. For this reason, our behaviour changes. Also what we eat and what we think affects our behaviour. Food also takes on the qualities of *sattva, rajas* and *tamas*, and our behaviour balances on what we eat.

The *sādhanā* of yoga has to be done so that our body, organs of action, senses of perception, mind, intelligence and consciousness, all these aspects make a journey from *tamas* to *rajas* and finally from *rajas* to *sattva*. The *citta* finally has to be shining with the luminosity of exhalted intelligence. The *citta* at this stage is recognised as *sattva* since it is totally changed with *sattva-guṇa*. It is in a pure and illuminative state.

For example, *yogaḥ cittavṛtti nirodhaḥ* (*Y.S.*, I.2), the cessation or restraint of movements of the consciousness, is a force or the vibrant quality of *rajō-guṇa*; as restraining is the function of *rajō-guṇa*. Without the *rājasic* character, cessation or restraint is hard to achieve. When *citta* remains without *vṛtti*, *rajō-guṇa* of the *sādhaka* disappears and the nature of *sattva-guṇa* dawns.

Q.- I have heard that you describe yourself as a *rājasic* teacher. Is that true, and why are you not a *sāttvic* teacher like so many other yogis?

'Vibrant' is the word. *Rajas* has a tremendous vibrancy. I am vibrant while teaching and I have a reason for it. If I'm very soft, do my pupils make progress? I have to be fiery to create fire in the students. Basically, students are *tāmasic* while doing *sādhanā*. In order to make them alert and vibrant, tell me whether I need *sattva* or *rajō-guṇa*.[1] Have I to be vibrant or luminous? I may have knowledge and wisdom, but when I have to give my knowledge and wisdom to you, does it not require vibrancy? When students are doing the *āsana*, how many times do they collapse? Is collapsing the way to master the *āsana*? Don't they need to charge their body and mind? The state of *saṁyama* is a tremendously energetic state. If one loses that state, *saṁyama* will not be there. In a split second the *saṁyama* disappears. That is why I have to be so *rājasic* to move the students from the inert towards the active state. You have seen me when I am practising. Am I vibrant? No. Why should I be vibrant at that time? I have to introvert my attention because I have to see what is occurring in my practice. While I am teaching, I have to give what I've got. How can I give when I get introverted in my teaching?

---

[1] See table n. 8, p. 120: The Evolution of *Citta*, in *Light on the Yoga Sūtras of Patañjali*, Harper Collins, London.

While doing *sādhanā* one has to be looking within. This "looking within" is the quality of *sattva-guṇa.* While teaching and imparting yoga to others one has to give them the same experience. This "giving of experience" is the quality of *rajō-guṇa,* which is necessary to bring the quality of movement, motion or vibrancy in *sādhanā.*

The so-called *sāttvic* yogis are make-believe people. The *guru's* job is not to remain on top but to see that his students come up to his level. He has to enlighten his students. He has to light the candle in them and keep it burning forever. You call me vibrant or fiery, aggressive or intense. This does not matter to me at all. Only know that I can't bear to see indifference of the students and to see them unlively! My fiery actions are meant to electrify my pupils. If I withdraw and remain passive, then one may say, "What a wonderful teacher! He never loses his temper." But does it help my pupils if I put up that appearance?

Vyāsa in his commentary on Patañjali says that the *guru* should be as soft as a petal and as hard as a diamond. What does it mean? When hardness is required, the teacher has to be hard. When compassion is required, he has to be compassionate. This does not mean indifference. Compassion and indifference do not go together. Indifference is negligence. So to some extent it may turn into *tamo guṇa.* Compassion is *rājasic,* vibrant. The *rājasic* nature is essential for illumination or for the *sattva guṇa* to shine.

Q.- Do you still do your *āsana* practice? Or do you feel that, because you have perfected the *āsana,* you no longer need to do them? Many yogis claim that they perfect the *āsana* and then only need to do *prāṇāyāma* and *dhyāna.*

Sorry, I cannot speak of other yogis. The question itself is self-contradictory. If somebody says that he has given up the *āsana* practice due to his mastery over them already, then one can give up *prāṇāyāma* or *dhyāna* too after perfection. So if one gives up, is it perfection or weakness? Who knows, they may be covering weaknesses or their inability to perform, so they say they are advanced. I am practising *āsana* even today. The other yogis may not practise, because they may be out of control, or they are incapable of practising. They have fallen from grace. For me it is the practice of *āsana* and *prāṇāyāma* that brought me to this state of understanding my body, my mind and my self. How can I discard that which showed me light. So I practise and I shall continue to do so even in the future.

As a result of accidents, I had lost my grip on *āsana,*[1] but I don't say that I've fallen from grace. I'm studying every day. I don't know what made me practise in the early days and what is

[1] The author met with an accident in 1979, whilst driving a scooter. The whole spine was damaged. He corrected the injury with the practice of *āsana,* without undergoing any medical treatment or surgery.

making me do so today. I try to do my maximum even today. Of course, my maximum of ten years ago is not my maximum today. But today's maximum is my maximum, and I have a choice to accept that or to give up. To give up is easy but to continue is difficult. So I find out the opposing force within myself, eradicate those oppositions and practise continuously. If I fail, then I say laughingly, "Yes, I tried my best. I will not give up now because I have some problems. I have faced them in early days and why should I become nervous now?" Then I try to find out where the hindrance is, where the energy is not flowing, where it is blocked. In fact, that gives me a better understanding. And now you see what change it has brought in spite of having these injuries. I have regained myself.

As far as the second part of your question is concerned, the eight aspects of yoga are not separate from each other. Tomorrow, say for instance, if one perfects in *dhyāna,* will one give up *dhyāna* or the other aspects of yoga? The question is what has to be given up. Does one practise yoga to give up yoga later? Then, why practise? After you have graduated from college, do you say that you will give up your education? Instead you use that education to build up your way of thinking for the better. At the same time you do not stop writing or reading. Similarly, here too, it is a continuous process. The devotee or a *bhaktan* does not give up repeating – *japa* – the name of God even after seeing or realising God. In fact, the saints pray to God to grant them further lives so that they can keep on reciting the name of God forever.

If you read the *Bhagavad Gītā*, Lord Krishna says "Whatever I do, that very thing men do taking Mine as an example. Whatever standard I set up, men follow. As a matter of fact, there is nothing for Me to do, since nothing remains unattained by Me. If I give up the action, then men will follow Me and give up the action. If I cease to act, the world will perish, and I will be considered the cause of destruction of people of the world."[1] If the Lord Himself says so, who are we to give up? So those who claim that they have perfected themselves, ask them whether they are greater than Lord Krishna.

Q.- Why don't more Indians do yoga?

Do you know why? In olden days, everybody was practising. Then the country was full of spiritual development, but they were never prepared for wars or invasions. That culture of spiritual growth was destroyed by countless invasions, and the British completed it by making us economically

[1] Whatever a great man does, other men follow him. Whatever standard he sets up, mostly others follow the same – III.21. – Arjuna, there is nothing in the three worlds for Me to do, nor unattained by Me, yet I continue to work – III.22. – If I do not engage myself in action scrupulously, Arjuna, men follow Me and harm will come to the world – III.23. If I cease to work, the worlds will perish. Then confusion sets in and destruction engulfs the world – III.24

poor so that we had to accept any work to survive. They encouraged us to learn English and tempted us with jobs if English was known. When the people of India could not get even two meals a day, was yoga important, or was it more important to get a meal? We are still fighting poverty, even though the British have left. This is the main cause for India to be indifferent towards its heritage.

Yet, it will be wrong to say that Indians do not practise yoga. They were not exposing their practice. The media did not give much exposure to the *sādhaka*. Hence, the subject became individualistic. But after independence, we are catching it and I am proud to say that yoga is gaining popularity.

Q.- In the first chapter of the *Yoga Sūtra*, Patañjali mentions that one must repeat the *mantra ĀUṀ* while meditating on its meaning. Do you personally chant or meditate with *ĀUṀ* or some other *mantra?* If so, why don't you emphasise meditation more to your students?

The word *āuṁ* is *akṣara*. It means imperishable, indestructible, undecaying. In the word *āuṁ* three letters are involved. They are *ā*, *u* and *ṁ*. *Ā* is the beginning of the alphabet. Creation begins from here. *U* is the continuity of the speech, and *ṁ* puts an end to communication. All the alphabets and words melt into these three alphabets. Out of the fifty-three phonemes in *Sanskrit*, all others melt and perish while these three never fade or perish. These three are the principle cause not only for uttering the words, but also for communication and communion. Therefore, words being imperishable and eternal, the sages and yogis of India gave a divine touch to them. As *āuṁ* gets the supremacy over other letters, it is considered as the epithet of the Supreme – the God as well as the Self. *Āuṁ* being indestructible, the *ṛṣīs* took this as *bīja mantra* or seed *mantra* on God.

Repetition of a *mantra* or sacred prayer like *āuṁ* is called *japa*. As I mentioned before, the mind tends to fluctuate and become distracted. By bringing it back to a single point like *āuṁ* or by looking at a candle or a rose or some other object, the *sādhaka* silences the thoughts and becomes one with body and mind. For me focusing on the breath while in the *āsana* with total one-pointedness is meditation. It is with this steadiness of intelligence that one witnesses the presence of soul.

From the Indian point of view, *āuṁ* has a specific meaning. You open your mouth to say *ā*. To pronounce, you roll the tongue like *u*, *ṁ* stands for silence. In order to learn silence, you must close your mouth. These are the roots for speech, like the root mind or *mūla citta*[1] for

[1] See the author's *Light on the Yoga Sūtras of Patañjali*, Harper Collins, London, p. 234. Also see in *Aṣṭadaḷa Yogamālā*, vol 1, pp. 179, 185 and 209.

thinking, so they are considered as the divine sound. Patañjali wants you to do this with meaning and felt experience. Without experience you cannot understand the meaning; you cannot experience just by knowing the meaning of it. Feeling must be there. Remember that the *mantra* is a seed, and ultimately you want to be seedless, or beyond the seed. This seed method may work for some.

Patañjali wants, basically, the purification of body and restraint of *citta*. Therefore, my emphasis is on body and mind. For me *āsana* is the *mantra,* the breath is the *mantra* and I have to understand the meaning of each *āsana* and feel the life force – the self – moving in with the rhythm of body and breath.

Q.- In other words, if it works, use it; if it doesn't, don't bother.

That's right. It is not compulsory. The practitioner has to have emotional maturity. One should not impose from outside. It has to emerge from inside.

Q.- I have heard a lot of definitions of *kuṇḍalinī yoga.* Can you give your version?

Kuṇḍalinī is a divine energy. In ancient days it was called fire, and I have written in my *prāṇāyāma* book that fire and *kuṇḍalinī* are the same. *Kuṇḍalinī* is *prakṛti-śakti*. There is a connection between *kuṇḍalinī* and the *sādhanā* explained in *Haṭhayoga Pradīpikā*. The treatise proclaims that where there is divine energy, there is definitely *haṭha*. *Ha* stands for sun, the positive energy and *ṭha* stands for moon, the negative energy. When these two energies meet or join, it is yoga. It is also said that *ha* stands for the *puruṣa* – the soul – and *ṭha* for *prakṛti* – nature. Consciousness is a part of nature. The yogi wants to have a grip on it through yoga. People say *haṭha yoga* is physical yoga. How can it be only a physical yoga? Positive and negative currents are produced by practising the *āsana, prāṇāyāma* and *mudrā*. When these currents are brought together, divine energy is produced. The divine energy can only arise in divine personalities, who have conquered lust, anger and greed. If anyone says, "So-and-so has touched me and awakened my *kuṇḍalinī*", they are ridiculing this great divine power. If that were so simple, then why would we have to search for God?[1]

---

[1] Read *Aṣṭadaḷa Yogamālā* vol 2.

Q.- This leads to another question. When I've been doing *prāṇāyāma*, I sometimes feel out of control. Electric currents shoot through my body, and I shake all over. I wonder whether I should stop, or is that my *kuṇḍalinī*?

That shaking has nothing to do with your *kuṇḍalinī*.[1] If the body shakes, that means that you are unable to withstand the strain. If your body shakes, some *gurus* will say that your *kuṇḍalinī* is awakened. I say, your nerves are not strong enough to take it. Stop it for the present. Develop the strength in the nerves, stabilise them and then proceed. Otherwise you will be injuring your nervous system and end up in a mental clinic.

Q.- How do you feel about being both a practitioner of yoga and a householder?

I enjoy both. I practised yoga with six children to bring up. I don't feel the difference at all. I am a free man because I feel the fulfilment in life as a householder. Those who claim to be renunciates are often caught up in their minds with sexual desires. They flirt, but pretend to be celibate when they are not. But a husband who has survived his wife, as in my case, a husband with a wife, a wife with a husband, practise morality more religiously than others.

Q.- Patañjali says that we can eliminate pain through non-attachment. Do you feel that we sometimes have to go through pain without avoiding it?

I do not think Patañjali has said anywhere to eliminate pain through non-attachment. In fact he asks the practitioners to see through pain. He analyses what the pain is. If you talk of physical pain, this pain is due to the imbalances in the contents of the body which need to be corrected. Are not the obstacles in the path of yoga painful? Patañjali says that the obstacles and distractions have to be prevented by practising yoga. According to him everything is painful.[2] Even pleasure concludes in pain. So if one has to avoid the pains which are yet to come, one has to know the cause of pain and the practice of yoga begins there.

There are many types of pains – physical pains, mental pains, intellectual pains and spiritual pains. Physical pains have to be fought with physical alignment, mental pains with mental discipline, intellectual pain with understanding and spiritual pains through intelligence

1 Patañjali says *aṅgamejayatva* – the shakiness of body is an obstacle. It causes the distraction of mind. Otherwise, there alone he would have said that the divine energy is awakened.

2 *Pariṇāma tāpa saṁskāra duḥkaiḥ guṇavṛtti virodhāt ca duḥkham eva sarvaṁ vivekinaḥ* (*Y.S.*, II.15). The wise man knows that owing to fluctuations, the qualities of nature, and subliminal impressions, even pleasant experiences are tinged with sorrow, and he keeps aloof from them.

and consciousness. One has to face them all. We have to use the body to make the mind strong and mind to make the body strong. When I work with you, I make you face what you cannot face. The avoidable pains have to be known and understood so that one can avoid them with deliberation. So non-attachment is not the answer. The deliberation is the answer. You have to act thoughtfully. With prudence.

Q.- What if someone comes to you with an emotional problem or block? Do you feel that the yoga you teach helps that person?

Of course, yes! I have taught so many people who had mental and emotional blockages. You need to teach them with patience. You need to understand their problems. Their mind which is scattered needs to be channelled.

We have to divert their imprisoned mind by getting them to concentrate on body grips, which is the easiest method. It is difficult to concentrate on abstract thoughts or ideas, we have to get them to focus their attention on the concrete body so that the mind is connected to the body. As their concentration develops, the emotion, the blocking, disappears. These people are dreamers, whether they are awake, walking, standing or sitting. We bring them to be in contact with the body so that their empty minds are diverted to be fully conscious with their movements in body and breath.

Q.- May I ask a personal question? Is there anything you are afraid of?

Up to now, no. If I had fear, I don't think I would have mastered this art.

Q.- You have had some times in your life when it would have been easy for you to be afraid. How did you manage?

I asked myself, "Is this the end, or is my life going to go further?" And *haṭha*, or will power, brought me through. As I have mentioned before, my body is my strength. "I'll rise in this art or I'll fall in this art, but I will not surrender to anything" – that's the kind of determination I had. It was the will over matter. That's how I conquered fear. Now everything is fulfilled and there is no room for fear.

If you want something, then naturally you will fear. Attachment to life is fear. Love for life is sustained by its own force. This clinging to life is so strong that it affects the wise as well as the ignorant. Patañjali explains that each human being has the taste of death lingering at the back of the mind. This imprint of attachment to life is the seat of fear. This instinctive defect can easily be transformed into intuitive knowledge or insight through the path of yoga. While practising *āsana* and *prāṇāyāma*, a person can trace how the flow of intelligence and the current of life force become one. Then he attains the state of evenness in which he sees no difference between life and death as both converge together as life force. When we are practising the *āsana*, the intelligent current and the life force current are united and make us understand that life and death are one. We have no sense of life and no sense of death – which is the perfect state within the *āsana*. With this understanding, the yogi loses the attachment to life and conquers the fear of death.

HOW TO BECOME A YOGI?*

Q.- The first question I would like to ask, are you a *rāja* yogi?

We don't demarcate yoga. Yoga is one. I am a practitioner of yoga and I don't brand myself to any particular kind of yoga like you have in your mind.

Q.- What would one need to become like you?

How can you become like me? God blessed me to be like this. So, I am. But it is hard for one to explain the ways to become like me in the practice of yoga. To become like me you have to work like me – ten to twelve hours a day, irrespective of difficulties, upsets and upheavals of life. The goal I have chosen in life is full of inspiration and full of perspiration. Nothing can be earned without pain. One has to go with a certain discipline to reach a goal. This certain discipline to follow itself is painful. But nothing can come or can be achieved with comfort. For example, if you plant a seed in your garden, without caring for it, do you get the fruits? How long does it take to get the fruit? It depends upon the care you give at each stage. After a few days, when the seed sprouts into a sapling, how happy you are in your heart and mind! It is the same in yogic discipline and practices. When you begin yoga, it is like a seed, and you have to see that it grows into a sapling and then into a tree. You have to prune the tree very carefully to get the fruit or else it does not give it. Similarly, you have to work hard to trim the body and mind to reach the harvest of health and happiness.

---

* This interview was taken by Rod Hayes, Australia. It was broadcast on "The Body Programme" for the Australian Broadcasting Commission, September 1983. Transcribed and edited by Sandra Mulcahey. First published in the BKS Iyengar Yoga Association of Australasia Newsletter in June 1985.

Q.- You have written that there are four grades of pupils: feeble, average, superior and supreme. I feel and most of the people I know would fit into the category of feeble. You have written that it would be very difficult for those people to follow the path that you have taken.

I have not said that it is very difficult. I have only quoted one of the yogic texts.[1] Of all the different levels of pupils, only the very intense have the goal near to them. Those who are feeble and average reach the goal, but the time factor works on feeble and average grades of *sādhaka*. The feeble have to put more efforts to reach the grade of supreme. *Sādhanā* demands faith, vigour, memory and patient awareness[2] besides dedication, *tapas, svādhyāya, Īśvarapraṇidhāna*,[3] *abhyāsa, vairāgya*.[4] All these have to be adopted little by little by everyone. This is the reply to your previous question too.

It is steadfast determination that makes one reach the desired ambition to master yoga.

Q.- You have demonstrated quite clearly in your book that yoga has great benefits for the body and for the mind. Can you describe yoga?

I will explain it using some analogies. Many classics say that the body is the temple of the soul, but the yogis go one step further and say that the body is only the temple of the soul provided you keep it healthy and happy. Otherwise, it cannot become the temple of the soul, it becomes the devil's workshop. The body contains innumerable muscles and joints. We do not know how many minor muscles there are to help these major muscles to function and how to work on the linking tendons, which we never exercise. It is said that the lungs when stretched would cover the size of a tennis court. The heart supplies oxygen into the blood stream. It is also said that the nervous system if connected together stretches to 6,000 miles or 9,600 kilometres and blood vessels to about 60,000 miles or 96,000 kilometres. You can understand how intricate the human body is. How do we feed this entire system: the muscles, joints, tissues, tendons and on top of all that, the mind, the consciousness and the conscience? These are the layers of what we call the human soul. From the body to the self, we have different coats: the anatomical, the physiological, psychological, intellectual and the causal bodies. If you have a rusty sword and you have

[1] See in this volume, p. 183, also read footnote of that page.

[2] See *Aṣṭadaḷa Yogamālā*, vol. 2, p. 204 and vol. 3, p. 146.

[3] See *Aṣṭadaḷa Yogamālā*, vol. 1, the article entitled, "Yoga – A Fount for all Spiritual Paths", vol. 2, *"Aṣṭāṅga Yoga* – The Eight Limbs of Classical Yoga" and "Svātmārāma Shakes Patañjali's Hand", and vol. 3, *"Anukrama Sādhanā Śreṇi"*.

[4] See *Aṣṭadaḷa Yogamālā*, vol. 1, "Yoga and Peace", "Essence of the *Yoga Sūtras of Patañjali*" and "Pearls of Yogic Wisdom".

tremendous valour, is that valour useful to you? If the sword is sharp and you have no valour, what use is that sharp sword? The body acts as a sword and the mind acts as valour. So these yogic practices sharpen the body, and due to this sharpening of the body, tremendous concentration in mind and valour in body is created. In this way, the body and the mind are made to function equally with intelligence. This is the effect of yoga.

If your nation or my nation is not properly protected, an aggressor can enter. So second to second, moment to moment, you are to be aware and watch the frontier of your country or my country so that the aggressor may not enter. Similarly, in the human system, disease in the form of an aggressor awaits outside our skin, knowingly or unknowingly, waiting to occupy this territory of the body. If your inner mind is very careful and cautious and keeps the entire system, namely, circulatory, respiratory, digestive, nervous and uro-genital systems in complete harmonious function, naturally the aggressor known as disease cannot enter this healthy territory – the body.

Q.- Is yoga the only path to develop this?

To a great extent I say, "Yes", because yoga is effectively an interpenetrating art and science. Man is made up of hands and legs which are meant for action, head for clear thinking and heart to feel the emotional temperaments. Yogic *āsana* play a tremendous role in developing the firmness in body, cleanliness in hands to keep the actions pure, clarity in intelligence and stability in emotions. Yoga is also self-discipline through which a total change or transformation is brought out in the body, mind and intelligence in the practitioner.

In order to feel one's existence at all levels such as physical, moral, mental, emotional, intellectual and spiritual, yoga builds up that awareness to spread from the body to the self and vice versa. It is a cleansing process at all levels, contributing health, wellbeing and balance. In this sense, yoga is a holistic science since its practice needs a lot of concentration and reflection in performing it. All these are made to function in the process of practice. The capacities of mental aspects like reflection, action and thinking are cultivated together in the practice of yoga. In this sense I consider this path as the only path as it covers man from sole to soul and soul to sole.

Q.- You have written extensively not just about the *āsana* but about the eight stages of yoga. Can you describe what the eight stages of yoga are?

When you think of the human being, the hands and legs are meant for action, head for thinking and the heart for feeling. On these three basic points the eight aspects of yoga are evolved. They are called *yama*, *niyama*, *āsana*, *prāṇāyāma*, *pratyāhāra*, *dhāraṇā*, *dhyāna* and *samādhi*. The principles of *yama* are meant for the control of the organs of action – hands, legs, mouth, genital and excretory organs. *Niyama* controls the senses of perception – eyes, ears, nose, tongue and skin.

The *āsana* are meant to clean and purify the body – the temple. The practice of *āsana* irrigates the entire system and prevents calcification and stiffness of the joints and keeps every tissue in the body mobile and healthy so that the waste in the form of impurities of the body and the immoral and unethical dirt of the mind are removed by the practice of *āsana*. When the *āsana* are practised well, then *prāṇāyāma* or breathing practices that contain deep inhalation, inhalation-retention, deep exhalation and exhalation-retention in different forms regulate the flow of energy in the system. Having removed the impurities in the system, the *āsana* bring a unique interaction between the blood and *prāṇic* energy which is made to flow freely in the system without any interruption, and energise each and every cell. Having reached the perfection in the physical level, yoga deals with the mental apparatus. This is the process of watching the organs of action, senses and the mind. Then we go in and follow the vibrations of the consciousness towards the interior source. We have three bodies – physical, mental and spiritual. *Yama*, *niyama*, *āsana* and *prāṇāyāma* deal with the physical body. *Prāṇāyāma* and *pratyāhāra* deal with the mental body in order to make us know how to control the wavering mind that is oscillating from second to second. The method of controlling this oscillating mind is *dhāraṇā* and then to focus its energy and concentration, is called *dhyāna*. *Āsana* and *prāṇāyāma* are the concrete support to the mind – to rest on – to get a comparatively controlled grip. They help to a great extent to imbibe the qualities required for *dhāraṇā* and *dhyāna*. Then, the known comes to an end. Slowly as you come to know the known well, the mind turns towards the unknown, which is the return journey from the mind to the spiritual body. This is known as *dhyāna* or meditation. The state comes when a man forgets himself. It may be a split second or a split minute and that state gives a glimpse of the characteristic of *samādhi*. These are the eight aspects of yoga, which I explained to you in short[1].

Q.- It would seem that there are many obstacles in that path, especially in our community.

My dear friend, why say specifically in your community? It is in all the communities, . How can we differentiate man to man? How can we differentiate the human society? Maybe the environments are quite different but, as humans, we are not different. So naturally, yoga has to address the

---

[1] See the author's *Light on Aṣṭāṅga Yoga*, YOG publication, 1999, Mumbai. See also *Aṣṭadaḷa Yogamālā*, vol. 2, section I, particularly the first three articles of section I.

entire human system. When Patañjali wrote about yoga he explained it as a universal culture. He never said it is the culture of India. While explaining *yama* he has used the word *sārvabhauma* (*Y.S.,* II.31), which means the entire universe. If every human being decides and takes oath to follow the principles of *yama* namely, non-violence, truthfulness, non-stealing or honesty, celibacy or moral purity of mind and non-covetousness, will it not change the whole system of society?

Basically, our mind gravitates towards the worldly pleasures and we do not want to come out of it. If our mind gravitates towards yoga, the obstacles are lessened and then removed with practice. Therefore, the practice is important.

Q.- What are the major obstacles?

There are three obstacles which come in one's life. It may be due to planetary movements or it may be due to disharmony in the elemental actions, like cyclones, tides, heavy rains, drought, famine and it may be man-made disturbances. These are recognised as *ādhidaivika*, *ādhibhautika* and *ādhyātmika* obstacles. Man can make or mar his character the moment he is attacked by these obstacles.

As you sow, you reap. Man creates disturbances by overeating, overdrinking, or by overactivity in sex. They may be pleasurable for the moment but where do they lead one later? Other impediments that come in our way are; disease, mental laziness, doubt, physical laziness, sensuality or illusive thinking. Other obstacles such as changing our determined path, taking and leaving it in between, or having reached a certain stage, thinking that it has no further goal and allowing stagnation to set in, mental disorders, sorrows, heaviness of the breath or sickness of the body are more of the various illnesses and obstacles which come to man.[1]

Q.- To avoid these obstacles, do you need to remove yourself from normal life?

No, not at all. This is why eight aspects of yoga have been presented by Patañjali. Why would a monk or an ascetic practise yoga? He would have no bad disciplines at all. Nature alone would keep him healthy. Yet he needs yoga as he may not know when nature leads him to carelessness and heedlessness. As I said before, the yogic path that has been explained by Patañjali is applicable to one and all, whether married or unmarried, whether one is celibate or a monk, whether one is a saint or an ascetic or lives in busy cities or in the mountains. All have some or the other weaknesses pertaining to body or mind. A *sannyāsin* who thinks that he has sacrificed

---

[1] *Yoga Sūtra,* I.30-31. See also *Light on Aṣṭaṅga Yoga,* YOG Publication, 1999, Mumbai.

everything has to be doubly careful to see that he does not get caught again in the web of worldly pleasures. Whether he is a celibate, householder, retired or a renunciate, the pleasures and pains do bother him one way or the other. The body which easily deteriorates towards old age can get affected and attacked by disease. So yoga helps and shows ways of keeping oneself not only physically healthy but also mentally and spiritually healthy.

As I said, yoga is meant for the feeble, the average, and those who cannot go beyond a certain limit. It helps them to maintain themselves factually healthy. I am using the word factually healthy, not just healthy. Yoga makes you aware of what health is. When the impediments are conquered, there is no need for guidance. Hence, ardent and intense *sādhaka* can do on their own as they develop a sort of love and affection for the art which gave them that health.

The question is not at all whether one has to cut oneself off from normal life. On the contrary one has to lead their normal life as a yogic life. The principles of yoga are mostly applied to normal life, though it is difficult to explain what the normal life is. It may also be abnormal or subnormal. Normal life is that which shows how long one can enjoy the pleasures of life, how long can one remain soaked in pain, sorrow, attachments and hatred. The inner voice somewhere tells one to come out of all these things. There begins a normal life – a yogic life.

Therefore, in order to remove the obstacles, you do not go away from normal life. On the contrary you make normal life a yogic life, rather a supernormal life.

Q.- What is the danger of practising yoga in an inexperienced way and trying to do too much too quickly?

You have answered the question for yourself. Do you teach a child to run as soon as it is born? You allow the child to have support whether it can stand or not and you hold the child to take one step after the other and make the child to learn the art of walking. Each individual should know his own capacity and how much the body can take. You are not going to get into the lotus pose, *Padmāsana*, by the brain. You have to find out whether the knee cartilage is mobile and whether the knee can rotate very well. If the knee cannot rotate, you cannot do the *āsana* from your head. If you do it from your head, then the cartilage may get broken and you may have to limp and stay in the hospital. When I say, "doing from head or doing from brain", it means that without watching or observing, one thinks that one can manage. This leads to danger. One needs to study and judge judiciously how much movement there is in the knees, how much are the muscles extending to get the *āsana*. If one cannot sit in *Svastikāsana*, how can one perform *Padmāsana?* At least one can try to do one leg *Padmāsana*, known as *Bhadrāsana*. Know that there is a difference between imagination in thinking and factual happening in the legs for the *āsana*. Yoga is factual knowledge. It has to be studied from the level of the body, not from the level of the brain. It cannot be experimented hypothetically. It has to be dealt with practically. Then, no danger comes.

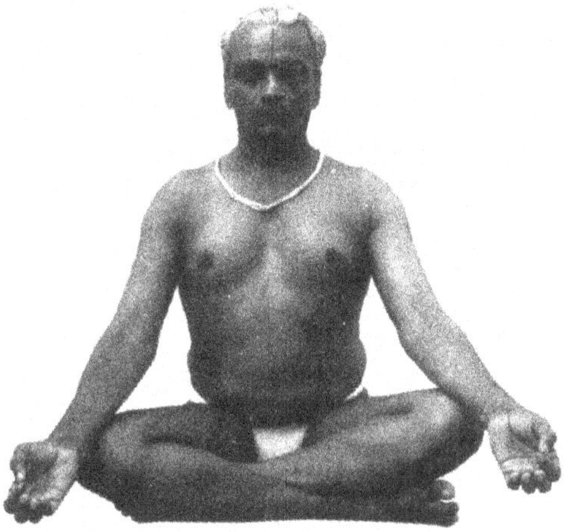

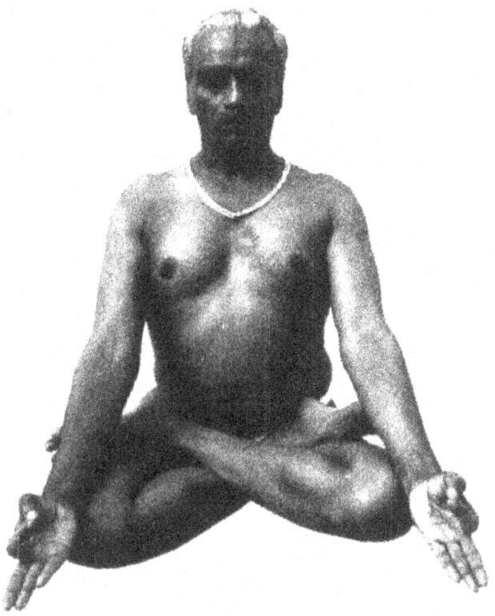

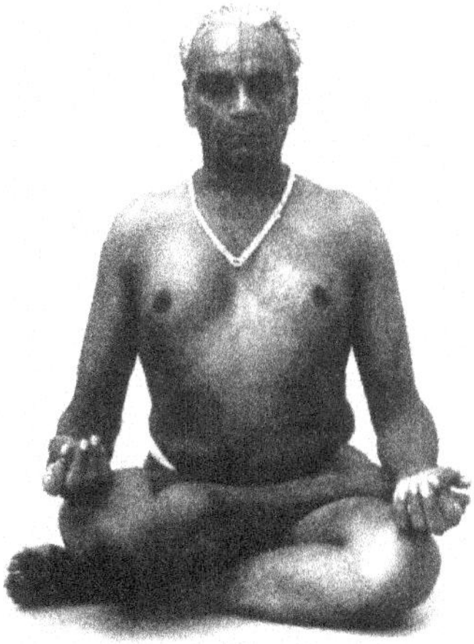

Plate n. 11 - *Svastikāsana, Padmāsana & Bhadrāsana*

Q.- The way yoga is taught and practised in Australia seems to be mostly a series of exercises without people understanding that there are other stages to yoga or that it is a deep philosophy. Most people seem to regard yoga as something to tone up their bodies.

In the West, those who practise yoga are excited on motion, but are not excited by action. There is a difference between motion and action. Suppose I go for a walk. The action is motion. When I am doing *Sālamba Śīrṣāsana* – the head balance, for example, going up into it is motion. But it takes tremendous action to watch each and every cell of the body, to see that they are co-operating, that they are doing their jobs and that they are not dull. In the Western countries, while practising the yogic *āsana* the inner penetration from the skin to the source body and outer penetration from the source body to the skin are missing. That is why Westerners demarcate physical exercise and spiritual exercise. Indian yogis do not demarcate because for them the body is the envelope of the soul. Each one has to keep his house clean and tidy so he can live in it comfortably. When we practise, we penetrate in that way so that each and every tissue, each cell of our body is kept tidy and healthy. That is known as action. If yoga is practised this way with mental application, then it is a total practice, where body, mind, intelligence and self are involved. But if there is a difference between the body and mind as two separate entities of a human being, it is not yoga, it is almost like a split personality. So, in the West, there is tremendous presentation of a dual personality of a single person while practising yoga. The practice of yoga has to be done in such a way that we communicate fully to make the body and soul a single entity.

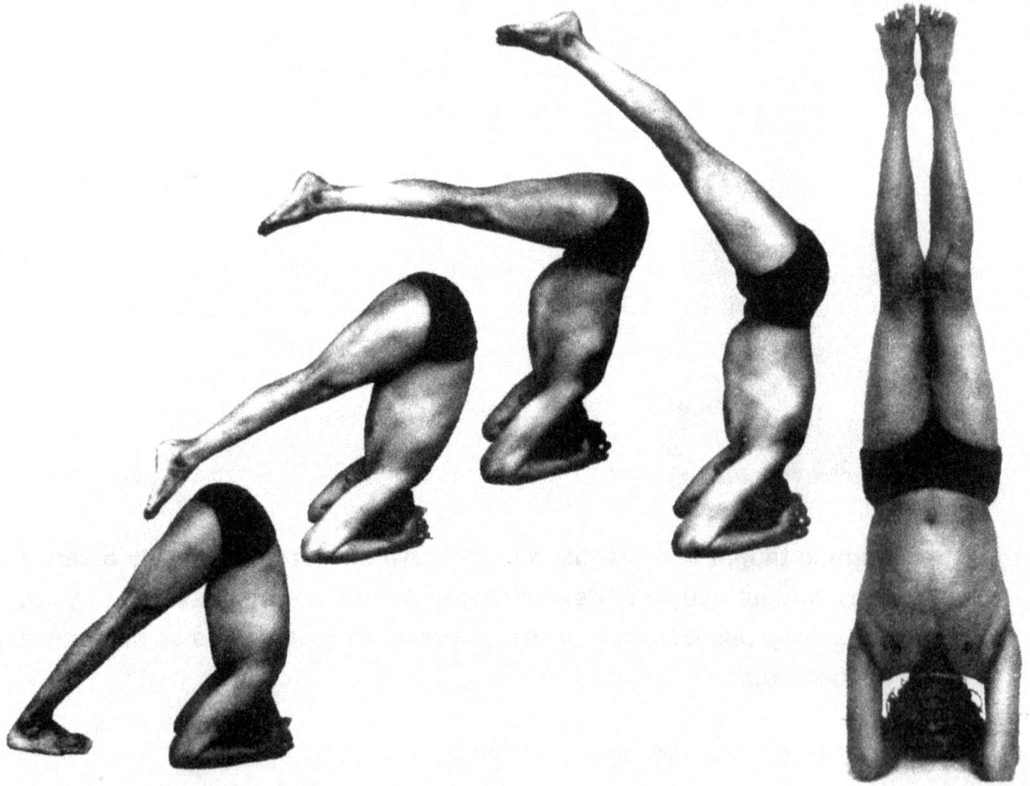

Plate n. 12 – *Sālamba Śīrṣāsana* – movement and action

Q.- In your writings, you relate to your Indian thought, philosophy and religion and to the notion of yoga being a communion of the human will with the will of God. I find the concept of the Universal Soul a difficult one. Can you explain the concept in a way that it might be better understood for the Western mind to comprehend?

This is as old as civilisation. If you read the early Indian philosophies, there is no mention of God. When man saw the universe and its functioning, he began to wonder what was the source of all that he was seeing or practising. He could feel the omnipotent energy that created the universe. Man could realise that pleasures and pains or sorrows and joys are beyond his control. Yet he could imagine the very source which could be beyond all these and free from any entanglements. Patañjali was the first yogi to define God clearly and distinctly as the ONE who is eternal, who is free from reactions to His actions and has no sorrows or joys. Man is caught up with pleasures and pains, afflictions and sorrows. God is not. God is existing but we cannot see Him. We can feel His presence because new ideas, new creations are happening every day.[1]

He is called *Paramātmā* – Supreme Soul. *Parama* means great or subtlest of the subtle and *ātmā* means soul. So *ātmā*, Universal Soul, exists everywhere. The Universal Soul has engulfed this whole universe which has been traced by some and what remains unseen which has not been traced by many. When we have not traced the other solar systems, does it mean to say that they do not exist? There are several stars, which we have not traced. Even certain planets were traced recently. Then how many unknown planets and unknown solar systems are existing? We do not know. The same is with the entity – *Paramātmā* or Supreme Soul, which we haven't perceived, haven't traced, as the Supreme is all pervading and beyond the expanse of known and unknown universe. If we cannot see it, it does not mean that it does not exist. For example, you have your back which you cannot see with your own eyes. Then do you say that it doesn't exist? As you feel your back but cannot see, similarly each individual can feel God even if he cannot see God. If you can feel your own back, your own self, your own being, your own presence, then I am sure you comprehend and conceive God. Religion or philosophy is not needed to see the Supreme. One has to realise and experience it. That is why you need to practise yoga.

---

[1] See *Light on Aṣṭāṅga Yoga*, YOG Publication. Mumbai, 1999, pp. 22-29, and *Light on the Yoga Sūtras of Patañjali*, Harper Collins, London, "What is Soul?", Introduction, pp. 11-12.

THE STRENGTH OF YOGA*

Q.- How did you come to yoga? Who was your guru? How did you start to work the way you do now? How did you come to develop the method you are now teaching?

It so happened that I was born with very bad health. At that time, after the First World War, there was a world influenza epidemic. Naturally, my mother had an attack of influenza and that affected my health from birth. Then, slowly, the doctors found out one illness after the other and at the age of thirteen, doctors traced that I was suffering from consumption. Then, after consumption, I developed malaria. Then, on top of that, I had typhoid. And naturally, after the typhoid, I lost my interest in life and began to wonder whether it was worth living. Somehow or other I survived to live like a vegetable.

It was then that my sister's husband, who was a yogi, said to me, "Why don't you do a bit of yoga? Come with me to Mysore." The doctors had told that I would not survive more than three years. Since I had nothing to lose, I took a chance. So slowly I started to practise yoga with my brother-in-law. It took me nearly four years to recover, just to live. Then I gained health and understood the meaning of health only after five years of yoga.

In 1936, I left Mysore, where I had learnt yoga from my brother-in-law, and established myself independetly in Dharwar, where I opened a school. In India, those days, there were no combined classes or co-education for men and women or boys and girls. However, being young a number of ladies wanted to learn from me, and refused to be taught by the elderlies, as my *Gurujī* and his senior pupils were in Dharwar at that time. I began teaching, although I knew nothing. It was a big responsibility destiny threw upon me and I had to develop this subject with double vigour in order to help them to learn well.

As you see, though I began practising yoga strictly for the sake of gaining my own health, when this responsibility fell on me, I had to find ways and means to convey the presentations better than what I knew up to then. This freshness in the art of teaching made me think deeply and experiment to get the best out of my practice, which helped me to impart with clarity and confidence. As the years rolled by, a certain refiness set in my teaching.

---

* Interview by Roger Raziel in Paris on 23rd April 1984. Published in the French magazine *Le Monde Inconnu*, no. 52, July 1984. Also published in *Victoria Newsletter*, May 1991.

Q.- The *Bhagavad Gītā* and Patañjali's *Yoga Sūtra* say that yoga is a means to arrive at, to master, to eliminate all the fluctuations of the mind, to become the master of the mind and of the self. And when you practise this method, according to Patañjali, you are in the path of *rāja yoga*. While *haṭha yoga* is the way to master the body. My question is: are you depreciating the value of *haṭha yoga*, or is it the same for you as *rāja yoga?*

You must know that in the early years of civilisation, there was no differentiation in yoga. These were known only as "paths", or "ways" to practise yoga. There were four ways of experiencing this:

- One is known as the path of knowledge, or *jñāna mārga*.
- The second is known as the path of action, or *karma mārga*.
- The third is the path of love, devotion to God, or *bhakti mārga*
- And the last is *yoga mārga*, the path of yoga, which you read about in the *Bhagavad Gītā* and the *Yoga Sūtra* of Patañjali.

These four paths are meant to realise the Self and hence they are one and the same though the means may be different. But unfortunately people started making differences and started showing the difference between *jñāna mārga* as *jñāna yoga*, *bhakti mārga* as *bhakti yoga*, *karma mārga* as *karma yoga* and as they could not define clearly the *yoga mārga* as *yoga yoga*, they showed division in yoga as *rāja yoga*, *haṭha yoga*, *tāraka yoga*, *kuṇḍalinī yoga*, *ghaṭa yoga*, *bhakti yoga*, *karma yoga* and so forth.

Yoga means union, or coming together – through knowledge, through action or through love, and finally coming together in body, mind and self. Together with whom? With the individual self, so that one understands the subjective Seer. We call it *ātmā*. This is the essence of *yoga mārga*.

Patañjali gives the first shock, with his very second *sūtra*, *yogaḥ cittavṛtti nirodhaḥ*, meaning, still the mind in order to understand. By controlling the fluctuations of the mind, one experiences something which is superior to the mind, known as the Seer or the soul. And this is yoga.

The author, Patañjali, does not mention, "I am explaining *rāja yoga*". He says, *atha yogānuśāsanam*. He does not say, *atha rājayogānuśāsanam*. It is the readers who have coined the name *rāja yoga*. Patañjali speaks of the soul, the Seer. He starts with the Seer, but it is not he who has called it *rāja yoga* but others. He calls the Seer *ātman* or *dṛṣṭā* and the approach to realise the Seer, he defines as *aṣṭāṅga yoga* made up of *yama*, *niyama*, *āsana*, *prāṇāyāma*, *pratyāhāra*, *dhāraṇā*, *dhyāna* and *samādhi*. With these eight aspects of yoga, he covers the ethical and moral principles, physical, vital, mental, intellectual disciplines to reach the ultimate - the eternal *puruṣa* that abides in all these sheaths.

Q.- Where is the place of this *rāja yoga* in the different paths?

That is what I just said above. What is the meaning of the word *rāja*? In *Sanskrit*, *rāja* means a royal king.

Who is the king of your body? Who is the king of your field – the body? Who is the fielder? You are the fielder. Take an example: consider a field like France. In the olden days, there was a King. But today there is a President. So, in modern terminology, the President replaces the King. The whole of France is like a field to the President. Who is the King/President of your field – the body? The Seer or the soul is the king of the body.

Through the instrument of the mind, you realise the Seer, because the king who is inside your body knows the entire system of your body, your mind, your intelligence, your consciousness – everything put together. Here, I use the word mind for your consciousness, the *citta*.

The word *haṭha yoga* was not used by the author. He called it *haṭha vidyā*. *Vidyā* means knowledge. Unfortunately many narrate this *vidyā* as the practice of *āsana* and *prāṇāyāma* and call it physical yoga while attributing the practice of *dhyāna* to *rāja yoga*. You know Patañjali also speaks of *āsana*; so does *haṭha yoga*. He also speaks of *prāṇāyāma*. Only the problem is that *haṭha yoga* explains *ṣaṭkriyā* or *ṣaṭkarma* such as swallowing of cloth – *dhauti* –, taking water through the nose – *neti* – and so on. However, it is clearly mentioned in the text by Svātmārāma, the author of the *Haṭhayoga Pradīpikā*, that these are purificatory therapies and not yoga.

People misunderstood this *ṣaṭkriyā* as yoga. For them, these purificatory measures became the main practice and they forgot the other aspects connected to yoga which are explained by Svātmārāma, and this is how the misunderstanding on *haṭha vidyā* got mixed up.

In *Sanskrit*, *haṭha* means "will". By using your will power, how do you conquer your body; how do you conquer your mind; how do you conquer yourself; that is what *haṭha vidyā* teaches. Patañjali actually uses the word "consciousness or *citta*", not "mind". His word *citta* is translated as "mind". For us the word that we use such as the "I", the "me", the "you", "I" did it, "he" did it, etc. means the self. So *haṭha* means the discipline that the individual self builds up to reach the Self. This individual self gets transmitted into *citta* as consciousness, intelligence and mind. The mind is the vehicle of the *citta*. It is inferior to the intelligence, which itself is an instrument inferior to the consciousness and again the consciousness itself is inferior to the conscience. And all these instruments are different from Self, which we call the soul. So, when you conquer the very conscience, the instrument of virtue, then the rest is all in your hands. Unless you conquer the conscience, you cannot reach the Seer.

Yoga means union. *Haṭha yoga* is the union of Self and consciousness. *Haṭha yoga* is not meant for physical fitness, but for the union of *prāṇa* with *puruṣa*. First, you should know the meaning of that word *haṭha yoga*. Union of body and mind, union of mind and intelligence, union of intelligence and self and union of *prāṇa* and Self is *haṭha yoga*. There should be a tremendous communication between the body and the Self, through these instruments. In totality this is yoga.

If you understand this meaning of yoga, then you understand what is *haṭha* and what is *rāja*.

Further, if you see the word *haṭha*, it has two syllables. You have *ha*, which means sun, i.e., soul, and *ṭha*, which means moon, i.e., consciousness. The union of these both entities is called *haṭha yoga*. Again *ha* and *ṭha* stand for energy. *Ha* is a positive current and *ṭha* is a negative current. In our body system, we know of two nerves: one is called the solar nerve, the other is called the lunar nerve. *Haṭha vidyā* calls it *piṅgalā* and *iḍā*. The balancing of these two energies is known as *haṭha vidyā*.

Again, *haṭha vidyā* makes the energy flow freely and brings about communication as well as balance. Due to our different patterns of behaviour, our moods and modes in our day-to-day life, our energy and our consciousness go in different directions or in different angles. We must learn to control these two energies not to let them go in various directions. We need to discipline them in order to take them in a proper direction. This is what Patañjali conveys at the very start of the traditional discipline of yoga – *yogānuśāsanam*.

Patañjali explains that those things that hinder the practice of yoga should be discarded. In *haṭha vidyā* if *ha* means *puruṣa* – the sun, *ṭha* means consciousness, which waxes and wanes like the moon.

In the *Yoga Sūtra*, Patañjali too has said, *yogaḥ cittavṛtti nirodhaḥ*, which leads towards *tadā draṣṭuḥ svarūpe avasthānam*. The restraint of the modifications of consciousness or *cittavṛtti nirodha* means to bring the fluctuations to cessation. When the fluctuations are restrained the *puruṣa* expresses itself spontaneously. The *svarūpāvastha* of the Seer is that he abides in his own grandeur. This is a negative action, a negative current. You do not do anything here, rather it happens. Later Patañjali says, *abhyāsa vairāgyābhyām tannirodhaḥ* (*Y.S.*, I.12). *Abhyāsa* is a positive method and *vairāgya* is a negative method. When you learn to bring these two energies together you become a master of yoga. So, how can we differentiate between *haṭha yoga* and so-called *rāja yoga?*

I'll explain to you further. Patañjali has written four chapters. The first chapter concerns those people who have already evolved in their spiritual life, those who have already reached a high level of culture, those who already have a "civilised mind". Their practice is described in the first chapter to start from *citta nirodha*. Here, he explains the ways to achieve control over the *citta*. It is because of the means suggested for the restraint of the consciousness that everybody started speaking that *Patañjala yoga* is *Rāja yoga* or mind control.

In the second chapter, Patañjali addresses those who have not evolved at all but are tempted to take to yoga as they are not initiated but are interested. Here, Patañjali starts from the discipline of body. He gives the method to purify one's body, speech, mind and consciousness.

Nobody pays sufficient attention. Patañjali says, "Control your mind"; that is his first word. But if I ask you or if I tell you, "Control your mind", will you be able to do it? The average person like you and me, who is in turmoil, disturbed, cannot achieve control just by asking. It is a discipline that imposes strain. That is why the second chapter addresses those who are not initiated, who do not know anything about yoga, but who are caught up in sorrows and afflictions. Here he shows the ways of how they can come out from this affected state.

Patañjali's *Yoga Sūtra,* like the *Bhagavad Gītā,* is an analysis of sorrow. Both analyse the sorrows of humanity, and by knowing the root cause of sorrows, both texts explain how the knowledge of sorrows teaches the philosophy of freedom. The very first chapter of *Gītā* speaks of *viṣāda yoga,*[1] the yoga of sorrows.

You must understand that when Patañjali wrote the *Yoga Sūtra,* humanity was living with a very high standard of intelligence. Then due to a mixture of races and wars, disturbances came. Mankind forgot its high standards of living, and the overall level of culture dropped. Civilisation lost the real fragrance of life. Culture of the self began to fade. Patañjali's language alone indicates clearly that civilisation was highly developed in those days. When the *haṭha yoga* book was written, only about 700 years ago, in order to make people understand, its author had to start from the body, not from the mind. That is why, nowadays, one says *haṭha yoga* is a physical yoga. Patañjali, in the third *sūtra* says: "You dwell in your soul". How can you understand this affirmation? So from the spiritual, Patañjali comes to the mental, from the mental to the physical, from the physical to the intellectual, from the intellectual to the spiritual, until freedom is achieved. This is the method shown by Patañjali. He speaks of the intelligence, then he speaks of the mind and its various oscillations and fluctuations. Then, after explaining the mental structure and mental behaviour, he speaks of the physical and mental sorrows, which come from our want of knowledge. Want of knowledge is the cause of all sorrows. The mother of all sorrows is want of knowledge. In order to make progress, what must one do? *Haṭha yoga* starts from the ethical discipline: *yama, niyama,* then *āsana, prāṇāyāma* and *pratyāhāra* for disciplining the body and the mind; *pratyāhāra* and *dhāraṇā* for intellectual discipline and *dhyāna* and *samādhi* for the steadfastness of the self. Patañjali first speaks of the mind in I.35.[2] After gaining a certain level of control, he directly moves towards disciplining the intelligence, in order to bring the intelligence to balance equally with the Self so that both are integrated as one. This is yoga.

---

[1] The traditional colophon of the first chapter is *Arjunaviṣādayoga* (The Yoga of Sorrow of Arjuna).

[2] *Viṣayavatī vā pravṛttiḥ utpannā manasaḥ sthiti nibandhanī* (*Y.S.,* I.35). The consciousness becomes favourably disposed, serene and benevolent also, by contemplating an object that helps to maintain steadiness of mind. See the author's *Light on the Yoga Sūtras of Patañjali,* pp. 82-83.

To summarise, you can say so much: from the spiritual to the mental, from the mind to the body, from the body to intelligence and from intelligence to the soul is yoga. *Haṭhayoga Pradīpikā* starts from the body, leading towards the power of *prāṇa* – energy, from *prāṇa* to mind, then from the mind to the intelligence and finally from the intelligence to the Self.

In short, if you still insist on the words *haṭha yoga* and *rāja yoga,* then *abhyāsa* is the procedure to realise the soul and *vairāgya* is to realise the soul. *Abhyāsa* indicates *haṭha yoga* and *vairāgya* indicates *rāja yoga*. The soul will be known only when you know the sheaths covering it such as body, mind, intelligence, consciousness and conscience (*antaḥkaraṇa*).

Q.- May I ask a question about the word "spiritual", as there might be a confusion: is that what you meant before by "conscience"?

For you, the word spiritual or spirituality comes from the word 'spirit'. The invisible and indivisible 'Being' is called spirit. The spirit is separated from the body and mind. These days the word spirit is used for the disembodied soul. Even we use the word *ātman* for the embodied as well as disembodied souls. Again, there could be the difference such as black spirit and white spirit, which we may call *duṣṭātmā* and *muktātmā*. *Duṣṭātmā* stands for the wicked soul and *muktātmā* stands for liberated soul. Well! That is unimportant. What is important, is the sheaths covering the soul. The embodied soul or empirical soul has sheaths such as body, senses of perception, organs of actions, energy, mind, intelligence, consciousness as well as conscience. Conscience is called *dharmendriya* or the sense of virtue. To know the soul you need to unsheathe it. You cannot discard or destroy the sheaths. Rather you need to know them in order to eradicate their identification with the soul. The identification of all these sheaths with soul itself is a kind of misidentification and misunderstanding. One needs right knowledge to remove this misidentification. For this, we have been given conscience, which is called *viveka* in *Sanskṛt*. We need to use the weapon of *viveka-indriya* along with *vairāgya* – desirelessness and detachment. This weapon is not handy, and hence it is not very easily available. In order to trace it and sharpen it, we need *abhyāsa* – practice. We need to use all the sheaths of the soul in a proper way to sharpen and illumine the *viveka*. *Viveka* is an instrument which accurately detects the soul from non-soul, the Self from non-self, provided we sharpen and awaken it. The conscience is a vehicle which introduces us to our soul. There, we begin to identify our very source of being.

So the conscience is an insight. A tremendous insight. Which is beyond intuition. We have the *Sanskṛt* word *viveka-khyāti* to express this, which does not exist in English. Spirituality for us, therefore, is the process through the practice and desirelessness which lead us towards the very soul, which you call Self-realisation.

Q.- According to Svātmārāma, everybody who practises sincerely can be a yogi, whether he is sick or he is young, reaches *siddhiḥ*. How is this possible?

If you practise regularly, how could you let disease come to you? How can the idea of old age enter your body? If you don't practise, then only you'll start saying, "I am old". It is not the body that says it. The mind says, "I am old". In *Haṭhayoga Pradīpikā*, Svātmārāma explains very clearly that the body is completely inert, dull. So it gets rusted very soon and makes your mind and intelligence inert. But if you keep the body healthy, clear, it helps the mind to be full of vibrations of actions and emotions, because actions and emotions belong to the mind and not to the body. The body itself belongs to an inert world. There is no action in the body. The functioning of the body keeps on occurring on its own. However there is a tremendous activity and the crowd of emotions in the mind. There is another level, which is higher than the mind, where there is only the rhythm in both body and mind. Here the intelligence is free from the contact of body and mind and hence it is free to move closer to the Self.

I'll give further explanation. The body is *tāmasic* – inert – and the mind is *rājasic* – active. Lastly, the soul is *sāttvic* – pure.

So, the goal is to develop the body to the level of the mind, and then lift the body and mind to the level of the soul; that is *haṭha yoga*.

You read Patañjali's *Yoga Sūtra*. In the second chapter he says, the organs of perception and the organs of action – the body, the intelligence, the mind – are all the servants of the soul. Patañjali clearly says: "These vehicles will be the servants of their master." Patañjali uses the word *svāmi* for the soul. *Svāmi* means a king. Here, the soul is the king. Now please know who is the *rājā* – king – of *rāja yoga*. Hope you understand now? How did the word *rāja yoga* come when Patañjali has not used the word?

How can others call it *rāja yoga*? I feel it is a wrong interpretation to boost their own intellectual egoism.

So, the mind and the intelligence, all belong to *prakṛti*, nature. They are parts of nature and when nature reaches the peak, its very top point, it becomes one with *puruṣa*, the soul. In fact, the conjunction of the Seer with the Seen is for the sake of Seer to discover his own true nature.

The 23rd *sūtra*[1] says that, as long as there is disparity, difference, between the intelligence and the Self, conflicts exist. Once you trim and control them, the disparity vanishes. Then the body, mind and intelligence work as the servants of the Self, so you remain a master forever and you reach the ultimate unbiased freedom. The right knowledge breaks the link that binds the Seer and the Seen. You are in a state of blissful freedom forever.

[1] *Sva svāmi śaktyoḥ svarūpopalabdhi hetuḥ saṁyogaḥ* (*Y.S.*, II.23).

Haṭhayoga Pradīpikā says, "The king of the senses is the mind, and the king of the mind is the breath".[1] So those who know the art of controlling the breath, or making it rhythmic, become the master of their nerves, mind and senses.

Like Patañjali's *Yoga Sūtra, Haṭhayoga Pradīpikā* has four chapters. The first chapter speaks of controlling the body; the second speaks of controlling of the vital energy; the third speaks of controlling the consciousness; and the fourth speaks all about *samādhi,* the highest state of yoga. What does it say? It uses an analogy; when salt is mixed with water and the solution well shaken, whether you taste from the top of the glass or you taste from the bottom, or from the middle, it is the same salty water. So also when you have reached that state in which there is a control over the body, mind, breath and consciousness, there is no difference: your body, your mind and your soul are one without any differentiation.

There is another analogy: when you burn camphor, the camphor and the flame become one. Similarly, your body, mind and soul become one, says the *Haṭhayoga Pradīpikā.*

And a third one: take a glass, it appears empty to you. Fill it with water; it appears full. So, when the Self fills the entire body, like the glass filled to the brim with water, then you cannot separate the water from the glass. Similarly when the Self covers the entire body, both become one.

Your intelligence acts as a bridge between the Self and the body; then your body is full. If the water is separated from the glass, it appears empty but it is filled with air. Likewise, when the body reaches towards the Self, intelligence appears empty and the body unites with the Self.

I'll give you one more analogy. If a vessel is launched into the sea, it will float and stand out, because it is empty, but filled with air. If you fill it with water, it will become one with the sea. Similarly, when consciousness fills your entire body, there is no difference between body and Self.

And one more example. If the sky is cloudless, the rays of the sun touch the earth without distortion. If there are clouds, the rays cannot touch the earth. Similarly, the rays of the Self cannot reach the frontier, the pores of the skin. If there are "clouds" – diseases –, the "sunrays" – soul – cannot pervade the "earth" – body.

This clears your queries as to how the practice of yoga gives such a potentially effective result that, in spite of all barriers, one can cross all these problems such as age, sickness and disabilities and reach the goal.

---

[1] *indriyāṇāṁ mano nātho manōnāthastu mārutaḥ /*
mārutasya layo nāthaḥ sa layo nādamāśritaḥ // (*H.Y.P.*, IV.29).

Q.- Do you practise these eight paths of yoga or do you concentrate on *haṭha yoga?* Teaching and practising yoga, are you practising the eight limbs of yoga or only the *āsanas?*

I answered you already that there is no difference between *haṭha yoga* and *rāja yoga* as they are complementing and supplementing each other. (See *H.Y.P.*, II.76).[1] I am sorry you are dragging an unwanted question every now and then. I practise yoga. I do not differentiate yoga as you do. Therefore, I say I do what Patañjali and Svātmārāma prescribe and explain on *yama, niyama, āsana, prāṇāyāma, pratyāhāra, dhāraṇā, dhyāna* and *samādhi*. I am not confused. You are the one who is confused. For me, all go together. It is all combined together. It cannot be separated.

For instance, take *niyama*. What is *niyama?* Patañjali says: "Cleanliness, contentment, austerity, self-study and self abandonment are the observances".[2] The first *niyama* is cleanliness - *śauca*.

What is cleanliness, in its modern sense? And what is the real meaning? To be clean. Today, to bathe regularly is cleanliness. But, at the time of Patañjali, some 200 years BC, did he mean this when everyone was having a bath? Cleanliness means health. And what does health bring you? Contentment. Delight. Health does not mean only to be free from disease: Health means well-being of body and mind, purity of body and mind. Is not health purity? Using today's word – cleanliness, do you think that taking a daily bath makes anyone healthy and content? Your skin may be clean, but does it convey the cleanliness described by Patañjali? How do you clean yourself? You cannot clean the cells, the intestines, the organs and the nerves, with mere water and soap! A true cleanliness or health, as stated by Patañjali, is to purify the body and mind from within.

That kind of health requires ethical discipline. The inner cleanliness gives you health and delight. Till you experience this delight, yoga does not come into the picture. Patañjali being a highly evolved intellectual soul, when he speaks of *śauca*, he expects detachment from one's own body as well as the body of others, teaching what ethical purity is.

Fluctuations in mind and sorrows are diseases. From a non-diseased status, you have to gain health and happiness. Though health and happiness is a pleasure and delight, one has to get the unalloyed bliss according to Patañjali. The real yoga commences after one acquires health and happiness and not before. What do we find in the third step of *niyama*? *Tapas* – austerity. What is the meaning of "austerity"? Hard discipline and burning zeal is *tapas*. Austerity

---

1 *haṭhaṁ vinā rājayogo rājayogaṁ vinā haṭhaḥ /*
na sidhyati tato yugmamāniṣpatteḥ samabhyaset //

Haṭha [yoga] cannot be perfected without *rāja yoga* nor *rāja yoga* without *haṭha [yoga]*. So both should be practised until the stage of *niṣpatti* – state of becoming one with body, mind and self [is reached].

2 *śauca santoṣa tapaḥ svādhyāya Īśvarapraṇidhānāni niyamāḥ* (*Y.S.*, II.32).

means to burn the impurities of the body and mind. Austerity in this sense means that you must religiously follow the one that has given you health and delight. Then Patañjali says that after delight and health you have to develop that tremendous discipline in order to comprehend, to know one's Self – *svādhyāya*. By understanding oneself, where do you reach? *Īśvara praṇidhāna*. In *niyama* he says, "You will be surrendering to God because you understood yourself". In the first chapter Patañjali says that the effect of *samādhi* is to be one with God, or the surrendering to God makes one experience *samādhi*.

You come to know your behaviour and yourself through *svādhyāya*. *Svādhyāya* means studying of one's own self, one's own behaviour. In modern terminology, is this self-study an ethical discipline, is it a spiritual one, or is it a combination of both? Today, "know thyself" is considered a spiritual *sādhanā*. But Patañjali says it is an ethical discipline.

Yama controls the organs of action: arms, legs, organ of speech, generative organs and excretory organs. *Ahiṁsā* is non-violence. For instance, your mind may say, "I want to kill", but your hand alone will not do so, then how can you kill? Do you understand what I am saying? *Satya* means to tell the truth. It is all in your organs of speech such as larynx, throat, mouth cavity, tongue, teeth, palate, etc., is it not? The mouth. Close your lips. How can you say the truth or the false? The controlling of the organs of action – *karmendriya* – is *yama*. You bring them under your grip. And *niyama* controls the organs of perception – *jñānendriya* – eyes, ears, nose, tongue and skin.

Then, *āsana* comes. Why after *yama* and *niyama*? Why only when you are "clean"? Remember, you are clean only in your organs of action and your organs of perception, but you are not "clean" yet in your liver, spleen, in your chest, in your heart, in your head. So you have to keep not only your organs of action/perception clean but also your liver, your spleen, your pancreas, your stomach, your intestines, your bladder, your chest, your head, everything should be kept clean. This is why *āsana* were introduced.

Then, everything may be clean but does the energy pass through the entire system? For this, *prāṇāyāma* was introduced to that effect.

Then, with all that achieved, due to our memory, we will be caught to enjoy through memory. So by-pass the memory. Don't depend on memory, otherwise the mind does become the slave to memory. To master the memory is *pratyāhāra*. I'll give you an example: suppose you come into my house. I offer you some fruit juice. Then you go to another friend's house. He also offers you a choice of drinks. Your mind says, "Oh, I tasted this at Mr. Iyengar's house. So I will try that". Then you'll have the imprint of these two drinks in memory and you make the choice through your memory and not with your discriminating mind. *Pratyāhāra* is the art of discriminating. So, in order to discriminate, you must by-pass memory. Here is another example: I am enjoying a cup of coffee. Two days later, you offer me a cup of coffee. My system says no, because it knows that coffee will excite it. But the memory, which has experienced the taste, says, "Never mind, have it!" One should not get caught in the web of memory. *Pratyāhāra* is meant to by-pass it so that the intelligence can function. Intelligence has the power of discrimination, but not the mind. Mind's function is to gather information. Mind depends upon memory.

Dhāraṇā is the concentration of the intelligence on whatever subject it has selected through discrimination.

Still further, when the power of discrimination has been concentrated, the subject I and the object of concentration become one. This state is known as *dhyāna* and *samādhi*. The moment the difference between the subject and the object, the Seer and the Seen, disappears, you are in *samādhi*.

Samādhi can be explained only in logical terms; it cannot be described psychologically. *Dhyāna* and *samādhi* at the same time are one, because the intelligence and the Self are one, but when *samādhi*, instead of "experiencing", is "seen", it means you have come to concentration again, because subject and object are appearing as separate entities. So chronologically if you maintain this state where there is no Seer and no Seen, that is *samādhi*.

Q.- Can you obtain complete relaxation if you practice only *prāṇāyāma*?

Is relaxation the only aim of yoga? One can relax even listening to music or reading. But that is not the aim of yoga. As I said earlier, the conscience has to be clean and clear. Why can a culprit not relax? Because the conscience pricks. In other words, if one has to relax, one has to cleanse the body, organs of action, senses, mind, intelligence, consciousness and conscience.

If your pores are closed, your nose or lungs are blocked and the mind is in the dark, then what effect can *prāṇāyāma* have? If the sky is cloudy, what is the effect of the sunrays? They cannot penetrate. Similarly, unless and until your body system, blood vessels, the nerves are completely clean inside, how can the energy pass through? For instance, what is the modern hypertension disease? The nerves are blocked somewhere, so the energy remains blocked in the head. Therefore there is hypertension in you. So unless and until the mind is pure and the nerves are clean, *prāṇāyāma* has no effect at all.

You know, if all the nerves in our system are joined as a single string, the distance would reach about 9,600km. And if you join the blood vessels, the arteries, the veins, the capillaries, they would make up a length of about 96,000km. How can *prāṇa* travel that distance if the circuits are blocked and not healthy inside? What is blood pressure? Is it not a kind of blockage? The arteries get completely coated inside, so that blood cannot flow freely; the arteries become narrow, lose their flexibility and need to pump heavily causing high blood pressure. Therefore, *āsana* alone will not help. *Prāṇāyāma* alone will not help. All put together helps. That is why Patañjali speaks of eight aspects of yoga. Yoga has to be adopted in this total sense.

Q.- According to you, what is the worst evil of our society?

Greed and lust. Lust and greed are the enemies of society. What is greed: "I should have everything." That is greed.

I clearly say this: Love is passive. Love is very pure. When love transforms into lust, it becomes the enemy of the self. Lust is indulgence, or overindulgence. Lust and greed keep on increasing in an ascending order. There is no line of fulfilment for these two. They are never-ending. When one remains disappointed, these two terminate in anger. So the evil of society is greed, lust and anger.

Q.- Do you think that yoga is a quick remedy to reach rapidly the largest possible number of people.

No! Not at all! It took long time for me to attract people towards this art and convince them about the importance of it. It was not an easy job. Now, the subject has become popular, so the people are attracted.

Yoga is not a quick way. It is a slow way. That is why tranquillisers and drugs have been invented. Sometimes, one may feel the effects soon and in many cases it takes time. Like certain seeds sprout fast and others take years to sprout. Some seeds require even tremendous fire to break their shell. You know that men sometimes burn the jungle, for the seeds to break so that trees may grow. Yoga is like that. Yoga is like a seed. So it requires the use of much fire to break the seed. Then growth is rapid. One has to wait for a longer time to see its effect.

Q.- What is the difference between the method of yoga that you teach and other methods?

This is a personal question, which I always hate to answer. I have not said or claimed that what I teach is different to what others teach. It is other people who differentiate. Therefore the question should be asked of them.

Please note that as life is dynamic and fresh moment to moment, yoga has to be adapted afresh and dynamic. So I have to dynamise my practice daily. Patañjali says that there are different standards and categories of pupils, and that *samādhi* is close to those who have intensity in practice.[1] They reach the state of *samādhi* soon. Maybe I belong to that category. Differentiation amongst aspirants comes from the soft, medium or intensive way in which they practise. There are three categories of people – soft, mild and intense. As far as I am concerned, I am intensive in my practice. That's why I penetrate, I inter-penetrate and outer-penetrate as well. Those who practise soft or mild cannot and should not comment on intense practitioners. These comments create differences but actually it is my superlative approach in my practice that presents differences or divisions with other methods.

Let me explain to you about my way of practice. I practise yoga in such a way that my intelligence stretches and spreads everywhere instantaneously. If my intelligence sticks at one place, I immediately work to see that it spreads equally everywhere. This means that when I do *āsana* or *prāṇāyāma* I allow the intelligence to flow to each and every part of my body, so that I know and I understand what practice conveys to one for re-study and adjustment of *prāṇa* or energy to flow evenly. This is how I learnt with attention and study and I developed a progressive sequential method. If my intelligence is stretching here in one finger, if it is not stretching in the fingers of the other hand, I have to think and work out for the intelligence to flow in the same area of the other hand. Years of practice developed in me the instant feel to observe at once even the subtlest of the subtle disparities in my practice of *āsana, prāṇāyāma* and *dhyāna*.

Q.- What is the theory of alignment that you teach?

Perfect alignment of body, mind and self. If I am intelligent here in the head, then I should be intelligent at the other places too. Say in my toe also. Equi-distribution of energy and equi-flow of intelligence within the frame of body and the banks of the body in each *āsana* is alignment for me. The awareness has to uniformly spread all over the body through the face or the profile of the *āsana*. Alignment is to bring balance between the flow of energy and intelligence to connect the body to a mind.

---

1 *tīvrasaṁvegānām āsannaḥ* (*Y.S.*, I.21). The goal is near for those who are supremely vigorous and intense in practice.

Mṛdu madhya adhimātratvāt tataḥ api viśeṣaḥ (*Y.S.*, I.22). There are differences between those who are mild, average and keen in their practices.

See the author's *Light on the Yoga Sūtras of Patañjali*, pp. 71-73, Harper Collins, London.

Q.- You say that the diaphragm is the window of the soul.

No! I said that the diaphragm is the medium between the physico-physiological and psycho-spiritual bodies. What I said was that if the eyes are the windows of the head – brain –, the ears are the windows of the heart – mind. If any emotional or intellectual upheavals take place, the first reaction is on the diaphragm.

– *Why?* –

Why? Suppose you are suddenly frightened, then what happens to your diaphragm? What shape does it take? It shrinks. Suppose you are full of delight, how does the diaphragm move? You lift your chest. Don't you lift your diaphragm also? Don't you feel the exhilarating sensation, while in sorrow depression is felt?

When one is afraid, often one says that the solar plexus gets gripped due to the fear complex. But it is not the solar plexus that gets gripped. It is the diaphragm that suddenly contracts, thereby applying pressure on the solar plexus when you are nervous or get frightened.

Why do the yogis have a calm mind? Because they don't allow the diaphragm to become tight or to become hard, or to expand excessively; they do in such a way that the elasticity of the diaphragm is maintained permanently.

(Gurujī pretends to strike the journalist lady in the abdomen) Look, I just pretended to strike her; what happened to the diaphragm? Instinctively she got scared, she gripped her diaphragm.

Though the diaphragm is a physical organ, it is in direct contact with the mind, consciousness and the self. If it is balanced and stabilised, it brings a sort of freedom to the mind, intelligence and self. So, *prāṇāyāma* is mentioned by Patañjali so that, through the control of the breath and energy, control of the diaphragm too takes place. As you win over the diaphragm, control of your mind too sets in.

Q.- Why does the skin have such an importance in your teaching method?

Skin is an organ of perception. The sensory nerves of the skin gives us the feeling of touch. Skin is highly sensitive and receptivity is its main quality. We the practitioners of yoga need to develop the sensitivity of touch to a great extent. We need to have this sensibility. The motor nerves are the organs of action. Yet the sensitivity of skin depends upon the motor nerves. The senses of perception take the help of the organs of action. The motor nerves and sensory nerves have to co-operate with each other.

While doing the *āsana* or *prāṇāyāma* you do some action; you may stretch your hands or extend or expand the chest. The action takes place through muscles and bones. The motor nerves are activised. But when you are asked to recheck the actions or movements, the brain, which I call another organ of action and receiver as well, gets involved. There comes the sensitivity. The skin receives the message from organs of action, the muscles and nerves. Obviously, there is a feel of "inner touch" in the action. This feel of action, which is conveyed by the skin, is very important to understand. The.skin has this special sense of touch which is nothing but the touch of the inner intelligence. The intelligence flows like a river and brings message to the skin to let you know whether the inner organs of action, the cells, work correctly or not. Then you can call up your brain to help understand the *āsana*, or correct your position.

Q.- Certain contemporary sages from India, after having practised *haṭha yoga* themselves, criticised *haṭha yoga* because it is a means to develop certain powers. Do you agree with this criticism?

What about Patañjali's yoga? What does the third chapter say? Does it not contain *vibhūti* or supernormal powers, *siddhi* and attainments? The *Haṭhayoga Pradīpikā* does not talk about powers though *haṭha yoga* does give powers, provided that you are a honest pupil, an honest student of yoga. These powers come to the *sādhaka*, to the aspirant, to let him know that he is in the right path. And if he is not caught by the successes or the achievements of these powers, his practice will make progress.

But often what happens, the aspirant is caught up in the successes of supernormal powers or supernatural powers. He takes pride in his newly acquired power. He becomes so busy exhibiting his power that he forgets about his practice – the *sādhanā*. Here is the downfall, which *haṭha yoga* texts and *yoga darśana* emphatically warn not to fall into the net of powers.

These powers, no doubt, appear supernatural to an average observer. For the aspirant, they are distractions, destructive distractions! So, when they come, do not pay attention to them. Continue your practice. Do not blame either *haṭha yoga* or *Pātañjala yoga*. These are not two separate *yogic* sciences. Blame the ego, the pride and the ignorance of the *sādhaka*.[1]

These supernormal powers are described in *Vibhūti Pāda* of *Yoga Sūtra* from verses 16 to 45, where Patañjali explains various effects of achievements. It is possible that not every yogi gets the same powers, it's an individual matter.

---

1 See *Aṣṭadaḷa Yogamālā*, vol. 2, section I, "Svātmārāma shakes Patañjali's hand", and section II, *"Haṭha yoga* and *Rāja yoga"* and *"Haṭha yoga* and *Pātañjala yoga"*.

Q.- Is it possible to practise yoga and the modern form of gymnastic, aerobics, at the same time, or are they incompatible?

Yoga *sādhanā* is the feel of every action and thought in physical, moral, physiological, psychological, mental, intellectual or spiritual sheaths of the *sādhaka*. Yoga is the base or foundation to lead the life knowing all these sheaths so that one proceeds to practise with philosophical thoughts. It is a base, an art and science to train the physico-mental apparatus in a right way to reach the goal – the steady blissful state.

As far as gymnastics, athletics, aerobics, sports and karate are concerned, yoga is not antagonistic to these physical activities. On the contrary it helps to perform better all these activities. However, yoga goes beyond all these.

Since your question is aiming at *āsana*, even if we think of this one aspect, know well that it goes beyond all these activities. All above mentioned physical performances may need some seriousness in practice, will power, strength, discipline and so forth. But the expanse of *āsana* is farther than this. *Āsana* teaches one to use the body-mind apparatus in a rhythmic balanced way. The stretches, extensions, elongation of muscles and relaxing of the muscles are balanced in the practice of *āsana*. The intelligence is spread in each and every cell. Every action is attempted consciously with awareness. The effortfulness and effortlessness are balanced. The very purpose of practice of *āsana* differs from gymnastics and aerobics. The practice of *āsana* is not meant for performance or exhibitionism. It is meant for the search of the Self. The other above mentioned activities are antagonistic to yoga in this sense. But practice of *āsana* is helpful for the better performance of those activities.

Q.- Can yoga, as you teach, be assimilated, or associated, or compared to therapy, as some people have been cured of bad diseases in a spectacular manner?

You know, whether you read *Haṭhayoga Pradīpikā*, Patañjali's *Yoga Sūtra*, *Āyurveda* or any other texts, they speak of three types of diseases. They are known as *ādhidaivika*, *ādhibhautika* and *ādhyātmika*.

According to our ancient science, the terminology *ādhidaivika* is used for certain diseases which appear when there are such disturbances as cyclones, tides, famines, droughts, floods, virus, genetic defects and so forth. With today's modern terminology, these natural disturbances cause different diseases. Genes cause spastic children. Children have not done anything wrong, how is it that a child is born spastic? Similarly, suppose one of the couple gets AIDS because of immoral and unethical behaviour. Both become AIDS patients. Then these AIDS patients give birth to children, who carry AIDS without being involved or having committed any sin.

Ādhibhautika diseases: Each man is made up of five elemental principles – earth, water, fire, air and ether. When these five elements are balanced, the body and the mind are healthy. If there is a slight variation or disturbance or imbalance, then diseases like constipation, gastric troubles, burning sensations do appear. Gastric troubles and burning sensation are governed by fire; constipation by earth; dribbling of urine by water; flatulence, gastric problems by fire, rheumatism, joint pains and flatulence by air, and swelling in the body by ether.

Patañjali quotes that these five elements are the servants of the soul. Intelligence plays a dual role, one with nature and the other with the self. Achieving a balance between these five elements by an individual through yoga brings what one calls emancipation. When that emancipation comes in the *sādhaka*, he experiences oneness not only with *prakṛti*, which is the vehicle of the Self, but also with the Self.

Ādhyātmika diseases: These are the third group of diseases that spring from self-abuse and self-amuse. These are invited by one's own action. And this is where *pratyāhāra*, which I have already explained, the conquest of memory, comes into the picture along with the practice of *āsana* and *prāṇāyāma* to protect one from *ādhyātmic* diseases. This abuse and amuse is the result of the imprints in the memory. The memory triggers the sensation of pleasure enjoyed earlier and tempts to seek the same pleasures again and again. The body and mind indulge in these past experienced pleasures easily.

So, he who conquers the three types of diseases and is a healthy man, becomes the king of the body; he is the king of the mind; he is a king to himself; he is a king to the universe. That's why he is called a *rāja yogi* because he is a master of everything. Not because he is practising a certain method. It is when you reach that mastery that you are a *rāja yogi*. Till then you are a yoga practitioner using your will power which is the root of *haṭha yoga*.

So, if the medical professionals or doctors of today give a little thought to this ancient wisdom, they can make a rational approach in health study. However, yogic therapy cannot bring a quick cure. It is a slow cure. Because the patients have to practise themselves. "Heal thyself" is the motto of yoga. In order to get a grasp on "heal thyself" they have to get involved in the yogic procedure through the practitioners and teachers of yoga.

Know that yoga undoubtedly has a therapeutic value. The element of cure exists in it provided we use properly and prudently the yogic medicines such as the five elements and the seven ingredients – chyle, blood, flesh, fat, bones, marrow and semen – as well as the intelligence and the consciousness as intelligent surgical instruments precisely to achieve the therapeutic value of yoga.

MEETING B.K.S. IYENGAR*

B.K.S. Iyengar, as the saying goes, needs no introduction. Probably the leading haṭha yoga *master in the world, he has been in the forefront of yoga teaching for more years that most of us can remember. He was in London in May in the course of a British tour and* Yoga Today *had the opportunity to make his acquaintance and ask a few questions. This is a two-part report.*

Q.- It's a great pleasure to be able to meet you at last, Mr. Iyengar. Somehow our paths have not crossed all these years. You were last here in 1982, if I remember rightly.

Yes, that was the year we met for the first time for a very short period. Therefore, I think you shouldn't use the word "at last" because it was a very short stay. There was no time-space to grant an interview.

Q.- Your name has virtually become a legend in your lifetime as a teacher of *haṭha yoga*. I should imagine that in most countries you have centres and groups?

Yes, almost all the five continents, including Japan and Middle East.

Q.- And I understand you are retired now or about to retire?

No, no, no! Your understanding that I am retired is not correct. Having known and met great people of the world who say that one should learn the art of detachment, I thought that when God made me reach this height in the field of yoga, I should now learn to develop non-attachment

---

* Interview in London in May 1984, and published by *Yoga Today* (now *Yoga and Health,* U.K.) in two parts: vol. 9, no. 3, July 1984 and vol. 9, no. 4, August 1984

from the world so that I resign myself from public attention through non-attachment and detachment and be close to the sense of the supreme. I have held this top place for years, and if I continue as a teacher, then I live like a dictator in this art. I thought that the time has come for me to retire and I am building that temperament in me so that sooner or later I remain in the background and people forget me while I am alive. For the present, I do not retire, but guide the youngsters to pick up the missing points in their practice and teaching and explanations so that the link of continuity is maintained for a long period of time. So I want to tell you that at present I am not retiring, but like to remain in the background and help my students take the lead. Now I am an assistant to my students whom I have trained as teachers. This gives me a chance to observe their ways of teaching and obliges me to guide them wherever needed, so that they do not break the traditional links while teaching.

Q.- In an advisory capacity rather than as an active one?

It is yes and no. It is not on the advisory capacity or the control of them, but a means to uplift them in the art of teaching, showing the humanity and spirituality involved in it. Though I am on the way of detachment, I do teach sometimes. When my pupils are explaining, and fail to explain clearly, then I take the lead and oblige them by correcting their explanation and the missing points. After showing the right ways of explanation I advise them to lead the class upon those guidelines given by me. In case they misinterpret, then again I may intervene and teach, asking the teachers to do and observe what I said is happening in their practice or not. This way I build up so that the teachers learn to maintain the continuity without deviation. In fact, it is much more than active participation, but as a witness I keep the closeness of teaching on the teachers. When I am teaching the teachers, I show what I say so that not only the students are witnessing, but the teachers too witness and then I make them act. This helps both the teacher and the student for a better understanding of the subject. My responsibility doubles up since I have to convey to both the groups – teachers and students.

The clarity and purity of the effort of my work may be maintained as far as possible before it gets adulterated or polluted. I act as an advisor, actively demonstrating how to maintain this clarity and purity. If I retire totally, then I consider this as unethical detachment and disrespect to the art which is infinite. To maintain the clarity and purity of the art, I like to work till then and caution and oblige them to pick up the thread of teaching as it should be conveyed. When this qualitative confidence is built up, then I retire from teaching, but intensify my *sādhanā* to trace what is still missing in my own practice. This is retirement from the public and total involvement in my own *sādhanā*.

Q.- Do you think that the adulteration occurs?

Who knows, as the spokes of the wheel go up and down, while the spokes of yoga may now point to a higher level, they may face downwards if my students lose that attention and awareness. It has happened in almost all the fields of the art. That's why I say, let me build up the youngsters so that they can maintain that quality that it may not wane soon.

- To leave behind somebody who is really qualified to teach your way. -

It is the job of a teacher to make the pupils qualified. It is of course a duty of the teacher to bring the students to his level. Therefore I try and guide them so that no loopholes remain. It is not a question of qualifying them. My duty is to uplift them.

Q.- Not only has your name become known in the world, but also your yoga, so people speak of "Iyengar Yoga". I believe you don't accept this distinction.

How can I give my name to a universal art? Because they learnt from me, the pupils began to identify my teaching compared to others and started naming my work as 'Iyengar Yoga'. As yoga has spread like wildfire, my students shortened the terminology by calling my work as 'Iyengar Yoga'. But how can an individual name prefix this great art which is existing since time immemorial? Only I must have revitalised this art by new adaptations and made it palatable, attractive and educative by linking up what was missing in the progressive sequential practice in this chain of yoga. I was blessed by the grace of God, as well as by my *guru*, to find out the various missing links in each movement of motion and action in the body and the flow of the breath. With my *sādhanā*, whether it is *āsana* or *prāṇāyāma*, I not only observed the movements but the moments also while I practised which gave the depth of understanding of the *āsana* and *prāṇāyāma*.

God and my *guru* graced me to look, think with understanding and feel while in the *āsana* and *prāṇāyāma*, about the state of the body, mind, breath awareness, intelligence, existence of consciousness and presence of the self.

First I started learning the physical aspect due to my ill health, but the tremendous inner urge inside me made me feel that energy flowing along with the consciousness. I started uniting that infinite flow within the finite body, which is the frame for the flow of life's elixir. This new method of uniting the energy with the consciousness, which I gave to people, brought a new awareness on yoga and for convenience sake they call it as Iyengar Yoga. Unfortunately, it shouldn't be called that way at all. I cannot stop people, though I have shown my uneasiness by protesting against it.

Q.- I think what is meant is the approach to the teaching, which is felt to be somewhat strenuous, rather more strenuous than is used in other schools of teaching.

My dear friend, it is not a question of strenuous practice but inner intensity as the mind, intelligence and consciousness have to move in the darkest part of our bodies. I think it is unfair to the father of yoga to say that there is a smooth method and there is a strong method. Patañjali divides four types of students. He gives four types of *sādhaka*, aspirants. He says, one who practises intensely with intensity, for him the goal is near, and for him, there is no time bar. An intensive practitioner is called *tīvra samvegin*. This means he has conquered time to a very great extent. Then the other categories are mild – *mṛdu* –, average – *madhya* – and keen – *adhimātra*. These are the four kinds of aspirants. My journey in yoga was through all four categories of yoga since 1934. In the days of 1935, yoga was not in vogue as it is today. As a young boy, I naturally approached those who were masters of yoga then, to get the qualitative aspects and subtle hidden wealth of yoga. But I did not get any clue from them to work for re-discovery in its approach. So I undertook to work on my own to find out what yoga can present, and worked like a farmer in my field, the body, mind and consciousness.

I thought yoga is like a gardener gardening: if there are weeds, what does he do? Does the plant grow if weeds are there? So the gardener removes the weeds. He digs deeper and deeper to remove those hidden weeds again which are deeply rooted and grow faster than the seeds he sows. When the weeds are removed, the seeds that are sown by the gardener begin to grow. This is the same that happens in yoga. The slow and soft movements neither clear the impurities that remain deep in the body nor flush the impurities of the nervous system or freshen the circulatory and respiratory systems. If you read the yoga texts, they all give the effects of yoga more than the technique or the method. If the effects were of that magnitude through yoga, then certainly the slow and dull process cannot achieve these effects. In my early days, these effects dealt in yogic texts made me work intensively which made me go into the depth of each *āsana*. This intensity of approach makes people presume that my way of practice and teaching are strenuous. My goal is to see how far one can interpenetrate to reach the depth with dynamic intelligence in each *āsana*. If this intensity is misunderstood as strenuousness, I cannot help. It is easy to use the example which Svātmārāma gives in the *Haṭhayoga Pradīpikā* that in the state of *samādhi*, the mind and consciousness dissolve as the salt dissolves in water.[1] But when it comes to the practice of *āsana*, *prāṇāyāma* or *dhyāna*, the practitioners of yoga do not know that like salt, body and mind are to be dissolved in the self, so that everything becomes the self. People who do not want to get intensely involved in *sādhanā*, label it as strenuous. However,

---

1 *Karpūramanale yadvat saindhavaṁ salile yathā /*
tathā sandhīyamānaṁ ca manastatve vilīyate // (*H.Y.P.*, IV.59).
As camphor in fire, as salt in water, the mind directed towards reality merges in it.

Patañjali and Svātmārāma both demand this discipline. I bring this discipline in *sādhanā* giving the understanding of total absorption.

This method of intellectual interpenetration is now called the Iyengar Yoga system, which is not so. I started doing and observing, using my will to feel what is coming from the external to the internal and from the internal towards the external in my *āsana* practices. For instance, if I do *Tāḍāsana*[1] I make the intelligence of my legs to feel the surface of the floor. If I turn my right foot out in *Trikoṇāsana*,[2] and left foot inward, I see whether the width and length of my right foot is equal to the left or whether the left is affected to become short. This way I started adjusting my body, dividing the body from the centre to understand clearly. At the early stage it seemed to be a limbering process but later I found that I am not only digging into the body but my intelligence too. This penetration removed the weeds that were in my body and made my mind fertile to penetrate deeper. Having worked diligently with advertence in a needed way to remove these weeds, even now if anybody comes to me for guidance, I help in removing these weeds at once. Naturally one feels it as a stronger dose of yoga. People are so slow, dull and lethargic that they don't want to be quick. Actually it is not strenuousness or aggressiveness or strength but intensity and involvement in thought and work. Intensity and involvement bring not only dedication but devotion to the subject. In fact, it not only arrests the outgoing ripples of mind but takes them inwards.

Q.- Another question which has arisen amongst the yoga public is your attitude to *prāṇāyāma*. In the early days apparently you felt people should do *āsana* for quite a while before going into *prāṇāyāma* and then since you published your book *Light on Prāṇāyāma* your views seem to have changed somewhat.

No, I have not changed. May I request you to read again. When I wrote on *āsana*, the publishers wanted me to write on *prāṇāyāma*. As my practice was limited at that time, I said, I am very clear on *āsana*, but not on *prāṇāyāma*. I said then that I would think of the book on *prāṇāyāma* only when I get as much clarity as on *āsana*, till then I will not touch *prāṇāyāma* in black and white. The gap between *Light on Yoga* and *Light on Prāṇāyāma* is thirteen years. I might have written twenty to twenty-five times the same book. Even my *Gurujī*, Krishnamacharya, advised me: "Don't take to writing on *prāṇāyāma* at all. If you want to say anything, do so, but do not commit to write on *prāṇāyāma*." As the editor of my publisher was keen, I went on and on, writing and rewriting several times to do my best and to justify that it should be in black and white.

---

[1] See *Aṣṭadaḷa Yogamālā*, vol 3, pl. n. 27.
[2] See *Aṣṭadaḷa Yogamālā*, vol 3, pl. n. 25.

I have not seen any change at all. I said in *Light on Yoga* that unless and until one is perfect in the *āsana* one will never get the full effect of *prāṇāyāma*. I have nowhere in this book said that one can do *prāṇāyāma* without practising the *āsana*. Patañjali says that *yama, niyama, āsana, prāṇāyāma, pratyāhāra, dhāraṇā, dhyāna* and *samādhi* are the eight aspects of yoga. He has not said, practise *yama* first, then *niyama*, then *āsana*, then *pratyāhāra, dhāraṇā, dhyāna* and *samādhi*, as steps. However while explaining *prāṇāyāma*, Patañjali definitely and clearly mentions that only after mastering *āsana*, one should proceed towards *prāṇāyāma*. Read the *sūtra* 49 of *Sādhana Pāda*. He says, *tasmin sati śvāsa praśvāsayoḥ gativicchedaḥ prāṇāyāmaḥ*. The words *tasmin sati* indicate the step. "On achieving accomplishment in *āsana*", means there is certainly a gap of time.

Maharṣī Vyāsa while commenting on the *sūtra* says, – *sati āsana jaye bahyasya vāyorācamanaṃ śvāsaḥ, kauṣṭhyāsya vāyornisāraṇaṁ praśvāsaḥ, tayorgativicchede ubhayābhāvaḥ prāṇāyāmaḥ* – after the accomplishment in *āsana* or after perfecting *āsana* proceed towards *prāṇāyāma*. Here is the only place where Patañjali insists that *āsana* is the step towards *prāṇāyāma*. Unfortunately the *sūtra* is misinterpreted. The *yogis* think that "any comfortable pose would do for the practice of *prāṇāyāma*".

You sit five minutes in an *āsana*, and within a short period you change the position. How can a comfortable *āsana* become an uncomfortable *āsana* after a few minutes? In order to get firmness in an *āsana*, Patañjali says further, "When the effort ceases completely, then, that moment, that *āsana* has been mastered by one." Mastering the *āsana* is important to him and not sitting in a comfortable *āsana* which becomes uncomfortable after a while. When the *āsana* becomes firm, friendly and stable, consider that you have perfected that *āsana*.

Even Svātmārāma in the *Haṭhayoga Pradīpikā* says,

athāsane dṛḍhe yogī vaśī hitāmitāśanaḥ /
gurūpadiṣṭamārgeṇa prāṇāyāmān samabhyaset //
(*H.Y.P.*, II.1)

It means that after becoming well established in *āsana*, and having brought the organs of action, senses of perception under control and observing moderation in diet, start practising *prāṇāyāma* as taught by the *guru*.

Now, the question arises, how much effort has to be put in, in order to get that perfection? We have three hundred major joints, seven hundred major muscles, six thousand miles of nervous system to carry bio-energy, sixty thousand miles of the arteries, capillaries and veins to carry blood for irrigation, including all the vital organs such as liver, heart, kidney, pancreas and so on. Without penetrating the depth of the body through the *āsana*, is it possible to understand the functioning of the minor muscles, supporting the major muscles? We do not know how many unused parts we have entirely forgotten. The inner body is so much in the dark that our awareness does not penetrate there at all. That's why so many *āsana* were practised in those days with tremendous zeal.

While practising *āsana* we should attend to each and every part of our body, each and every joint, muscle and every cell so that they are looked after by themselves. When the quality of looking after themselves is developed, then my feeling is that *āsana* is perfected. According to my understanding of *Yoga Sūtra* and *Haṭhayoga Pradīpikā*, I am using these words, "the quality of looking after themselves", very meaningfully. We often say that we have to take care of our bodies; otherwise it revolts against the mind and self. Of course, the practice of *āsana* and *prāṇāyāma* do that job in maintaining the health of the body. This is a fact. But in our *yogic* practices what we need is that we have to bring the body to such a state that we are able to forget its existence without neglecting it. The body has to co-operate when our consciousness has to travel deep within. That is why I had to practise to go deep into various *āsana*. Without perfection in *āsana* the energy cannot flow. If joints are stiff or the bronchial tubes narrow, they have to be stretched in *āsana*. Otherwise how can one expect the area to be clear without developing elasticity in the lungs? With these in view I did not write much on *prāṇāyāma* in my book *Light on Yoga*. Perfection in *āsana* is a must if one wants to derive the full benefit of *prāṇāyāma*. Scratching a little here and a little there has no meaning. By stretching your hand, there may be circulation of blood in your hands. But that circulation does not reach the extremities. The stretch must make the blood to flow like the river, starting from the source to the sea which appears as one single unit, though it is flowing non-stop. While we do the *āsana*, the consciousness should reach as a single flow from the brain to each and every part of our body. This is how *āsana* have to be done according to the authoritative texts and that is how I am teaching. The practice of *āsana* is an essential need in order to perfect the practice of *prāṇāyāma*.

Hence, I say I have not changed in my thought and approach, your reading of my work is incorrect.

Q.- In *Light on Prāṇāyāma* you have quite a lot to say about meditation. I understand that meditation is actually not-done, or not much done in your classes, why so?

First of all is not meditation a diversion of ways of thought from a wandering mind to a tranquil mind? Is it not an effort to get completely engrossed in one's thought and action for a continuous, uninterrupted flow of attentive awareness while doing the *āsana* or *prāṇāyāma*? Is it not a deviation of mind from external movements into internal movements which is nothing but drawing the mind of the students indirectly towards meditation or *antara dhyāna*?

Here, I would like to show the difference between concentration and meditation. Concentration shows the difference between the object and the subject, and in meditation the subject is completely engulfed in the object or object in the subject and both lose their respective identities. *Dhyāna* or meditation is of two types, passive and dynamic. Passive meditation is to sit quietly in an *āsana* with closed eyes, watching the various rays of intelligence that move in the brain, and then to localise them to rest in the centre of the brain, so that all mental functions are brought to a state of stillness. This is known as *manolaya*. *Manolaya* is a passive state of alertness of brain and mind.

From this state of *manolaya,* one has to diffuse further to find out the seed of the consciousness – *hṛd* in the heart. This is not the physical heart. It is called *hṛd-cakra*. This *hṛd-cakra* is also known as *anāhata cakra*. I call it the seat of the soul. Here, the consciousness is brought from the petals of the brain to the stem of the brain and from the stem of the brain towards the seat of the soul. It is a state of balance and concord wherein the physical intelligence along with the vital energy are made to ascend from the seat of the perineum, while intellectual energy is made to descend from the top of the brain to meet at the spiritual heart. A kind of balance and concordance is established between these two energies. They finally intermingle with each other and unite in *hṛdaya* – the seat of the soul. This is meditation of one type.

The other type of meditation is electrical and dynamic. Here, each and every part of the body is looked after like a tree. The tree has the root, the trunk, the leaves, the branches, the bark, the sap, the flower and the fruit. We cannot see the whole tree at one time, but we see part by part of the tree separately, and putting all the parts together, we call it a tree. Similarly, while doing the *āsana*, the organs of action, senses of perception, mind, intelligence, 'I'-ness, consciousness and conscience seem to have the tendency to move in various directions, they are treated as different parts though they are connected to the root – the soul. It is the soul that is all occupying. In the beginning the *āsana* is performed observing all the separate parts of the soul. However, the root of the tree is underground and all the other parts are seen above the ground. But in a human being, though the various parts are recognised separately, they are all connected to the root, the cause, body or the soul. While doing the *āsana* we involve ourselves in it in such a way that all these components are connected to the root – the soul – as a single unit from one end of man to the other end. While performing *āsana* all actions are observed with reflection. This reflection in action is *manolaya*. With this reflective state of mind, *āsana* is re-formed and re-posed.

Therefore it becomes meditation while in an *āsana*.

People advise gazing at a burning candle for steady attention. If one can gaze at the candle, why should not one gaze at one's own toe? If I gaze at my toe you say it is physical, and if I gaze at a candle, you say it is spiritual. Is that logic? Is it an explanation? There your concentration is brought on the burning flame, here your attention is brought on the toe. For me both are same.

Looking at the toe, I at least see the defect and readjust. Hence, it is a living example, but by gazing at a candle what do you get? It is a dead thing, though I know both as I have done *trāṭaka.* I prefer to correct my defects and reflect on it, and that is meditation to me. In *trāṭaka,* concentration is from physical eyes whereas if I gaze at the toes or any other part of the body, the concentration comes with the mental eye.

I do not want my pupils to jump to that meditation, which leads towards dullness and laziness and which becomes unproductive. Meditation being exclusively subjective, it becomes a very difficult subject for common men. Especially today, in spite of very high intellectual development, the emotional instability is great. However, this intelligence is an objective one. Meditation requires subjective intelligence. The journey of the objective intelligence is outwards, whereas the journey of the subjective intelligence is inwards. Meditation is subjective intelligence with emotional re-adjustments. It belongs to the *anāhata cakra* where both intelligence and emotion meet. This is another type of electrifying dynamic meditation.

Meditation, being emotional, is an inward action. If one is weak physically and mentally, it leads to mental imbalances. For those who are introverts, meditation is meant to make them extroverts and for those who are extroverts, it is meant to make them introverts. Yoga bends either way. One who is in depression, dejection, mentally falling, yoga uplifts them. Those who consider themselves highly evolved and are proud of themselves, yoga trims their egoism. So the external meditation – outward attention – is for the introverts and internal meditation – subjective attention – for the extroverts as explained by Patañjali. Certain *āsana* like inverted poses and backbending *āsana* as well as *antara kumbhakā* – inhalation-retention, give the introverted people confidence, while *bāhya kumbhakā* – exhalation-retention – makes them nervous because their minds go further empty and this creates further confusion. So, what is to be given to each individual is to be learnt by experience through trial and error. For the extroverted, exhalation-retention is given to quieten the mind. It makes the mind become passive and pensive. This yoga has several methods to make the empty mind full and full mind quiet. That is why Patañjali says *prāṇāyāma* removes the dust of the mind and makes it ripe for meditation. He says that perfection in *prāṇāyāma* brings clarity in intelligence and makes the mind fit for meditation.[1] See how many years of practice are required to make the mind fit for meditation. That's why he explains meditation, *dhyāna,* in the third chapter after a hundred and two *sūtra.*

So, I introduce cognisable parts of the self, i.e. body concentration, while teaching *āsana* and *prāṇāyāma.* Instead of candle gazing, I ask to look at the body and mind totally in an *āsana.*

---

[1] *Tataḥ kṣīyate prakāśa āvaraṇam* (*Y.S.,* II.52) *Prāṇāyāma* removes the veil covering the light of knowledge and heralds the dawn of wisdom.
Dhāraṇāsu ca yogyatā manasaḥ (*Y.S.,* II.53). The mind also becomes fit for concentration.
See the author's *Light on the Yoga Sūtras of Patañjali,* pp. 158-159.

I ask to see from within as well as from without. While doing the *āsana* you learn to see one point and at the same time all points. This helps them to develop the art of concentration to go naturally towards meditation but not by induction.

Meditation is the art in which the consciousness is focussed both centripetally and centrifugally. Here the attention is made to ascend not only vertically, but also made to spread horizontally on all parts of the body maintaining one-pointedness throughout.

Now I hope you understand how I bring meditation indirectly while teaching *āsana* and *prāṇāyāma*.

Q.- It is felt that yoga in the West has taken on different forms, different approaches, from yoga in India. Do you feel this is true, do you feel there are differences?

There is no question of difference. It is a question of adaptation and adoption. Many try to simplify by introducing their own styles and in this simplification the fragrance of the subject is lost. I saw in *Yoga Today* the *āsana* of a man whose body is strong, toned and matured, presenting the *āsana* for beginners to start with. How can the majority of people whose bodies are not toned take to these so-called simple *āsana* which are not at all for beginners? A beginner has to start like a child who learns to write A, B, C at least a hundred times. Is that the end? Let people find still the simplest of the simplest path. But should it end there or should it be a springboard to go ahead, is my point.

Apart from this, when the teachers in the West adopt yoga with different approaches, it loses the core of the subject. The very purpose of the subject goes to the background and therefore chances of missing the principal points are bound to be there. People add different approaches to attract more students.

Yoga is practised for one's own progressive improvement and upliftment and not for limited and mild practice which leads to stagnation and boredom. Whatever the approach may be, one must keep in mind, while introducing them, whether they build up the quality of yogic discipline or not. When Patañjali says that the practice of yoga removes the impurities in various sheaths of the *sādhaka*, from body to the self and goes on to bring forth the essence of knowledge and wisdom,[1] I wish people keep this in mind when different approaches are introduced, otherwise only weeds grow and not filtered intelligence.

---

1 *Yogāṅgānuṣṭhānāt aśuddhikṣaye jñānadīptiḥ āvivekakhyateḥ* (*Y.S.*, II.28). By dedicated practice of the various aspects of yoga, impurities are destroyed and the crown of wisdom radiates in glory. See the author's *Light on the Yoga Sūtras of Patañjali*, pp. 132-134.

Q.- In other words yoga in the West has yet to mature, reach some kind of maturity?

Yes, one has to aim at maturity in understanding oneself. India is the motherland of yoga and it had reached its ripeness, but now it is a forgotten subject there also. Fortunately, there is again a sudden revival in my country. People have taken to it. However the depth has to further grow as they intensify their *sādhanā*. As the zeal has set in their minds, they want to know more and more of yoga. Let their zeal be more on the practical side to experience and not be contented with theoretical knowledge. Then *sūtra* II.28 of the yoga aphorisms is very meaningful.

Know that mere information of the subject is not enough, though it is necessary. One needs to take a dip into the subject. I feel that one day London is going to be the 'Ganga' of yoga, the holy river of India. The cities of London, Mumbai, New York or Tokyo are becoming the places for the Ganges of knowledge to flow as enthusiastic practitioners are very many. Secondly, yoga is an universal subject and culture. It can be adopted by everyone without having the boundaries of caste, religion, class, age, creed and gender. One can adopt according to one's capacity and intelligence. Only, the approaches must be constructive and creative and not showmanship.

Q.- Is there anything you would like to add, Mr. Iyengar?

There is no doubt that a major institute like the Iyengar Yoga Institute of London[1] may become a feeding centre for the other students who can evolve further in the field of yoga. We, as yogis, should not take pride in ourselves as personalities. It is the subject of yoga which is important. You know you are sometimes saying that Iyengar is very harsh, very rough and arrogant, but even Viśvāmitra, Paraśurāma, Matsyendranāth, Gorakṣanāth, Jamadagni and Ramakrishna were like that. Christ had spat on people too. If you are genuine students of yoga, these are not the things to be counted. Rather see the aspiration, dedication and devotion to the subject by the doer. As teacher, one puts on lots of physical, mental and intellectual garments while teaching which may appear crude, rude, gentle, abstract and so on. It is the spirit behind which has to be appreciated and not consider them as setbacks in yoga.

Everybody misreads yoga. Yoga has definitely accepted non-violence. Patañjali does not want anyone to be violent with somebody for no reason. He, in fact, guides how one has to adopt this principle. Patañjali speaks at what time you should show violence or non-violence. He wants us to analyse and understand all our defects, faulty actions, wrong notions and incorrect applications even while doing the simplest of the *āsana*. He wants us to be friendly, compassionate

---

[1] Situated in Maida Vale, London.

to the weaker side and indifferent to the side which prides itself as correct. While showing the compassion to the weaker side, he wants to use the weapon of *hiṁsa* to make the weaker side stronger. Suppose your right knee bends more and the left knee does not bend so much, be friendly to your left knee, be compassionate and teach that knee to get the movement as the right knee gets it. Calcification must have taken place on that knee, which may be painful. To break this calcification formation, some degree of violence is required, otherwise the disease increases. Is non-violent approach a friendly act on the left knee? This is yoga, where the scale of *hiṁsā, ahiṁsā, maitrī, karuṇā, muditā* and *upekṣā,* i.e., violence, non-violence, friendliness, compassion, joy and indifference towards pleasure and pain are balanced and worked out.

With all these, the main aim of yoga is for the realisation of the Self or uplifting of the body and mind towards the soul.

Q.- How far do you feel your kind of yoga has anything to offer to the person that is unable to move?

My dear friend, what my kind of yoga is, I do not know. I am really at a loss to know what my kind of yoga is. I practise what my *guru* taught me and I depend on yoga texts when examining my *sādhanā*.

If you come to the medical classes that I am conducting, then you may be surprised to know what I do for them. I go out of my way to find the source points of weakness – from there I build them up. It is not just do this or that *āsana*. Even if you do, you will not find relief, I see the weak points and help that person to gain confidence to recover successfully. I teach invalids, I teach spastic children. I teach people who are affected with paralysis and polio. I make people who cannot walk to walk. I teach those who are above eighty having all the old age problems. Until now I have not discouraged or turned down anyone saying that you cannot do yoga, or yoga is not for you. I may make them aware of their limitations but again show them how valuable the practice of yoga will be for them. For me yoga is meant for all.

Q.- Where does it help them most? In which part of their body does it help them most? Into the physical?

First remember that all cannot think of the mental plane or spiritual plane while they are raw beginners or an average *sādhaka*. Most people are affected in the body as they are closer and more affectionate towards their bodies. On account of this affection to the body there is a fear complex that they may suffer from ailments. So, first we have to begin from the body for them to have happiness by removing bodily sufferings. I start working according to their wants and needs through yoga. After satisfying their wants, then my job is to lift them to the higher level. If a student comes to me and says, "I want to spiritually evolve", I say, "Please start from the body, which is a part of the soul, and proceed. Otherwise please look for a *guru* who can take you instantly to the divinity," though this instant divinity is out of the question.

The body, which is the envelope of the soul, cannot be forgotten by any yoga students. Where can you divide the physical end, the mental end or the spiritual end of the discipline? They are all interwoven one with the other. One is coated with the outer body, the other is coated with the inner body and hence they are all intermingled, they cannot be separated.

I remember the words of Lord Christ who said, "If somebody asks you for bread, don't give him stone." If somebody comes to me with the problem of impotency, what have I to give? Have I to give philosophy or pay attention to his need? I have treated such cases and have given them new life and joy of life. Have I to make him potent or to speak to him about *brahmacarya?* I cannot say, what a lucky man you are that you can go in for renunciation as you have no potency for passion. In my life, through yoga, I have saved many married families who have suffered from impotency. Even their doctors were surprised to see how yoga worked on them. I would not have given help to anyone if I had a limited understanding of the *āsana* and *prāṇāyāma* A limited understanding only gives limited knowledge to others. It is better that the teacher works and goes beyond his capacity and gets unlimited knowledge and limited effects so that he can serve with deep love and affection and give his best to people. That is how I work. If I am mentally empty, I use the body as a concentration point and build up slowly to be mentally alert. This is how I adapt yoga to give first for what they came for and then process the practises to uplift them from body to the mind, from the mind to the intelligence, from the intelligence towards consciousness and from consciousness towards the seer.

Q.- So there wouldn't be any pushing into posture, or anything like this in their cases?

It's not a question of pushing. There you are wrong. It is a question of negligence as well as the lack of penetration, on which I work and push their mind a bit and not at all their bodies. While doing or being in the *āsana* you need to have the freedom of body and mind as well. It is a question of extension. It is the mind which puts a limit. If people think that they cannot do more than what they do, I help and guide them so that they can do more than what they think is possible. Here I create vastness or expansion for them to move their minds with freedom.

Read your sentence, you are not even sure of your own question. You think, you cannot do it, you're not sure of it. All these show your negativity and unwillingness. I have the power to awaken your mind to extend more. I make your mind positive so that you can look further for you to penetrate further in your attempts.

The stretches, extensions, placements of the various parts of the body in the *āsana* are not of stretching the flesh but the power of making the mind to move parallel with the movements of the body. It is the extension of mind that we emphasise. Your word "pushing" is wrong. "Emphasise" is the right word. If you cannot stretch, we do not use the horsewhip. We do not kick to make you fit. We make you correct it by repeated trials, we encourage you to do a little more, we give support and keep you moving towards progress. This means we extend your mind. We make you and your mind move with your body. This way we teach. The extension of the body is extension of the mind. We cannot say to the beginner to extend his mind, we can only advise him to extend the legs. We make him involve the body into action directly so that the mind unknowingly extends with the stretch of the body. We make the body and mind go together. To reach the leg means extension of his mind! *(Laughs)*. This is the teaching that's all.

Q.- About yoga for children, that has yet to develop. How to introduce?

I have taught in schools and colleges since I became a teacher. Not only in schools and colleges but also to the defence force. Unfortunately it is a loss for yoga that the authorities disturbed the continuity in the classes. I hope a day may come for yoga to become part and parcel of the educational curriculum. There are many countries that have got interaction of yoga with children as meditation. Definitely it is a wrong approach. A child is alert. The majority of children are very alert, and if they are not alert they go to sleep immediately. You need not tell them to go to sleep. You know, the moment they put their heads down, they go to sleep. That's why meditation isn't a right approach for them. At this point I am slightly against all yogis. I ask, why make a potent intellectual child an impotent intellectual child. Children demand variety. They like speed, they like competition and yoga is both competitive and non-competitive. I have been teaching for years in many schools and colleges. In 1937 I was the pioneer to introduce yoga in schools and colleges, and at that time the other yogis said that yoga cannot be taught to the masses and it's wrong to do so. Now, the same people are wanting that yoga should be introduced in schools and colleges. I just laugh.

If you give me a rough surface, I know what *āsana* to be taken in that rough area. If you give me a smooth area, I say what *āsana* are to be taken in that smooth area for children. I say let us have a general syllabus and not a fixed one. According to the feel of children, let us adopt, adjust and teach. I do not ask them to tear their skin. Children need competition, they need speed and variety. These are the three important things the youngsters demand. If you say go slowly in yoga, the child gets bored, you will never see that child in the class again. If you ask them to repeat, they say it is monotonous. In my classes, I take the same *āsana*, but I change the methodology and sequences in different ways, which they feel challenging, and they feel happy.

People who visit Pune have seen children from the age of six to the age of fifteen. We have once a week class on Sundays because other days they have school. Sunday is the only day which is a holiday for them, and children come to my class and never miss Sundays. I tell everybody, see how much interest is created in them. We play with them, and when necessary we admonish them. We as teachers join in competition. For instance, I may say, "Let me see whether you are quick or I am quick." Or as a teacher I may stand on the platform and tell them, "I think you are all very young, you are going to do better than me." I imitate as though I am stiff and I cannot do the *āsana*, and make them do it. Second time I say, "Hey! you have all done very well, I will also compete with you. Let me see whether I can." So I do a little better than them. I say, "See, I am better than you, can you do better than me?" This way I create interest in them. What I take this Sunday I will not do next Sunday. I change in order to show a new variety every now and then. I make them do the same *āsana* in a new way each time. I adapt different sequences, I jump from top to bottom, bottom to top, middle to end, so that they are made to love doing that. It challenges not only their bodies but helps them to develop quickness, memory, intelligence, co-ordination and synchronisation in movements. If you take classes like that, I tell you, the child will enjoy yoga tremendously.

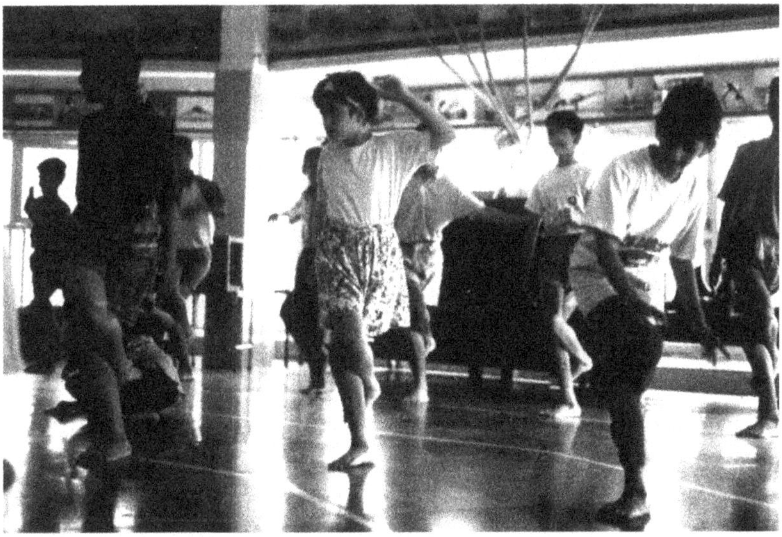

Plate n. 13 – The children's class

Let me tell you that I have taught hyperactive children so that they put reins to their hyperactivity. I have taught the children who are slow and dull lacking quickness and quick response. I have a class for those children who are physically and mentally challenged, epileptic, diabetic and polio affected. Of course the design of teaching differs for such children compared to the normal ones.

Undoubtedly we can introduce yoga in the regular education. We can divide yoga to fit into an educational curriculum. I have already put the suggestion before the Government of India, but I am only one, so I being a minority, nobody accepts.[1] I say, for a child it should go as a physical exercise. For a child yoga has to go from the physical level. You may like it or you may not like it. They need movements. When they are twelve or thirteen, then yoga is to be taught at the anatomical and physiological level. We need to tell them the movements of the joints, movements of the muscles, and how the muscles are controlled and how the joints are moved. We can teach them how to bring the effect on the organic body. When they go for graduation time, they are mentally ripe. At that time we teach how to use the mind in the *āsana*, how to use the mind while inhaling or exhaling, while in retention.

What is the functioning of the mind? When the mind is cultured, then, like the person going for one's doctorate, I say you can go to meditation. This way yoga can grow healthily. Unless the seed finds its sapling, how can it grow into a tree? So I say the fruit is the effect of meditation. The fruit on the tree is the meditation, the fruit cannot come the moment you put the seed. So you let the yoga tree grow, healthily and happily, so that the fruit of the joy, delight, will turn itself into spiritual blossom.

- *Very essential in this country, because as you know...* -

In all the countries.

- *But especially here.* -

No, no, in all countries, my dear friend, please accept my statement, I travel so much. I have seen the children.

---

[1] Refer to *Aṣṭadaḷa Yogamālā*, vol. 3, *"Yoga in Schools"*. See also in this volume, pp. 26, my answer to the questionaire sent by the Friends of Yoga Society on behalf of the Government of Maharashtra.

Q.- But the children, I am sure, get more exercise in other countries between those years, fifteen and eighteen. Children here, while they are doing their O levels and A levels, are just sitting the whole time and their bodies become stiff.

Yes, the period of adolescence and puberty is a very tricky period and I agree there. It has to be, that is nature's play. We need to make them use the body in a proper way for proper functioning of the mind. We need to teach them how to connect the mind with the body, how to connect the body with the mind, and that is the right time to be taught. When it is taught like this, I think tree of yoga just grows. As one takes care of the sapling every now and then for it to grow into a tree, we have to trim the children as good citizens. If you trim you can turn the sapling to any direction you want, but the tree breaks if you do it. So it is the same in yoga. If you start teaching the children, you can turn them in any direction you want. You can make them like flowers or you can make them like weeds. We do not want them to grow like weeds. Therefore, a right methodology is needed to teach them.

The programme of yoga education for children does not change whether they play or do the deskwork. For them, the *āsana* aspect has a great potency. They are not mere flexible physical movements. They have a good bearing in developing their nerves, breath, mind and intelligence both emotionally and intellectually. The method we adopt in teaching is such that they begin to gradually evolve. Though we begin from simple physical movements, they are made to proceed miles away from this starting point to reach progression in their way of living as well as yoga.

Q.- But if you're teaching them competition, will it not lead them towards unhealthy feeling and malice etc?

Here, competition means healthy competition, I do not create ill feeling in competition. Not competition where your energy is sapped in order to win a prize. It is neither to give incentive n or bring negativity. I say, "See he has done. Now you do like him." This makes them channel their efforts and they begin. It is not a kind of imitation of breathtaking or bloodsucking competition. It is meant to bring alertness and awareness in them. It is the way to break the lethargy and bring the new energy to surface for better action.

Q.- How is that different from normal competition?

In normal competition, "come what may, I should win" is the approach. But here I teach the healthy method of development. If he does better, I say, "You should also do like that". That is competition. I don't say, "You should do better than him." So the teacher's quality is not to boost the one that does well, but to boost one who doesn't do well. That is competition.

I have taught in my life many people of various ages, and believe me my ten fingers have touched many more people than any other yogi in the world and that's why I can grasp. The moment I touch, I can tell the person the quality of the skin as well as his moods and modes. This is known as compassion. I never sat at one place dictating. I use words exactly as I do, correcting them while they were doing. I say, "Do not do from here, do from here," and so on. I give them the source point of movement. When we develop from the source point of movement it interests them to practise more and more and in response to that and they begin to know more about their bodies. Each one wants to find out one's own source of action. By such competitive ways they find out from where they did. This is what we call *savitarka* – right analysis; without using the terminology to children. How to analyse, how to reason out, to find a synthesis between reason and action is the teacher's job. We do not want to confuse them. We say, "He found out and you didn't find?" Then we ask, "How did he find? How did he get it? He must have been knowing before." To one who says, "I don't know Sir", we show the correct movements, correct action. We show where there was lack of action and we cultivate healthy actions, healthy feeling in children in order to bring about progress.

It is very interesting. Sometimes we just flop. I say, "I also do not understand – where did you get it? Let me try to be serious now." So the pupils laugh. Then all of a sudden I let them see me do it very well. "Oh, now I see I have beaten you! Let's try". *(Laughing).* This way, I do and play with children. I do not dictate to them. They begin to see my efforts too and put in their efforts in order to achieve. If I get twenty children, sometimes I do with five children in the middle, sometimes I come with another five children. So they feel as if I am one of them and they are on a par with me, so that they can't treat me as a teacher. If I yell at them, that time only they know they have done something wrong. Soon I make them laugh and I even offer them sweets when they do well or achieve something new. This way, they mature totally at the physical level, psychological level, intellectual and spiritual level. There are no interferences or interruptions in between. The growth is steady and certain and the children become the wealth of the nation.

This is the way I encourage them to build up intellectual vigour and not at all competition.

IYENGAR, YOGA PROPHET*

" First this temple of the soul, the body, must be cleaned well
before one thinks of coming towards the Self.
Eat sweets and be sweet "

His vitality is as contagious as it is intoxicating. He eats with gusto and never throws disapproving looks at your plate. He does not have a long face nor does he only like to talk about transcendental things veiled artificially in empty mysticism. When he pulls your jacket to show you the glass vase, which was just given to him in Venice the day before yesterday, he even inspires tenderness. He is a child who inspires joy and friendliness through those vibrations, which only can be transmitted through wisdom. This is Iyengar, a yogi and a brāhmin, officially recognised as the best yoga teacher in the world. His official residence is in Pune, India, but he has schools in every part of the world, even in countries in Africa with hundreds of thousands of students. He has been teaching yoga for exactly fifty years and he doesn't know "for how long he will still have to learn it".

We met him yesterday morning in a splendid and serene villa in the hills of Fiesole where he has come to visit a dear friend. Surrounded by a group of yoga teachers and students, honoured by a tasteful vegetarian lunch, he willingly accepted an open conversation.

"There is one basic concept in yoga", says Iyengar, "it allows one to become master of circumstances and not a slave. Everyone talks about happiness and serenity but only limits this to talking about a concept or a desire without passing into action or putting this into practice. Yoga is action. How can we expect to give tranquillity to the brain if we don't make our muscles work well and our blood circulate to supply the cells uninterruptedly? If we don't use every part of our body fully and totally, physical health is bound to miss and mental health will remain only as a pure utopia. Physical and mental health have to go together as well as the tranquillity of brain with the tranquillity of mind."

---

* Published by *La Nazione*, Tuesday, June 5, 1984.

Q.- Should we all convert to this Indian conception of man?

That which I teach - *answers Mr. Iyengar smiling happily like a malicious gnome* - is universally known, it is only that few people want to work seriously with the body. Christianity, for example, says that the body is the temple of the soul, but the yogi adds that before the soul is thought of, this temple of the soul - the body - must be cleaned well. The Ten Commandments are similar to the principles of Indian religion. The fact is that all these must be put into practice and then, that's that - *exclaims Mr. Iyengar with a winning smile.*

The nicest thing which I observe - *says the yogi playing with a very patient pen* - is that at one time people thought about God when they were old, and now I see thousands and thousands of people who do yoga and think about God are young enthusiasts. Yoga brings intellectual clarity and emotional stability. The spiritual light glows only after a long time of practice. The world certainly changes for the better if this tendency continually increases. Physical and mental health, in fact, opens the doors of the soul and when the soul is free from entanglements, society will transform positively.

As far as the conversion to the Indian concept, as per your question, is concerned, I would like to tell you that whatever is exclusively good in ours, I share with joy with others. It is not fair to hold good things to oneself. Then it becomes selfish motive. Please do not divide these good concepts, and do not consider these concepts as if they were Indian. Much of what I say, who knows, you may be able to trace in your scriptures also. If I put these with Indian expression, do not think it as a conversion towards Indian thought. For the progression of man, thoughts coming from any science are good. Fortunately yoga is meant for humanity and all human beings have the right to it. So, I think it is good to share it with one and all irrespective of whichever country or religion one belongs to.

Q.- Iyengar, what is life?

Life is like a river, a flowing energy, energy is life. Breath is life. Life and breath are vibrant which makes us conscious beings. And consciousness is nothing but awareness in understanding.

(He almost whispers while he eyes contentedly some coffee with cream which kind hands have prepared for him.)

Q.- Why do many different schools of yoga exist? Doesn't that risk creating confusion?

Yoga is one and it fits everyone to whatever religion or country one belongs to or whether one lives in India, the U.S. or the Congo. It is spring of nectar from which everyone can drink, be he a Christian, a Buddhist or a Hindu. As there are many roads to reach God, each one may create one's own pathways through yoga to reach the Ultimate. However one has to follow it consciously and conscientiously. *(After a pause)* I feel each and every road ends finally at the same place.

Teachers who are after name, fame and money may label their approach or pathway as their yoga. If the teachers are honest and have a proper knowledge, they realise that all roads end at the same destination.

Q.- What is a checkpoint to try to know if we are or are not headed for the finish line that is offered by complete yoga?

You see, the finish point is a long journey. A beginner cannot see a finish point that easily. In order to reach the finish point, one needs to have a complete transformation. This transformation occurs in seven stages namely, rising consciousness – *vyutthāna*, restrained – *nirodha*, calm – *śānta*, one-pointed – *ekāgra*, sprouted – *nirmāṇa*, with pores – *chidra* and divine – *divya* or *paripakva*. Finally, the sequential and successive mutations of the three qualities, namely *sattva*, *rajas* and *tamas*, come to an end point. I know that for a layman this does not give the correct idea. Therefore let me answer in such a way that a common man understands.

The skin gives us the exact quality of our physical and psychological health. It must be relaxed, lengthened and extended as extension means freedom; freedom is knowledge and knowledge is the window on to God – which means on to harmony. But, I will repeat it again once more, the first step is to get physical health. We have to defeat the dictatorship of the brain. The intellect, which has its own power has to be pure. Intellect should not be confused with intelligence. If the intellect is from the acquired knowledge, intelligence is the imprint from the impressions by right action. Faculties like knowledge, sensitivity, feeling, awareness, develop only through the felt intelligence. So the practitioners need to work on physical, physiological, biological, cellular, psychological, moral, vital, mental, emotional and intellectual health and then transcend towards the divine life. This is the finish line.

Q.- Iyengar, I have been told that you enjoy food, is this true?

It's true, it's true. Food is God. One should enjoy without indulging in it. I enjoy the food with purity of mind – *he admits happily, almost dancing.* But you too enjoy eating, I've noticed. Eat sweets and be sweet.

IYENGAR ON *PRĀṆĀYĀMA**

Q.- Could you explain the difference between *prāṇāyāma* and deep breathing?

You know, when I picked up this rose just now to draw its fragrance, many of you laughed. But the question is very appropriate in the way in which I smelled it. This flower has a tremendous fragrance. If I take it inside like this *(sniffs forcibly)*, I can't gradually take or feel the fragrance of the flower, is it not? But gently I draw the fragrance with my breath. I get the fragrance moving through the carpet of my nostrils tickling my membranes. This is the same with deep breathing and *prāṇāyāmic* breathing.

Deep breathing is normally done through the physical reaction from the body when the breath is taken. As being is eternal, so is nature. The spirit, the self, the soul, is immutable, whereas nature is mutable and changeable. Now, our bodies are made up of five elements: ether, air, water, fire and earth. When we do deep breathing, we forget the subtle element, the ether, and start from the other end, the earth. When you breathe in or inhale forcibly, the earth is activated first. Then act on the quality of earth, which is nothing but the movement of the muscles. When you breathe out or exhale and the breath comes to an end, you experience the space within the body. So, in deep breathing, the initiative comes from the earth. But in *prāṇāyāmic* breathing all the elements are kept passive to experience the vibration and space. The quality of ether is vibration or sound. The sound of the incoming breath should be so soft, so delicate, that the sound, which vibrates comes from the inner interior space to touch the place, the body of the chest wall. Then it forms into a shape, the right lung, the left lung, the spine, the various chambers of the muscles so that they take a certain balancing shape. You have to control and feel the quality of fragrance of the breath, how it is moving in, when it touches the extremities of the body, which is the element of earth, then that becomes *prāṇāyāmic* breathing. Similarly while exhaling, the breath is not to be pushed out. Whatever shape the body or the chest has taken in the inhalation process, it has to be maintained throughout the exhalation. You have to feel the

---

* From *Iyengar Yoga Institute Review*, San Francisco, vol 5, no. 2, October 1984.

fragrance of the breath that is moving out without disfiguring the earth element to catch the ether element. If the body is jerked faster than the breath, it is deep breathing. In *prāṇāyāmic* breathing, the breath is channelled, directed. In deep breathing there is no direction. Here the air is just pulled in or pushed out. In *prāṇāyāma*, the body remains unmoved and tremendous space and place are created for the drawn-in breath without disturbing the chest box. So by channelling, the breath is made to find its avenue in the torso that is not visible to these physical eyes. But the practitioner feels the channels or pathways very clearly. If it is done in that way, that is yogic *prāṇāyāma*.

If you keep a vessel under the tap, the water which flows, touches the bottom of the vessel and moves to the sides to accommodate the water as it comes. Unless and until the first water which dropped into the vessel finds a surface, the vessel does not fill at all; there will be air gaps. So if you open the tap very heavily, it will seem that the water has come to the top, but if you slow down the flow, the water descends to find its level. If the water gushes from the tap, the vessel cannot be filled at all to the brim. It is the same in deep breathing. Though it appears that one has filled the lungs, the vessel of the breath remains empty. Secondly, if the tap is opened fully, the force of water from the tap makes the vessel vibrate and distorts its position. The same happens for the torso in deep breathing and one will not know whether the drawn-in breath is absorbed or not by the lungs.

If the tap's opening is narrowed, the water that drips into the vessel does not disturb, and when the vessel receives the water, the level rises smoothly, rhythmically, covering the surface of the vessel evenly. So also in *prāṇāyāmic* breathing you make the upper palate open in such a way that the air that is drawn in is not made to gush but flow into the narrow passage through the half closed palate.

One can measure how much one wants to open or close the upper palate to allow the breath to go in smoothly through the windpipe to fill the lungs. The windpipe bifurcates into two branches, which further branch off. The tissues open out tremendously in *prāṇāyāmic* breathing. This way the drawn-in breath goes toward the extremities and feeds the alveolar cells. The alveolar cells absorb the drawn-in air without any disturbances, vibrations, or leaving any gap between the air cells and the bronchioles. The drawn-in air is not released without feeding those areas. In deep breathing, they do not feed, because the walls harden. The intercostal muscles of the chest become hard, therefore that breathing does not supply the needed energy to the extremities.

If you see the surface of water in a lake or sea, you can observe how gently, how subtly the water wets the sand, without disturbing it. So our inhalation has to move in such a way that the energy, which is drawn, wets the air cells so that they can absorb the energy. In channelling and controlling the drawn-in breath, one gives sufficient time for the air cells to absorb and use the full residue of the energy which is still in the lungs before releasing the breath in the form of exhalation. Whereas in deep exhalation one expels the energy along with the unwanted energy before the absorption takes place in the system. In *prāṇāyāmic* exhalation, there is no expulsion of the energy that is drawn-in, but still maintained in the system for further support as a feedback system.

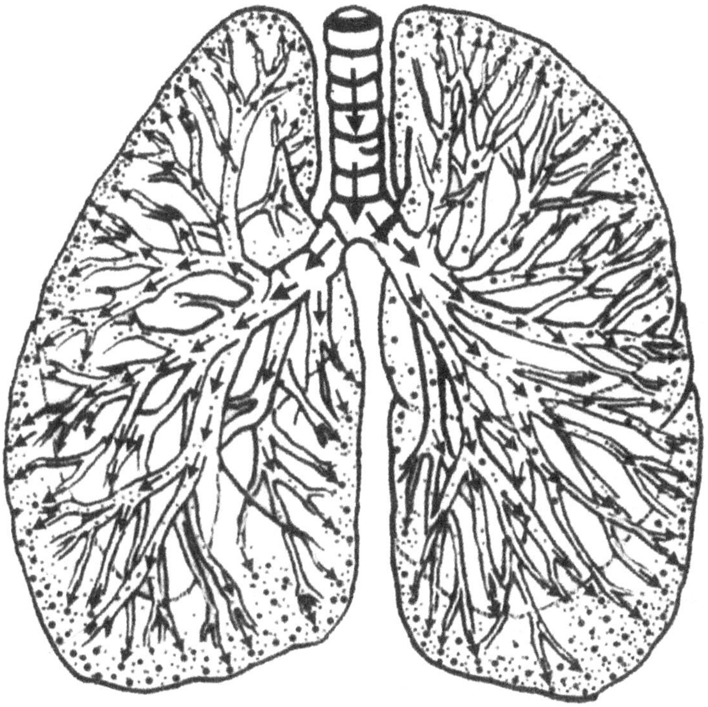

Plate n. 14 – The drawn-in breath goes towards the extremities

When the vessel is filled with water, it touches from the bottom and comes to the brim. So also in the torso, when the breath is drawn in, one has to fill the drawn-in air, energy from the floor of your torso to the top of the chest. For an asthmatic, the top may only be the upper sternum. For a thoracic breather, it may only be the bottom of the sternum, or the diaphragmatic area. For those who have got a tremendous elasticity in the diaphragm, it may be even from the bottom of the navel. And if it is still soft, then the floor of the torso becomes the girdle of the pelvis. In deep breathing, due to the volume and velocity of the movement, the breath does not touch from the pelvis to the top. In *prāṇāyāmic* breathing, it taps the floor – the pelvic girdles – and from there the breath is filled up to the top without strain.

When you start to go to *Sālamba Śīrṣāsana*, do you go on your head at once or do you feel the crown of the head? You keep the crown of the head on the blanket very carefully and delicately. If you suddenly go on the head, you feel heaviness and rushing of the blood.

When a vessel is filled with water up to the brim and if you suddenly make it topsy-turvy to empty out, how does the water come out and with what sound? Tremendous vibrations, tremendous jerks take place, is it not? But if the vessel is gradually slanted, the water flows gradually, it does not make a sound and there is a smoothness in the flow. Then it is not forcing out the water but releasing the water from the filled vessel. If you turn the vessel topsy-turvy, it is as if one hates that water. But if one gradually slants, one is still attached to that vessel, that water. Also when one waters the plant, one does not pour the water. With compassion, one allows the water to touch that plant very carefully. If one pours the water directly on a plant, what happens to that plant? The plant does not receive the water. But if one wets it gradually, the surrounding area of the plant gets wet and feeds the plant to grow. In *prāṇāyāma* too if one learns this art, then that becomes a yogic *prāṇāyāma* and not deep breathing. Unfortunately, the yogis of today do not read the original text to learn the art of using the method shown but interpret in their own ways and call it yogic *prāṇāyāma*.

(Gurujī demonstrates the way of prāṇāyāmic breathing taught these days, and then says that for him it is deep breathing and not prāṇāyāmic breathing.)

They do with the support of the element of earth and neglect the other four elements: water, fire, air and ether. Only they make one feel the skin, the flesh, moving up and moving down. Let not the so-called ordinary deep breathing be called as *prāṇāyāmic* breathing since the technique of *prāṇāyāma* dealt in ancient texts differs from deep breathing.

Prāṇa is the vital energy which modern science names as bio-energy. In *prāṇāyāma* this energy has to seep to spread into the air sacs. In deep breathing strong physical movement is expressed wherein the intake and output of breath is very little. This forceful movement only irritates the nerves but does not draw in the *prāṇa*. In *prāṇāyāma* the energy is distributed to spread, and absorbed so that energy of the nerves is maintained and not wasted as happens in deep breathing.

Q.- *Gurujī*, when first starting to practise *prāṇāyāma*, is it inevitable that some strain will be felt? If so, are there places where strain should be particularly avoided?

Suppose you are gazing at a burning candle, what happens to the eyes after some time? You feel the strain. But what do teachers say? They tell you to continue. But I don't say continue. *(Laughter)*.

You have to know that in any disciplined movement there is a certain stress and strain. Discipline means regulation. Do not take the colloquial meaning of discipline as regimental dictation, like training soldiers in the army. We know only that side of the meaning. But discipline means regulation. The entire system moves zigzag for want of knowledge and understanding. As it has to be regulated, a certain stress and strain is felt, is it not? You have to measure that stress and strain to know whether the stress is creative or obstructive.

I spoke yesterday at the demonstration[1] about discrimination between aggressive stretch and non-aggressive stretch. Here, there might be lots of lawyers. Let me explain in their language. When you are getting stress on one side, and not on the other side, one side becomes a plaintiff and the other becomes a respondent. Each one wants to win over the other. In legal cases, you know you want to win the case and the other person also wants to win the case. You don't know the method, so you engage a lawyer because he knows the law. This is like calling a third person – the intelligence – to discipline the flow of breath, the movements of the intercostal muscles, balancing the spine straight without hardness and so forth. In your body, you should know the laws of your own system. And when you know the law, you judge according to the law. The intelligence has to watch the movement of the right and the movement of the left, the rhythm of the right, the unrhythmic movement of the left, or the healthy movement of the spine on one side, the unhealthy movement on the other side while inhaling and exhaling, or the air filling freely on one side and with a little strain on the other side: these disparities are known as plaintiff and respondent. So you have to be a lawyer within yourself. The lawyer says, "Let me study your case and then let me give my views." You as a lawyer within yourself have to study your case. The question is always the same. You say, "My point of stress on one side is strong, but my point of stress on the other side I do not know." If you use the discriminative faculty, the reasoning faculty of the intelligence, then you say that the stronger side, the plaintiff, is probably too strong and is annexing the property belonging to this part of your lung. So you should get back, is it not? The lawyer says, "You go on telling your points, let me listen." So also the intelligence which is the seat of judgement becomes a judge. The judge sits there quietly. He does react or interact, since he is not supposed to favour either side. So the intelligence tells your acquired knowledge, "Do whatever you want to do. Let me impartially observe. Let me think within myself." You do what you want to, so you act, one side this way, one side that way, a little more, a little less in your presentations. The intelligence remains cold inside to watch with the insight between this side and that side of the lung while you are inhaling, or between this party and that party which are known as the fibres, muscles, ribs and what not. You have called the witness to the court. The muscles of your ribs, the ribs, the fibres on right and left sides, are the witnesses to tell you either

[1] Lecture-demonstration, Davies Hall, San Francisco, July 1984.

the truth or the untruth. So when you feel a certain movement, the intelligence, as the judge notices carefully. The judge, your intelligence, observes whether the right or the left of the lung is filling and moving or not. One side does not move, the intelligence knows that the witness is a false witness. He is hiding something. The truth may be little but he wants to overdo the truth. The intelligence has to measure the movement of the breath on the left side and the right side, and then you have to go on balancing without allowing the weaker side to become weaker or stronger side to become stronger. If extra power, extra attention is thrown by your intelligence on the side that is weaker, then it is a stress. Release the intelligence from the stronger side and shift it to the weaker side, then that stress is non-stress. The *puruṣa* inside too should guide the intelligence to look at both sides of the chest box to see who the plaintiff is and who the respondent is. The *puruṣa* sends the message to the intelligence to listen to the plaintiff as well as the respondent – the two lungs. The intelligence listens to both sides. Then the *puruṣa* says to the intelligence to weigh, so that both the sides receive the energy evenly. This is like settling the case outside of the court. *(Laughter).* I hope you have understood. *(More laughter).* Learn to have the dialogue with your own intelligence. Often, make an appeal and demand for the judgement.

The most important point to note is when you are inhaling, the first inhalation acts as the key point of the behaviour of your entire human system, from the entire cells to the self and vice versa.

You know, the first breath should be like your meeting with a stranger for the first time. Somebody comes and introduces you to me or me to you. You say, "How do you do?" At that time, what is your state of mind, what is my state of mind? *(Somebody from the audience answers, "Aloof union".)*

Yes! Aloof union! Aloof union means neither close nor far. Our minds are at a distance, yet we say, "Hello". There is neither prejudice, nor friendliness nor animosity. Hence, there is a freshness. Freshness in the consciousness of both. Is it not? We don't know each other. Both are completely new to each other. As there is no background, there is no room for prejudices, so both see with freshness. There is a tremendous newness and purity in the first meeting. Impurities come when the contact becomes closer as we study and judge the other with our own frame of mind. The strain comes when one studies another according to one's calibre, and you study someone according to your frame of mind. If we do this, we both are wrong. How can we judge someone through one's tainted mind? How can one judge another by one's own standard? Your standard is different; somebody's standard is different. We have to learn to look with aloofness. If we look moment to moment, day in and day out, year in and year out, and maintain that first state throughout, are we not ever fresh, aloof in friendship, aloof in understanding, in a state of oneness without prejudice?

Similarly you have to follow the sequence of breaths, keeping in mind the behaviour of the first breath. The first impression is what is important, and all future movements, cultivated or cultured, refined and progressive, should be based on that first contact, because that first movement which is done unconsciously is very pure. When you start, the self is aloof, the intelligence is also aloof, the breath is aloof, the cells are aloof. After three to four breaths, if you feel strain, then your mind should go back to the first breath. You have to question yourself how was it in the first breath, you did not get strain. How did this strain come now? What mistake did you make? Where were you? Were you aloof, or did you get caught up in a certain fluctuation in the self? Which part became friendly to you? Which part did not become friendly to you? It is for you to notice. So as you are inhaling on one side, you have to keep the other side also in contact. If you can balance this, then your breath will be the same forever; there will be no stress, no strain, no pain, no exhaustion. If this quality of attention and observation is maintained, then there is no strain in the performance of the *āsana*, and there is no strain in the practice of *prāṇāyāma*.

When you do the *kumbhaka,* when you hold the breath, have you seen in the beginning how fresh it looks, the fragrance of the movements of the cells which act as a friend? But later, within a few seconds, you realise that the cells press the body; the body presses and pushes itself on the skin; your mind grips the breath; your mind hits the body. The clashes and the quarrels commence inside.

These unconscious movements should be observed by you. You should avoid such movements. Without getting the movement and the breath distorted, see whether you can maintain that unknown purity knowingly, in a purified form. This is known as the culture of the breath, the lungs, the intelligence, or culture of the self. Cell is also cultured; self is also cultured. That is how you have to learn and differentiate between stress and non-stress. Stress and non-stress are both wrong. There should be no positive tension; there should be no negative tension. You have to balance the positive and the negative; only then the energy is produced. If one of them becomes stronger, then short circuit occurs as it does in the flow of electric current. In yoga some people say there should be no stress at all; some people say there should be stress. If I want to look at this flower, I have to open it very little, is it not? If I give stress more or force more, it gives way. The petals will drop. You have to measure the zero state of feeling in the nerves and mind while breathing.

This is the centre of the chest box; these are the sides. *(He points out at the thoracic chest.)* If the skin moves, you think you are inhaling. The positive current in the centre moves very fast; the negative current on the sides does not move at all. You have to feel that the negative and the positive are in line with each other. Then there are no shocks in your movements. When there are no shocks, there is no stress. That's how you have to master the breath; that's how you have to master the *āsana*. That is how you have to master the *prāṇāyāma* from the zero state of energy and consciousness.

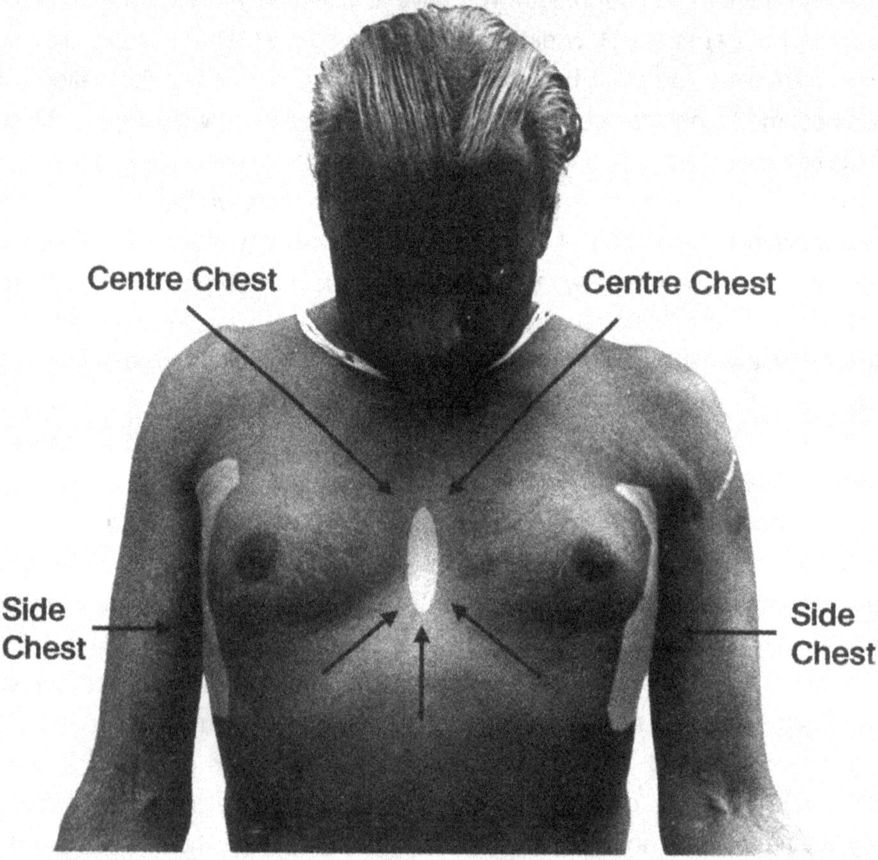

Plate n. 15 – Centre chest and side chest

B.K.S. IYENGAR – YOGA EXPONENT*

Today the famous B.K.S. Iyengar, yoga expert of Pune, is known all over the country and in most parts of the world. He has Iyengar Yoga Institutes all over Europe, the United States of America and many other parts of the world including South Africa, Australia. Some time back Shri Iyengar had gone on a two-month tour of the U.S., chiefly to preside over the "First International Iyengar Yoga Convention" at San Francisco, California (Aug. 24 to Sept. 2, 1984). This is a get-together for yoga teachers and pupils from the world over, who come and discuss the art of yoga, and listen to doctors' theories about the medical effects of yoga. They also see the master of them all, Shri B.K.S. Iyengar perform some yogāsana *himself. This incidentally was Shri Iyengar's 35th trip abroad, from the time the great violinist Yehudi Menuhin introduced him to the West in 1954. Justifiably I was awed by Shri Iyengar. But I was pleasantly surprised to meet a humble, modest, kind and cheerful man full of jokes and good humour. He took great pains to put me at ease.*

Shri Iyengar was born on 14th December 1918 at village Bellur in the Kolar district of Karnataka. From his birth he was a weak child, and suffered from a severe attack of typhoid when in school. It took a long time for him to recover. In 1934-35 at the age of sixteen he weighed about fifty to sixty pounds and was just 4 feet 10 inches in height. He learnt yoga from his Gurujī Shri T. Krishnamacharya – his own brother-in-law, who was Director of a yoga school at the Mahārāja of Mysore's Palace. Shri Iyengar started teaching yoga in 1936 at the twin cities of Dharwar and Hubli in northern Karnataka. In those days the practice of yoga was unheard of and the payment Shri Iyengar received was not enough to secure even two square meals a day. The bus fare from Dharwar to Hubli was two annas (twelve paise). Shri Iyengar could not afford that and hence had to trek twelve miles up and down each day. Those were the days of struggle and they did not end in a hurry. When he came to Pune for the first time in 1937 he literally had to live from hand to mouth. As he put it, "I used to subsist on bread and tea from Lucky restaurant in Deccan Gymkhana and sometimes used to just drink water from the taps to appease my hunger". Those were gloomy days of grinding poverty and opposition from people

---

* Interview by Rahul Chandawarkar. Published by *Maharastra Sunday Herald*, October 7th, 1984

who did not appreciate yoga. Shri Iyengar got married in 1943 to a sixteen year old girl called Ramaa and she provided him with the emotional support and courage that he then lacked. Times did not change immediately. As the early fifties approached, with yoga being reintroduced in schools,[1] *etc., and general recognition for the art increasing, Shri Iyengar started gaining stability and some sort of security. He met the world famous violinist Yehudi Menuhin, who later became his disciple and also took him abroad for the first time in 1954. In his most illustrious career as a yoga instructor he has taught and is teaching people ranging from the commonest hawkers to the very richest strata of society. He has taught many famous people: Yehudi Menuhin, the late Dowager Queen of Belgium, Aldous Huxley, Clifford Curzon, Jacqueline Dupré, Julie Felix, the Scaravelli family, famous Indian violinist Lalgudi Jayaraman, Leela Naidu, J. Krishnamurti, Smita Patil and politicians such as the late former Vice President of India G.S. Pathak, Jaya Prakash Narayan. But he still is modest in his 66th year because he has seen it all – the grinding poverty and the luxurious riches. It makes absolutely no difference to him because, as he put it, "Body is my temple and the* āsanas *are my humble prayers".*

Q.- What is yoga?

From the practical point of view yoga means to keep the body and mind healthy, free from diseases, so that the practitioner has the benevolence of freedom. Philosophically it is to unite the individual soul with the Universal Soul or God. Scientifically it is to bring the body, which is lazy – *tāmasic* – to the level of the vibrant mind – *rājasic* – and then to bring both of them on par with the illuminative soul, which is pure – *sāttvic*. That is yoga.

Q.- What is its importance in modern life?

There is a tremendous stress, strain and speed in the modern world. There is a tremendous load on each individual, hence a tremendous want of bio-energy, which is eaten away by stress and strain. This leads to the constriction of the entire nervous system and narrowing of the blood vessels which in turn lead to hypertension, diabetes, emotional diseases, high blood pressure, cardiac attacks and so forth. Practice of *yogāsana* and *prāṇāyāma* creates tremendous elasticity and mobility in the nerve current so that it can take any load of modern stress, without becoming a victim. This effect is more important today than decades back.

---

[1] The author introduced yoga in schools for the first time in 1937.

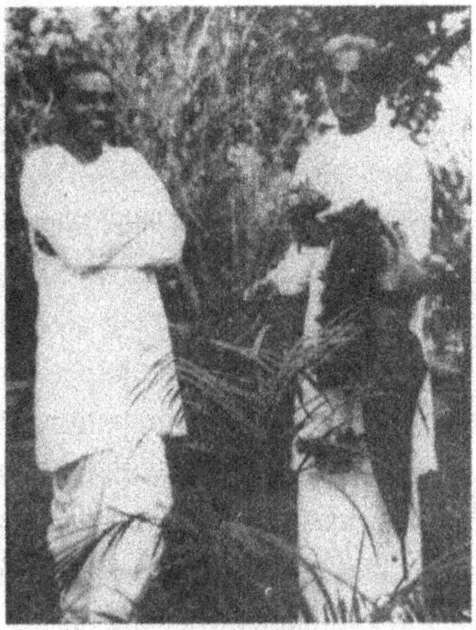
J. Krishnamurthy

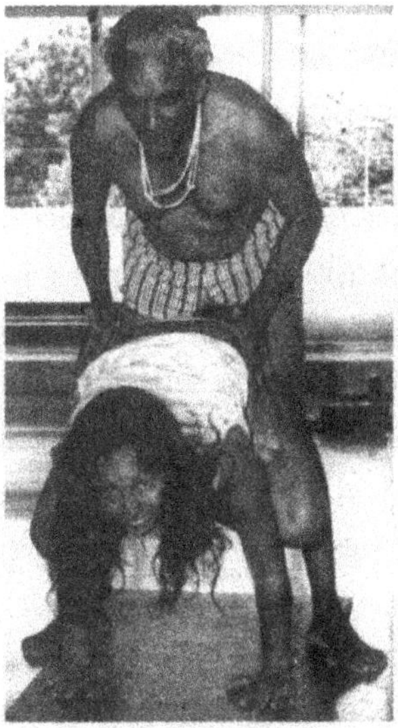
Julie Felix

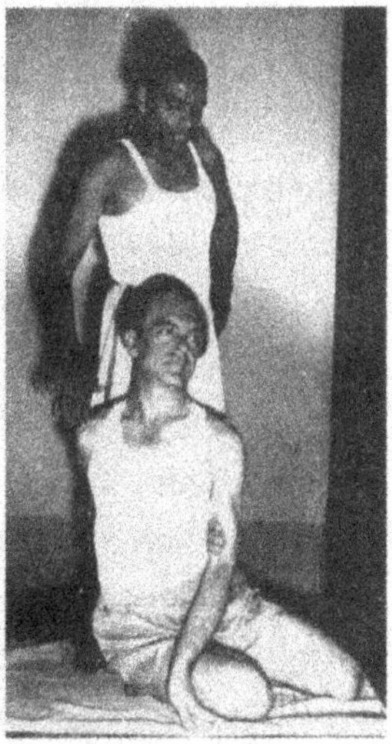
Malcuzinski

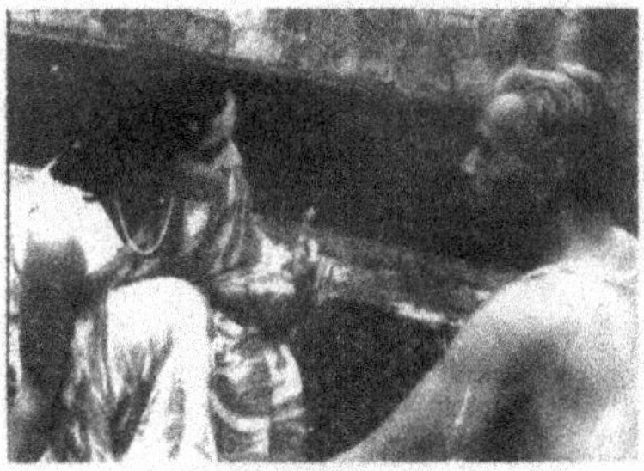
Leela Naidu

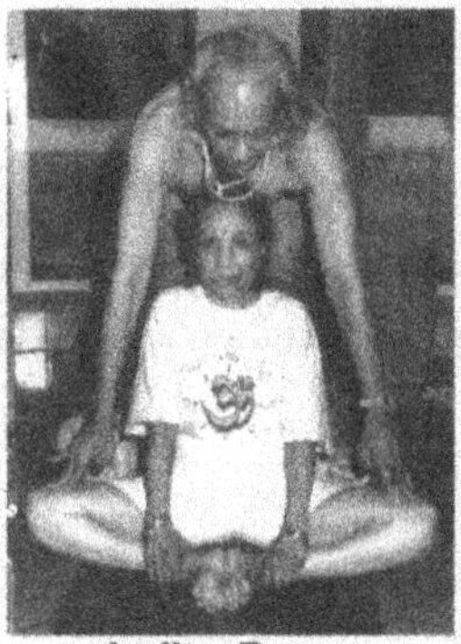
Lalita Pawar

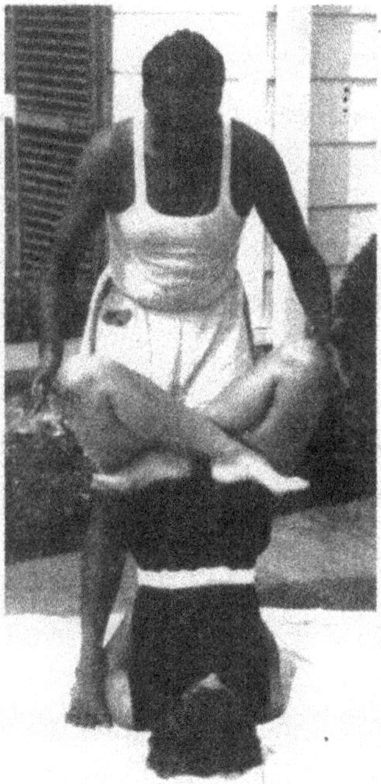
Mrs. Harkness

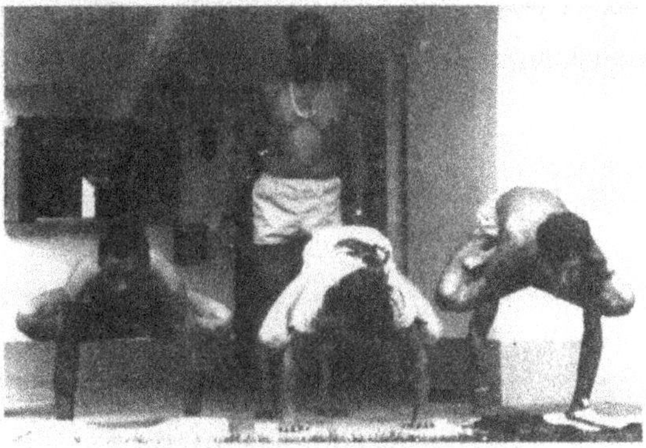
Scaravelli Family

Plate n. 16 – Some of the famous people taught by B.K.S. Iyengar

Q.- Yoga has been upheld as a science in a century where all remedies for modern ailments and diseases can be found. Your comments?

As I told you in the second question, there are two gates of the human system – the respiratory and the circulatory systems. If there is any defect in any one of these two, the whole system is upset. In yoga there is tremendous emphasis on these two systems, as a lot of vital ingredients are supplied to the body by these two. If there is any weakness in the physical body, especially in the physiological body which includes various systems such as respiratory, circulatory, urinary, excretory, glandular, digestive systems and so forth, the body becomes an abode of physical illness and mental sorrow. Practice of yoga increases the defensive mechanism in the system to such a degree that it does not allow the aggressive qualities in the form of diseases to enter the body. The practitioner of yoga therefore possesses a perfect physical body, stability in mind and clarity in his intelligence. Hence it acts as a preventative system while it can also act as a curative system because there is tremendous emphasis on the extension and expansion of the muscles and organs which supply energy and blood to the affected area.

It is heartening that yoga has been accepted gradually by the people in the medical field. Undoubtedly, science has made great progress in curing many of the complicated diseases. Yet, yoga is beyond physical health as it deals not only with the body but mind and intellectual health. Slowly one learns to deal with oneself – the core of the being.

Q.- Who founded yoga?

It exists since time immemorial. It is as old as civilisation. It was in the ancient *Veda* but Sage Patañjali, between 500 and 200 BC, codified the scattered subject into a treatise and called it *Yoga Sūtra,* though to some extent the evolution of yoga had been established before Patañjali.

Q.- Can you trace the evolution of yoga in India and around the world?

Due to historical invasions and disturbances in our country, people were scattered and ran away to different places out of fear. Hence the link or continuity of yoga was lost due to this historical fact and communication hardships due to geographical displacements. It was only after independence that the Indian arts of yoga, music and dance regained a foothold. The world has come much closer, with improved communications. So naturally yoga, which is meant for peace and happiness, started attracting the West in the early fifties. Today it has become their own natural subject to penetrate into their hearts, for further evolution.

The fact is that now the modern facilities, books and communicative devices help people to the introduction of yoga faster. At the same time charlatans in yoga too have grown.

Q.- What are the different types of *āsana* and the concept behind these *āsana?*

There are varieties of *āsana*. The ancient *ṛṣi* had known the details and depth of the body which influence one's mind, ego, intelligence and consciousness. In order to penetrate into the depth of one's consciousness, they had to invent varieties of *āsana*. Being close to nature and nature's environments, they respected nature - *prakṛti* - and introduced into the body systems by imitating nature's creations in the form of *āsana* to improve our inner environment. Hence, with this concept of nature, different types of *āsana* were invented.

It is also necessary to know that limited *āsana* do not maintain the inner stability. Though we all know that the immortal Self cannot be measured, it is also difficult to know the depth of the mortal body. Innumerable *āsana* were discovered by the yogis to feed the inner remotest parts of our body with sufficient nutrients, which in modern terminology is called the biofeedback process. With these innumerable *āsana* one gets the full benefit to keep the body, mind and soul in a healthy and happy state.

Q.- What is *haṭha yoga?*

Haṭha, in one word, means stubbornness or vehemence in *sādhanā*. So, it is the yoga of will power. Will power over matter or conquest of body and mind with will power. Traditionally, *ha* stands for *prāṇa* and *ṭha* stands for *apāna*. Unification of *prāṇa* and *apāna* is *haṭha yoga*. In the same way *ha* also stands for the sun or cosmic vital energy, and *ṭha* stands for consciousness, intelligence or the moon. This means *haṭha yoga sādhanā* brings a perfect understanding between the cosmic vital energy and mind so that they are evenly blended and balanced throughout the human system. *Ha* also stands for the soul and *ṭha* for the consciousness. When the consciousness is purified to an exhalted state of intelligence for it to be equal to the pure state of the soul, it is termed as *haṭha yoga*.

Haṭha yoga gives the practical methodology to purify the body, mind, vital energy and intelligence so that they are all cosmicalised to the level of the cosmic soul.

Q.- What then are *jñāna yoga, bhakti yoga, karma yoga?*

In the early days all these three were known as *mārga* – paths, and not as 'yoga'. *Jñāna* means right knowledge, *bhakti* means right compassion and *karma* means right action. God has given us legs and arms for action, emotional seat for love and intellectual head for knowledge. In order to have perfect knowledge, action and love, the path of yoga was treated as a base or fountain. But the modern intellectual giants coined the 'paths' as different yoga and hence misunderstandings and misgivings have arisen in this field with terms like *rāja yoga, haṭha yoga, kuṇḍalinī yoga, mantra yoga, japa yoga, tāraka yoga, ghaṭa yoga* and so forth. Yoga is like God – one. As people call God by different names, so also yoga has started getting different names.

Q.- Who have been the great yogis of our time?

We have had the good fortune of having seen three great yogis in India, in our time. Shri Ramana Maharshi of Arunachalam, a great *jñāna yogi* who had a ripe intelligence of knowledge of the soul. Then we had Shri Aurobindo, a great *bhakti yogi* whose heart was filled up with love and compassion and the Father of the Nation, Mahatma Gandhi, who was a great *karma yogi,* man of action.

Q.- When did you start teaching yoga abroad?

The world famous violinist Yehudi Menuhin introduced me to the West in 1954. Mr. Menuhin, whom I taught, presented me a watch with the inscription: "To my Best Violin teacher B.K.S. Iyengar from Yehudi Menuhin, Gstaad, Switzerland, Sept. 1954". In 1961 I began teaching local people in England and in the 1970s the educational authorities there introduced my art which caught on very well and spread. In 1974 the United States too introduced yoga into the "Y" as well as in the community, colleges and universities.

Q.- What is the duration of a normal course? What sort of students do you enrol and what are your charges?

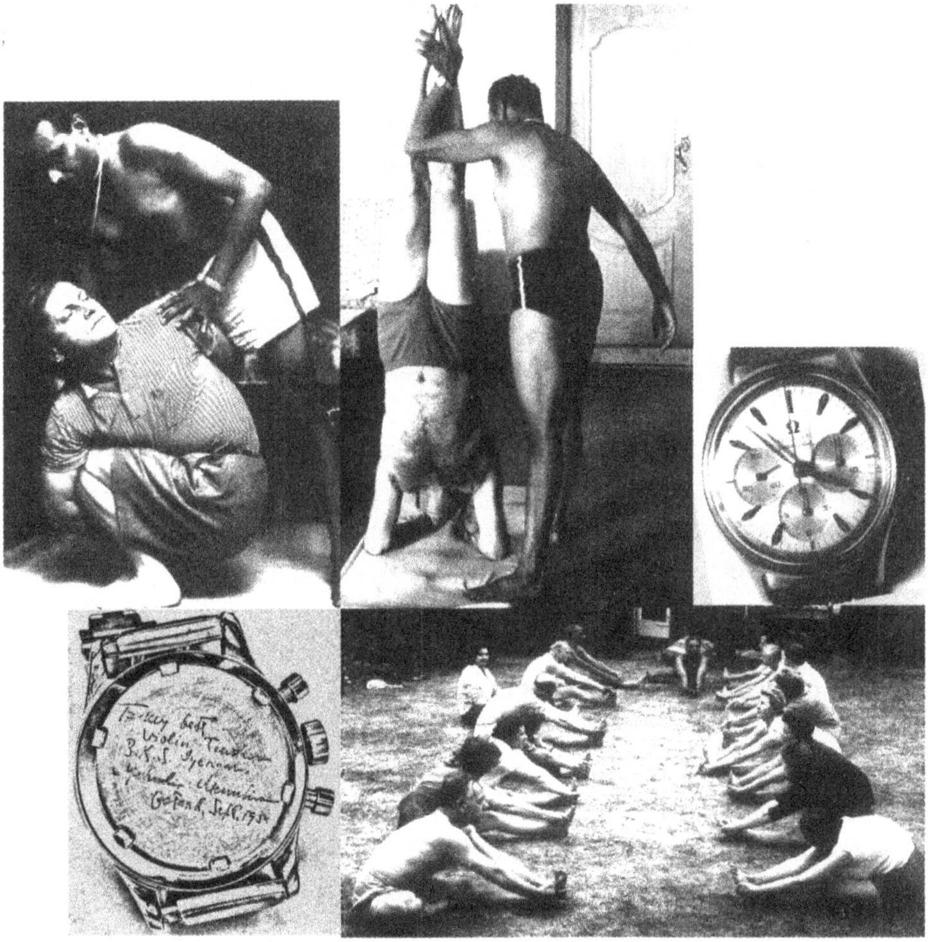

Plate n. 17 – Teaching abroad & the watch given to Iyengar by Yehudi Menuhin

One should join for three months at least just to know the practical use of the subject. However, the learning of yoga is endless and it has to be continued. There is always a beginning to an art but never an end. Art also is meant for evolution, hence I admit all types of people from the poorest to the richest and from the ignorant to the effulgent. I take twenty-five rupees as admission fee and twenty-five rupees as monthly fee for once a week training at my Institute.

Q.- In what way do you think you are different from other yoga teachers?

Well, the only reason could be that I am totally devoted and dedicated to the art of yoga. I am not and I was not ever angling for name or fame. I started in 1936 when nobody had heard of me and my *sādhanā*. Those were the days when I could not afford two meals a day, and yet I have gone into the very depth of yoga and I came up on the strength of my very own hands and legs. In a way I feel I am the pioneer of making yoga popular to reach people with ease.

Q.- Does the teaching of yoga necessitate calm and quiet surroundings?

Not at all. If it were so, then how could yoga cure ill effects of stress and strain? You can practise yoga even in Piccadilly Circus in London. What I mean to say is that the commotion within our body and mind can be channelled perfectly by yoga, anywhere. You are twice blessed if the surroundings are calm and quiet.

Q.- What do you think of these God-men in our country?

Oh, they are a load of rubbish. They have become so called god-men because they have succeeded in exploiting innocent people of their money by instructing them to renounce everything in the name of God. What has happened is that these so-called hoaxes have become richer and richer by cruel and non-ethical methods.

Q.- We have heard of *sadhus* performing such acts as sleeping on a bed of nails at places like Hardwar and Kashi.

That has got nothing to do with yoga. Yoga is for purification of body and mind so that the soul shines. Yoga is not sleeping on a bed of nails, walking through fire, swallowing acids, etc. Yoga sees that the nails of jealousy, lust and hatred do not grow in the mind and body.

Q.- Rakesh Sharma, our first man in space, performed yoga aboard Salyut-7.

I was very happy to know that yoga was performed in space. I do not know which *āsana* Rakesh performed in space, so I can't comment. But some newspaper reports said that the blood circulation was from leg downwards to the brain. That is particularly interesting because I find a clue to the whole thing. Now I know why the ancient sages gave so much importance to standing on the head in yoga. For the practitioners of yoga, the inversions are very important since the blood flows from the legs to the brain. It is not only meant for good circulation but it maintains the discipline of mind, checks hunger and thirst, strengthens the nerves and eradicates the fear of space and loneliness.

Q.- Should a yoga student be a vegetarian only?

Not necessarily. But as you sow, so you reap, and hence as you eat, so is your mind! I do not condition them to be vegetarians. But as the pupils practise, their system rejects such non-vegetarian food and changes them towards vegetarianism. The discipline emerging from within is better than imposed and forced from outside.

Q.- How much time should a busy man give to yoga each day?

Twenty to thirty minutes minimum in a day is good enough.

Q.- Could a mistake in performing a particular *āsana* bring on ill effects?

If you are walking carelessly on the street, you are bound to trip and fall. So also in yoga, similar ill effects are possible if not done properly.

Q.- Can people learn yoga from books?

A good book is better than a bad teacher. So it is up to each person to find a good book to practise from if a teacher is not available. Often, people want books prescribing easy methods of practising yoga. They have to search for the books that are genuine.

Q.- How many books have you written?

Four. One is a life-sketch called *Body Thy Shrine Yoga the Light* (taken out as a memento on my 60th birthday in 1978),[1] *Light on Yoga*, published in eleven languages, *Light on Prāṇāyāma*, published in eight languages and the last one, *Art of Yoga*, is still in the press.[2]

---

[1] A completely revised edition is now available under the title *Iyengar: His Life and Work*, Timeless Books, USA, 1987.

[2] A current list of the works by this author is given in the beginning of this book.

PRĀṆĀYĀMA UNVEILED*

Q.- Mr. Iyengar, you have a school of yoga in the city of Pune, India. There are more and more Iyengar Yoga Centres opening up all over the world. How is it all organised? How are these teachers trained? And we are mostly interested to know how you came to open a school and to have a centre in Pune.

Though I started teaching yoga before I came to Pune in 1937, I could not build an institute or a centre until 1975. I was teaching yoga in educational institutions from 1937 to 1940 but later when the institutions terminated my services, I began teaching individuals and small groups. Only in 1975 did I start the centre. My teachings and my practices must have impressed a great deal on the students who came to learn from me, whom I encouraged to go back and teach. They went back to their countries and started teaching yoga. I not only taught them the art, but also trained them how to teach and what to teach and adapt according to the needs and circumstances, for this subject to become attractive, effective and loveable to students.

Actually, mine is not an organisation at all. Yoga has organised my pupils. It has caused them to become deeply rooted in their practice of this art. The essence of this art has made them come together to form centres for local people to take advantage of yoga as taught by me.[1]

Yoga definitely transforms each individual morally, physically, mentally and spiritually, the moment one takes to its practice. That is how yoga became popular in various countries. Please know that they are called "Iyengar Yoga Centres" or "Iyengar Yoga Institutions" and not "Iyengar Yoga", as many brand my teaching as "Iyengar Yoga". I just gave a new look, new colour and a new touch to the art which is as old as civilisation and hence for this distinctive sake calling this by my name. It is nothing but pure, traditional yoga. For the sake of convenience, my pupils began calling this "Iyengar Yoga", but it is not at all to be called by my name. Please know that yoga is yoga and has no brands.

---

* Interview in Paris by Roger Raziel. Published in the French magazine *Le Monde Inconnu,* October 1985.

[1] see plate n. 2 pp. 41.

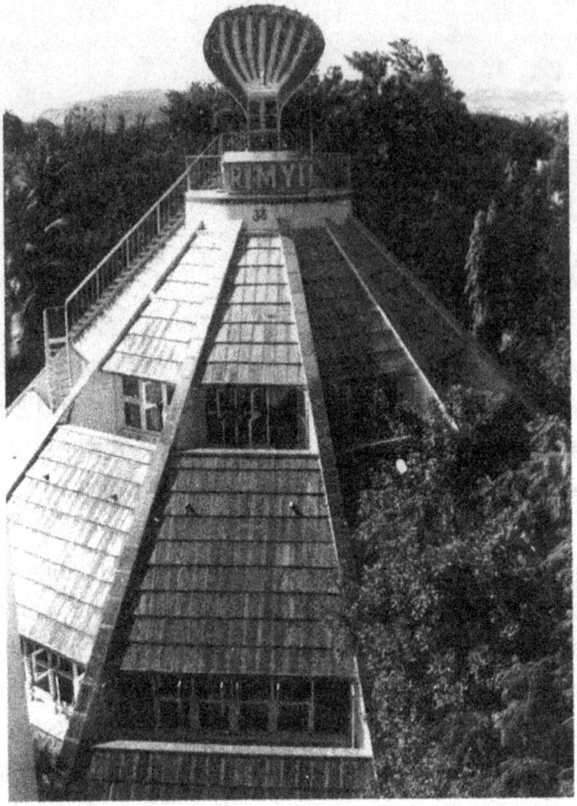

Plate n. 18 – The Ramāmaṇi Iyengar Memorial Yoga Institute, Pune

The early students who became teachers started training their students as teachers with the help of the syllabus that I made by splitting the course that was in my book *Light on Yoga*,[1] and I made them train teachers so that a uniform construction is maintained. First I introduced three categories of gradation as Introductory, Intermediate and Advanced. Later I had to break the courses down further as a safety lock for teachers to teach with comfort so that no untoward injuries take place. They are divided into two Introductory levels, three Junior Intermediate, three Senior Intermediate, three Junior Advanced and two Senior Advanced levels.

As the numbers of teachers and students increased all over, I requested they form regional associations for administrative convenience and issue of certificates. The trainee teachers are examined and assessed with moderators by the association of the respective countries. The associations organise all these matters and when the teachers are certified they teach according to the certificate levels they hold. I do not organise but the associations organise.

---

[1] Harper Collins, London.

Q.- We know that at your Institute in Pune you don't give teachers' training courses. But you try to educate the real yoga practitioners who may one day become yogis. Who is a yogi, according to you?

A yogi is one who can remain silent inside and outside and at the same time not allow any thoughts to touch him. For example, a lunatic speaks outside. An average man, like you and I, speaks internally whereas a yogi does not speak internally or externally.

In our centre I regularly teach yoga. When I am teaching, I give so many points in order to convey the subject matter to the students in totality so that the students are trained to become good teachers. I do not find it necessary to have a teacher training course as my teaching combines throughout both the art of practice and art of teaching at the same time.

Q.- Mr. Iyengar, you wrote five books on yoga which are published in different languages. Of the five books, there is *Light on Yoga*, which is translated in eleven[1] languages and which is known throughout the world as "the Bible of yoga", and *Light on Prāṇāyāma* which is translated into four languages.[2] How, as a traditional yogi, did you come to write pedagogical and didactic books on yoga? Because normally all of the books written on yoga are written by Western people who like too much to speak and write. What was the purpose for you in writing these books?[3]

I had never thought that I would be an author. I had never thought that I would be a yoga student or a yoga teacher. The reader of Allen and Unwin, Mr. Gerald Yorke, saw my practice and told me that he was waiting for a practical book on yoga by a practitioner from the land of yoga which he was keen to publish. So he encouraged me to write if that would be possible. As I had the script already in hand, I showed it to him. On the whole, it took me six years to write *Light on Yoga*. After I had written it about half a dozen times, I gave it to him. He said, "You are a practical teacher", and advised me to write the theory practically and directly without depending on the quotations from the books. Having taught yoga to people who were completely innocent, uninterested, unintelligent and dull as well as those who were eminent philosophers, scientists and artists, I learned human psychology from scratch as I had dull students to highly developed students.

[1] This classic has now run into over seventeen languages - Dutch, English, French, German, Gujarathi, Hindi, Italian, Japanese, Kannada, Korean, Marathi, Polish, Spanish, Russian, Ukrainian, Hungarian and Hebrew.

[2] Now published in thirteen languages: English, French, German, Hindi, Italian, Japanese, Kannada, Korean, Marathi, Persian, Polish, Russian and Spanish.

[3] Both books are published by Harper Collins, London.

This helped me to write with a practical presentation and, on the theory of yoga, in a way which could be understood by the uneducated as well as the elite. And I thought that a good book is better than a bad teacher. Hence, I thought I should give the best of what I knew by reflecting on my own practice and teaching into this book which many consider as 'The Bible of Yoga'.

However, while writing these books, I never intended that these books would guide the yoga teachers too. Being basically a yoga teacher since the day I began yoga, the clarity and explanations came which in turn turned out to be the best guide book for those who wanted to become teachers to teach in the right way.[1] And that is why it seems as though they are pedagogical and didactic.

Q.- How can one practise yoga? How must one begin to practise yoga and what is the aim that he or she must follow in the search through practice?

The aim of yoga, according to Patañjali, is to cleanse the body and the mind so that the impurities of body and mind are eradicated, vanquished and sublimated. This allows each individual to have the vision of the light of the soul with illuminated wisdom. At the same time, it is important to live in innocence; that is, without arrogance and without pride. This is the aim of yoga. In order to achieve this goal, one must start from the body because the body is visible. The body is cognisable, that which can be felt. Hence, the *āsana* were given to understand the movements and functions of the body. Then, from the development of the *āsana*, one is educated to bring the mind in contact with each and every part of the inner body and then towards the self so that the body and self move as a single unit. This way you live in life with balance, harmony, concord and beatitude. In short, we begin with the cult of the body and end with the culture of the soul. This is true and real yogic practice.

Q.- You told us that yoga must be practised according to your teaching of the eight limbs explained by Patañjali. What are these eight limbs? And what is the connection with the practice of yoga?

It is not according that to my teaching the eight limbs of yoga are to be taught, but according to Patañjali's, there are eight aspects of yoga. They are all interrelated and interwoven. They are known as *yama* and *niyama*, or what to do and what not to do. This comes under the ethical

[1] Now the author has published *A Basic Guidelines for Teachers of Yoga*, YOG Publication, Mumbai, 2002. (Co-authored with Geeta S. Iyengar)

discipline. Then comes *āsana* so that each part of the body is not only known but kept healthy: the joints, muscles, circulation, respiration, glandular secretion and excretion. Next comes *prāṇāyāma* so that the energy, which is hidden in the air, is made full use of when drawn in into the system. *Pratyāhāra* is discipline of the mind where the intelligence is made to supersede the memory, or the art of superimposing the memory so that the intelligence comes to the surface with an intensive power of discrimination. These are really the five practices of yoga to begin with. Though there are eight aspects altogether, it is important to understand that the first two, *yama* and *niyama*, are as old as civilisation itself. They are common everywhere and known as the universal way of moral living. Then comes *āsana*, *prāṇāyāma* and *pratyāhāra* for physical perfection, mental poise and intellectual maturity. These three are gained by *āsana, prāṇāyāma* and *pratyāhāra* while *dhāraṇā, dhyāna* and *samādhi* are not practices but the effects of the practice of the earlier five aspects of yoga. These are the properties of yoga which come automatically when these evolutionary methods are maintained with precision and perfection. Hence, *dhyāna* and *samādhi* are the wealth of yoga. They come by themselves, they reveal themselves without effort. That is how we have to practise yoga; to enjoy life's real happiness, peace and poise.

Q.- Now I would like to hear you speak about your last book in French, *Light on Prāṇāyāma*. What is the word *prāṇāyāma?* What does it mean and how can it be practised?

It is very difficult to define *prāṇa*, though I have, to some extent, succeeded in understanding and explaining what *prāṇa* is. When two stones are hit together, there is a light, which sparks out, and that spark is the *prāṇa* of those two stones. Similarly, in the air, there are lots of hidden energies. The air includes also ions, which are necessary for the chemical quality of the blood. The circulatory system maintains the supply of energy through the blood supply to the various parts of the body. This process is enhanced by the practice of *prāṇāyāma*.

Prāṇa means energy and *āyāma* means distribution or spreading by extension and expansion. So in order to distribute that *prāṇa,* the lungs take in the energy that is drawn in through the breath. The air is made to move to the extremities of the lungs so that the air-cells or air-sacs or alveoli, which are known as *vāyu-koṣa* – where the air is received and stored –, draw this inhaled energy to pump into the blood. The inhalation therefore is done in such a way that through this process of respiration the energy is spread to the nooks and corners of the body. Between each inhalation and exhalation there is a pause and that is known as retention. This retention is enhanced in *prāṇāyāmic* way. This retention is to see that the drawn in energy is made to move farther and farther into the system so that each cell gets a chance to rejuvenate itself to do its job. This is known as retention of breath. Then comes exhalation. Exhalation is to remove the unwanted air, which cannot supply energy. Here, the breath is released gradually, so that the residue of the energy can be absorbed by the organs before the exhalation is complete. This allows time for the cells to reabsorb the energy and hence it is called deep exhalation. After exhalation there is again a pause. This pause is again extended so that the energy is further taken and received by the entire system. Let me compare this to our food-processing within the system. We eat food. Inhalation is like eating the food. Inhalation-retention is like digestion. Exhalation is like absorption and exhalation-retention is like assimilation.

There are various types of *prāṇāyāma* and these varieties are meant to irrigate the energy like water supply to each area. In *prāṇāyāma* the *bandha* are introduced which are like dykes or dams.

In short *prāṇāyāma* is like the process through which the energy is generated, organised and distributed so that the whole human system including the mind, intelligence and consciousness is made full use of to function with concord and harmony. Hence, *prāṇāyāma* is very important to each and every individual in order to live a happy and relaxed life.

Q.- According to the *tantruṁ* or *tantric* texts, the aim of *prāṇāyāma* is the awakening of *kuṇḍalinī*, the snake-shaped energy, which is in the basis or root of the spinal column. This awakening, this stimulation of *kuṇḍalinī* – isn't it dangerous and doesn't it cause bad effects on the practitioner who is not ready?

It is true that when the body and the nerves are not strong enough, any extremes, whether they are good or bad, are bound to affect the personality. In *prāṇāyāma*, we are all aware of the *iḍā* and *piṅgaḷā* which are known as the lunar nerve and solar nerve which carry lunar and solar energy respectively. They are on either side of the spine, and the *cakra* are hidden within the spinal cord.[1] Due to this deep and finer filter method of drawing in breath, energy is able to accelerate in these two nerves which are connected to the *cakra* and criss-cross at each *cakra*. These *cakra* are wells of stored energy. They are chambers in our system. When the energy is made to move through *iḍā* and *piṅgaḷā* with *prāṇāyāmic* practice, this energy gets charged into a very subtle and powerful form with its various attributes; then it is allowed to pass through the special nerve or *nāḍī* called *citrā* which runs in the interior of the *suṣumṇā*. This newly generated energy gives a new life – a nectar of life or an *amṛta* of life known as the *kuṇḍalinī*. When two stones are struck together they produce light. Similarly, these two nerves, *iḍā* and *piṅgaḷā*, come

[1] See in the author's *Aṣṭadaḷa Yogamālā* vol 2, the articles *Viṇādaṇḍa*, "Physiology of *Cakra*", and "*Cakra, Bandha* and *Kriyā*".

close to each other and remain in a well balanced state due to the practice of *prāṇāyāma*. That is how a new energy is produced. This new energy then circulates in the system and pervades all the cells of the body. It circulates not only in the gross body but in the subtle body too. If it is worked out gradually, there is no danger. But people with motivation struggle very hard to charge this life force without knowing their own capacities; without knowing whether or not they can hold this divine energy when produced within. Instead of paying attention to produce this energy, if they concentrate on the correct way of doing *prāṇāyāma* to improve their physical, mental and moral health and bring their senses of perception under control with renewed intelligence and awareness, then there is no danger at all of what you have asked.

Often, people have a wrong notion that to awaken the *kuṇḍalinī* they have to force their body and breath. Therefore, they use wrong methods to do *prāṇāyāma*. Any forceful action has to lead to some danger. That is why *prāṇāyāma* is said to be very dangerous – for the simple reason that people go for the effect before they have mastered *prāṇāyāma*. In order to enjoy food you have to cook, which is laborious. Similarly, you have to learn *prāṇāyāma* well before you want to savour the nectar or essence of *prāṇāyāma*. You take the fragrance of a flower carefully with inhalation. When *prāṇāyāma* is done, it is important to feel the fragrance of the breath, not the force of breath which, in fact, can be dangerous.

Q.- It has been said that yoga develops the powers. In one word, can you say what these powers are?

When you are happy with someone or you like someone, do you not give yourself to the person? Similarly when you conquer the elements of the body, mind, senses of perception, *prāṇic* energy, emotions, intelligence, consciousness, conscience along with its constituents of *sattva*, *rajas* and *tamas*, they do present you their special and specific qualities and powers. In yogic terms, these powers are known as *siddhi*.

You know that Patañjali in the third chapter, has definitely said that thirty-four powers come through the practice of yoga. Actually, these powers come to the *sādhaka* as a guide to know whether or not he is on the right path. It is not necessary to get caught up in their effect, and Patañjali clearly mentions that these powers appear as supernatural to others whereas for the practitioners they are hindrances towards meditation and *samādhi*. Hence, like astrology, which tells about future events and warns one to be careful and plan accordingly, similarly, the accomplishments of these powers are meant to know that the practices are correct. Therefore, one can proceed further towards the ultimate goal, the liberation. Beyond this, they are of no value at all. If we are caught in these powers, we are worse off. We become worse than non-yogic practitioners in our behaviours.

Q.- We always talk about the fact that to practise yoga, one must leave the world, become completely detached and observe asceticism. And yet, in your case it is completely different. You are a householder. You have your wife and children. You gave them a good education. You practise your yoga without stopping. So how did you come to arrange the situation in this way?

The question is long but my answer will be short. You know, if I renounce the world, why should I practise yoga? If there are no ups and downs in life, which is the life of a *sannyāsin*, then why does yoga have to be practised? So this was the idea in me to live like all other people and still benefit from yoga. Was yoga meant for only *sannyāsin* or was it meant for ordinary people? So I determined myself to live the life of a householder as the *ṛṣi* like *Yājñvalkya* and *Vaśiṣṭha*, to face the upheavals of the world and at the same time to continue practising yoga with poise. And I say that I have succeeded. As I have succeeded, I am preaching and teaching that yoga is for a common man more than for a *sannyāsin* or a renunciate.

THE ART OF TEACHING*

Q.- *Guruji*, it's three years since a Canadian group came to Pune for an intensive. During those three years you've done a lot of travelling. Would you speak about the changes that have occurred during that period – both in your personal work and the work that is being carried on in your name all over the world.

In me, the change is maturity in yoga. My experience in this field and in my own practice has helped me to go to the core of the subject. I cannot say anything more than this.

As far as the second part of your question is concerned, I think the work has been carried out very well by my students. My only fear is that people emphasise things where very little emphasis is required, and do not pay attention where attention needs to be paid. If this barrier is taken off and work on a missionary zeal for propagating yoga, the work will have a better background. Otherwise, I am afraid that it may get stale soon. It should not get stale. The change is that many more have begun to believe in yoga and are coming forward to learn.

Q.- Have you seen this happening?

Yes, I have seen many getting attracted towards yoga. Therefore, the teachers too need to refresh their knowledge. For example, there is a proverb: "Out of sight, out of mind". People who come here regularly and hear the same words hammered in again and again, naturally develop a grip and then they begin to understand the depth of it. Unfortunately others come only once and go away without asking themselves whether they have understood or not. For instance, India is a hot country. Even in winter a little rest here does not disturb the body. The blood current continues to flow to the extremities, so we can afford a little more relaxation. The cold is severe in many Western countries and here the explanations are too long and hence the warmth of the body

---

*Interview by Shirley Daventry French, Leslie Hogya, Jim Rischmiller and Karen Fletcher, from Canada, and Caroline Coggins and Peter Thompson from Australia. Published in *The Yoga Centre of Victoria Newsletter*, May 1986 and September 1986.

disappears which may take time to get recharged. This is one of the ways to think and adapt between the East and the West. In the West, the teacher should be careful to see that the body remains warm. If the body is cold, even when the correct technique is given, the body does not respond to it soon, therefore the explanations lose their charm. You have to demarcate and balance words of explanation to go into action without getting cold in the body, but maintain warmth. Never take more time than needed.

I am also seeing that teachers try to explain so much in one day that they exhaust themselves as well as their pupils. Teachers should break their sentences, see whether the student and his body mechanism have absorbed the instructions. Explain the key point for the student to catch, then add a few more words of explanation at a later time.

In the West teachers are not differentiating between untrained beginners and someone who has been practising for years. Teachers should observe how much the pupil can absorb; otherwise what is the use of expressing pride and boasting of intelligence? It's of absolutely no value unless the pupil can receive it. When we run classes we give our technique and present how the *āsana* should be done because we know the subject, but at the same time we see what mistakes are happening. This is the feedback system. A teacher has to capture the weakness of the pupils and build points from there for them to get better; this will make the teacher a good teacher, and also help the pupils to become good *sādhaka*.

Maturity in the pupils comes as the teacher matures. That is what I say is lacking here and when that develops, I say, "Wonderful".

Q.- There's more patience in India than in the West.

It is not just enough to have patience. Do you mean to say that there is no impatience here? Though patience is a must, it does not solve the problems. One has to put in an effort to work out ways to find means to eradicate problems. Impatience and restlessness do not.help. Enough patience is needed to think right and act right. In India your brain may say, "I want to get this *āsana* today", but can your body take it, can your knee take it, can your spine take it? If your arm is injured and you cannot lift it, what is the use of saying I want you to lift it? The range of movement must be understood – that range may be too much or too little. This study of range of movement has to be co-ordinated. It is not impatience, it is skilfulness in understanding.

Unlike anatomy, *āsana* have to be taught to living bodies and practised by living bodies. Although many western people have an intellectual knowledge of anatomy and physiology and name different parts of the body, they don't really understand their functions. Only *āsana* can teach this. We cannot depend on anatomy alone to teach yoga because it does not give the whole picture.

The practice of *āsana* makes you feel the body from within. It creates a special intelligent sensitivity in the doer. It makes one analyse one's own movements, one's own actions. *Āsana* makes one feel and experience one's own body.

Analysis and experience have to go together. Teaching is analysing the students' physical and mental calibre. Then the teacher has to discover and find out the ways of bringing their deficient part at par with the other part of the body which is healthy and smooth in presentation. The teacher's mind has to think how to use the background of knowledge, use the right skill and find ways to work on their mind.

Sometimes an ignorant man does better than an intelligent man. Why does this man without having intelligence present well? Why does the other with such understanding commit a mistake? Compare the bodies. This is the art of earning factual intelligence from which you gain knowledge for better teaching and build up good relationship with the taught.

- *That's the science of yoga.* -

Yes, that's the science of yoga. I know the *āsana*, I know the technique of the *āsana*, but I also have to know how this technique is going to help the individual, because technique for me is science. What I say about *āsana* is applicable to all other aspects of yoga.

I have been teaching for years; people love my work, although they were criticising before. It has withstood the test on account of dedicated students. I am happy that this good work is going well on account of students like you all.

Q.- In the intensive, Geeta's explanations are very clear and I've appreciated the focus on each step and the progression. She is really emphasising the correct order of practice. Are you taking more time to emphasise this?

There should be rhythm in yoga. In music, unless there's tune and tone, do you listen to the music? What is the body, after all, but an instrument of yourself? And the vibration like the sound is the tune. The vibration in my body must synchronise with my movements. That is why *āsana* are done in a certain order. They are known as cycles. We can group these cycles, but for certain persons they may not work at all. So we have to show another group of cycles according to their body. You know that in cars they have four or five gears. Can you change the gear without coming to the neutral?

- *No, you'd grind the gears.* -

It is the same in yoga. We lose our tempers when we see people suddenly do the back arch, or suddenly they go back over the rope. What happens without coming to the basic and neutral *āsana*?

- *Injury*. -

Now, what is neutral? If you do a back arch, you cannot immediately do forward bends. *Bharadvājāsana* is a neutral gear. How many people know the neutral gears? Three or four standing *āsana* and in between you are made to do *Uttānāsana* which acts as a neutral gear. I am telling people now to trace the neutral gear. When they make a mistake, I bring them back to the cycle. This prevents injury to any part of the body.

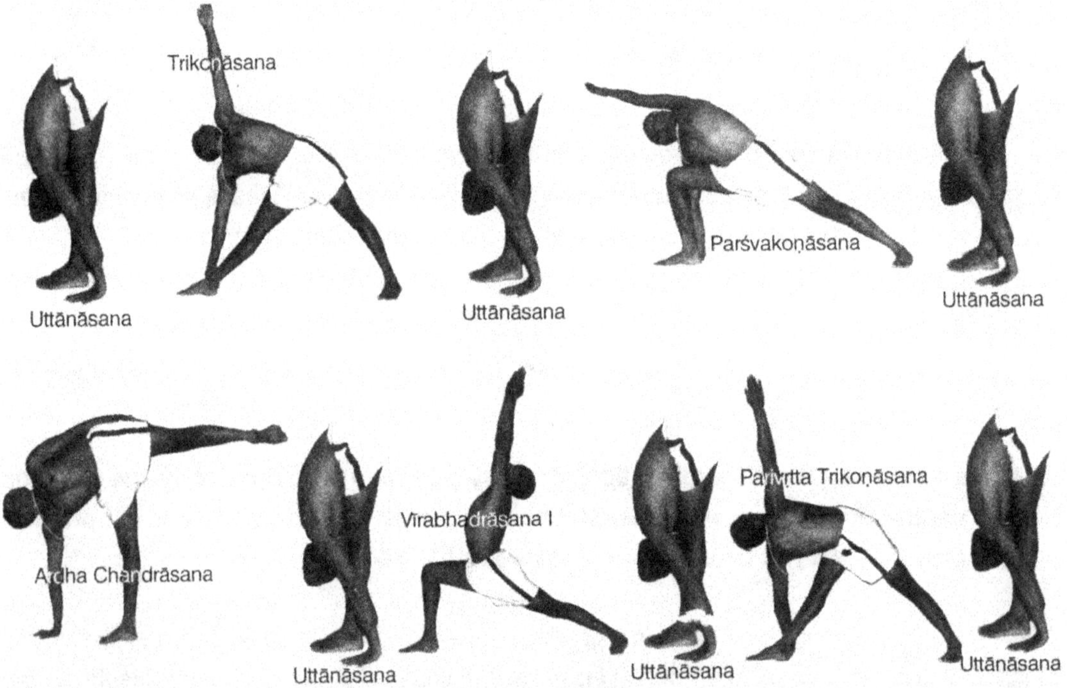

Plate n. 19 – Standing *āsanas* with *Uttānāsana* as a neutral *āsana*

First the teacher should demonstrate the *āsana* two or three times, then stand and take the class. If the pupils have not understood, show it again twice more, and then the third time do it with them saying, "Look at me. Look at my leg. Look at my hand. Look at my other leg." In the beginning if the teacher works thirty minutes, the pupils have to work only twenty minutes. After one month the teacher will be working twenty minutes, the pupil will be working thirty minutes.

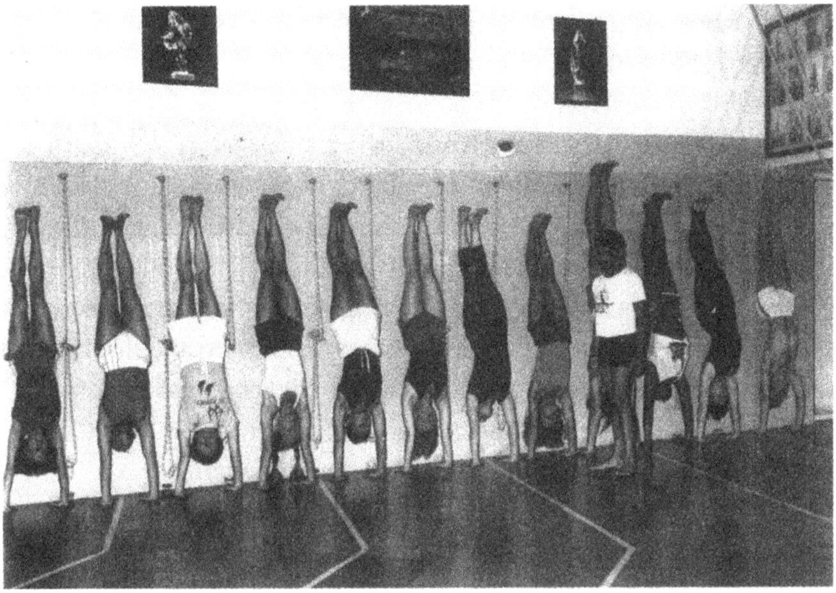

Plate n. 20 – Class in full-arm balance

When I am doing the *āsana* with my pupils my practice improves, and also I know what as the area that has to be attended to throughout in the practice of that *āsana*, then from that point I can see the whole class, from one end to the other end with ease.

Teachers should also be very mobile. There are two types of teaching. First you should know the technique of the *āsana*. Secondly you must understand the intellect of the heart or the emotional feeling. Take *Sālamba Śīrṣāsana* – head balance. Technically I know the *āsana*, but according to emotions, I change. The thick muscle of the thigh, you have to make thin. Technique cannot be given there. The technique is from my experience, and the change in the technique here is from the student's presentation. "What techniques do I have to adapt in order to change the position of this person who is presenting differently"? That is what the teacher has to think. A technique can be created on the spot because that has to happen on the pupil's body. That is what the teachers have to learn, and if they learn, these teachers will be on top in the art of teaching. Take it from me, these teachers cannot be shaken. Even what little they know, they present very well. They will be better teachers than those teachers who say "I can teach this, I can teach that". One can teach variety but to teach skill is very difficult and challenging too.

If only you can put all this together, then you will understand how to lessen and remove the pain if any. One link can pull the chain down. We have hundreds of links in our body which help the body to function. One muscle is dependent on the other. We have to come to the basic end root to find where this muscle is holding. Then you develop in the art of teaching and become a good teacher with this sound grip. Then the foundation in you becomes stable and cannot be shaken by any means. This is what I want.

Intellectually you are all very good, but what about emotionally? Human beings live 90% emotionally. Can you stay one day in the Himalayas in a lonely place alone? It is a known fact that you cannot because you are all living emotionally. You want someone to share the experience. Mind is connected to the emotional feelings: brain has an intellectual feeling. A balanced personality is one whose intelligence of the heart is connected with the intelligence of the head, and the intellectual seat of the head with the emotional seat of the heart. In yoga, when we are doing the *āsana*, we have to connect the intelligence with emotion and synchronise these two with the body. We have to use the *āsana*, otherwise the mind becomes empty.

The following has been given as an explanation by the author:

Observe the first two *Śīrṣāsana*, **(a & b)** if you look at the direction the body is moving, how the various parts of the body are positioned in relation to each other you can see if its focus is in the centre or core of the practitioner.

For many it never meets in the core/centre. The upper-body – arms and shoulders – work well, but the lower-body – thighs and shins are working in different directions. Though the *Śīrṣāsana* (a) looks as well balanced . . . if we reverse the image, as if she is standing in *Tāḍāsana*, you can then understand how it would be impossible to stand like that. The students *āsana* is not working according to a rhythmic inner sense of balance, the efforts are not equal throughout. The awareness and consequently the work in the *āsana* only reaches up to the waist, as a result the legs are loose, the pelvis and tailbone are going backwards and the thighs are forward. The various parts of the body in the *āsana* do not have their link and placement in balance with each other. The effort in the *āsana* is unequal. The practitioner has concentrated her awareness more on the upper-body, but not on the pelvis, legs and feet.

Again look at the next four *āsana* – **(c), (d), (e)** and **(f)** – in one way or the other there is some part of the *āsana* that is not working in a unified way. The struggle to maintain the *āsana* vertically is coming from the head, but all the parts of the *āsana* are not equal to each other. The resolution of all the forces of the *āsana* have not yet met with the intelligence of the heart.

In (g) though a raw student, we can see how with awareness the different parts of the *āsana* can be brought to a more unified whole. The perceptions of the *āsana* from the inside are equal to how the *āsana* is working from the outside, the student has worked rhythmically, evenly with both the intelligence of the heart and the intelligence of the head.

What is the difference between *āsana* and *dhyāna?* Don't you experience calmness and tranquillity in a good head balance? Don't you experience serenity when you are resting very well in *Sarvāṅgāsana, Halāsana* or *Setubandha Sarvāṅgāsana*? (see page n. 245) That means you are doing meditation even though you are in the *āsana*. You are connected to the body and at the same time you are detached.

Meditation, as it is ordinarily taught, leads you to emptiness. There is a disconnection between the body and the soul and in-between there is emptiness. But when you do *Halāsana*, the mind is not distracted from the body or from the soul and that is known as fullness.

In other methods they are controlled by the heads. But I give a free hand to each and every one of my students to study and understand how to co-ordinate the mind and the brain while doing and teaching. You people have to come and work together in order to maintain good friendliness or rapport. I can only be a guide but I cannot control. It is against my principles.

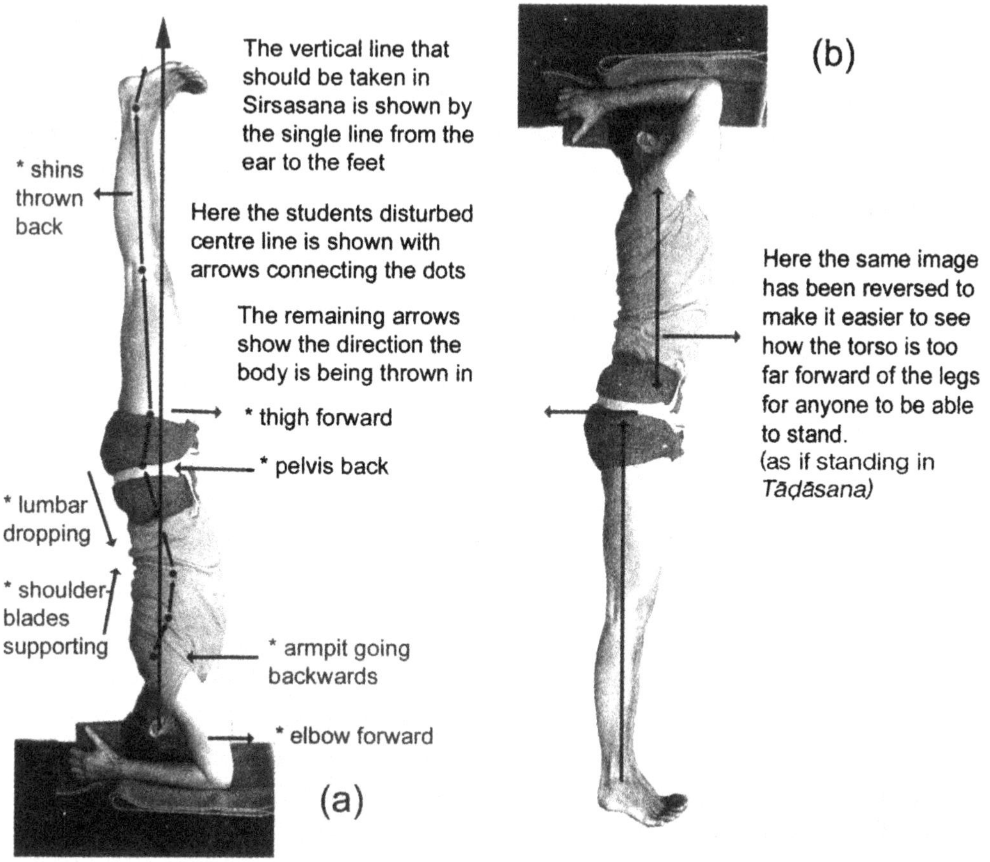

Plate n. 21 – Intelligence of the head and heart

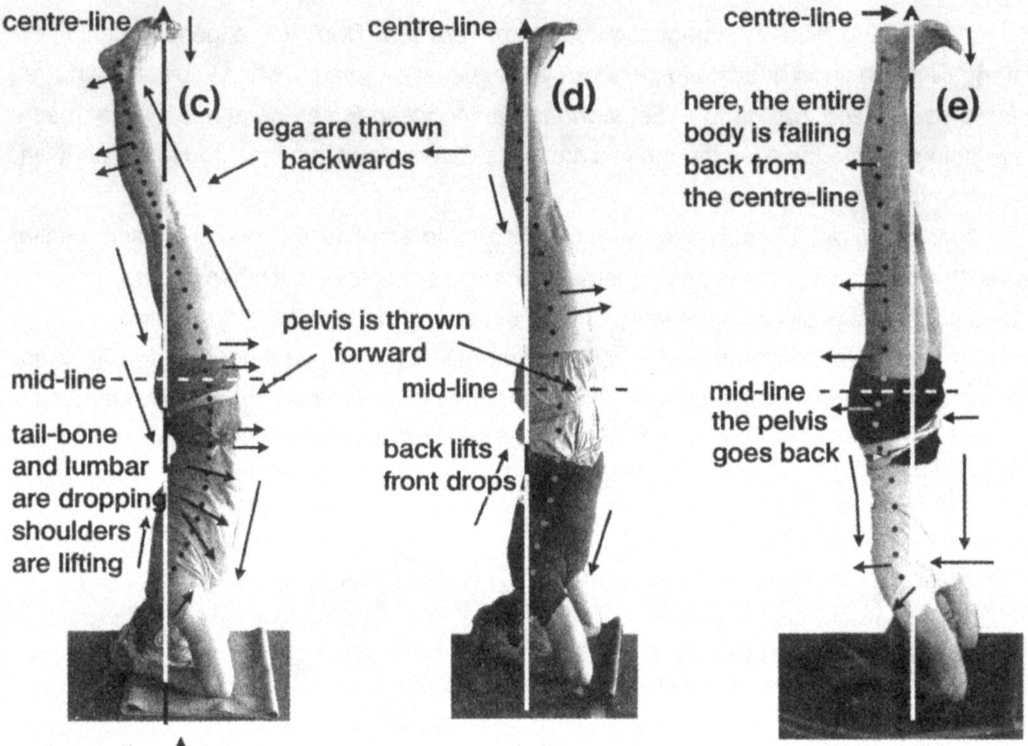

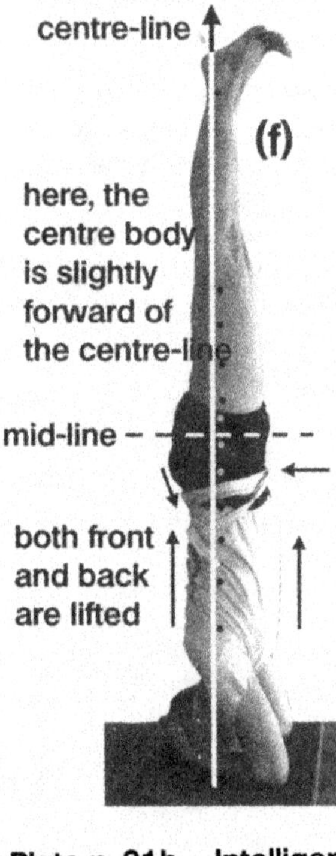

(In the *Śīrṣāsana,* the centre of the ear has been used for the axis of the centre-line, for the *Sarvāṅgāsana* it is from the centre of the arm-pit)
From (c) to (f) there is a progression as the student learns to balance the outer border of the body with the core of the *āsana*
in (g) the centre and the core are rhythmically maintained

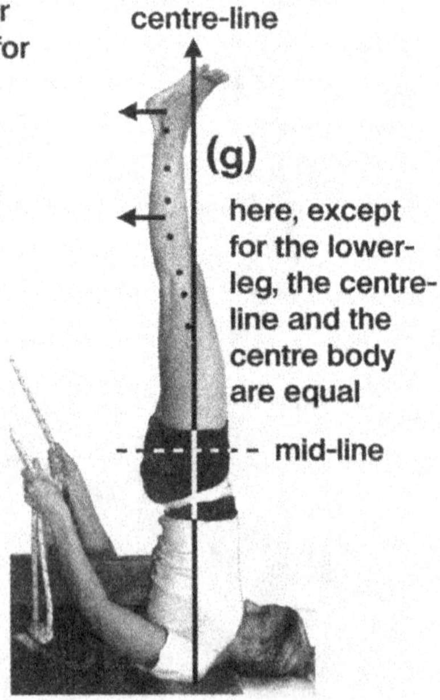

Plate n. 21b – Intelligence of the head and heart (cont.)

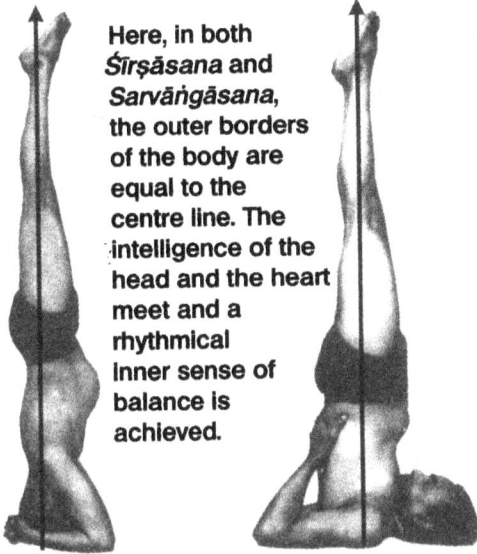

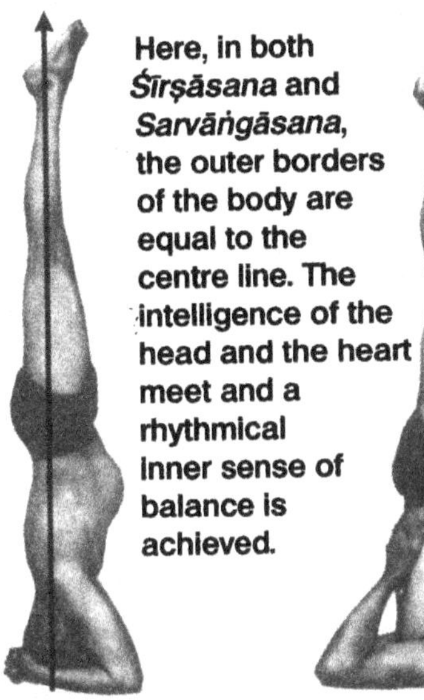
Here, in both *Śīrṣāsana* and *Sarvāṅgāsana*, the outer borders of the body are equal to the centre line. The intelligence of the head and the heart meet and a rhythmical inner sense of balance is achieved.

Plate n. 21 – Intelligence of the head and heart (cont.)

My control is in the *āsana*. For me this art is God, and my job is to correct you in that art. If you go wrong in your way of living it is my job to guide you; but what more can I do, tell me?

Q.- What do you mean when you talk about people abusing your name?

As people respect my work, many use my name saying that they are following my way of practice. How true it is I do not know. Is it not in a way abuse? This way I feel the art gets a bad name and the art is God. For me

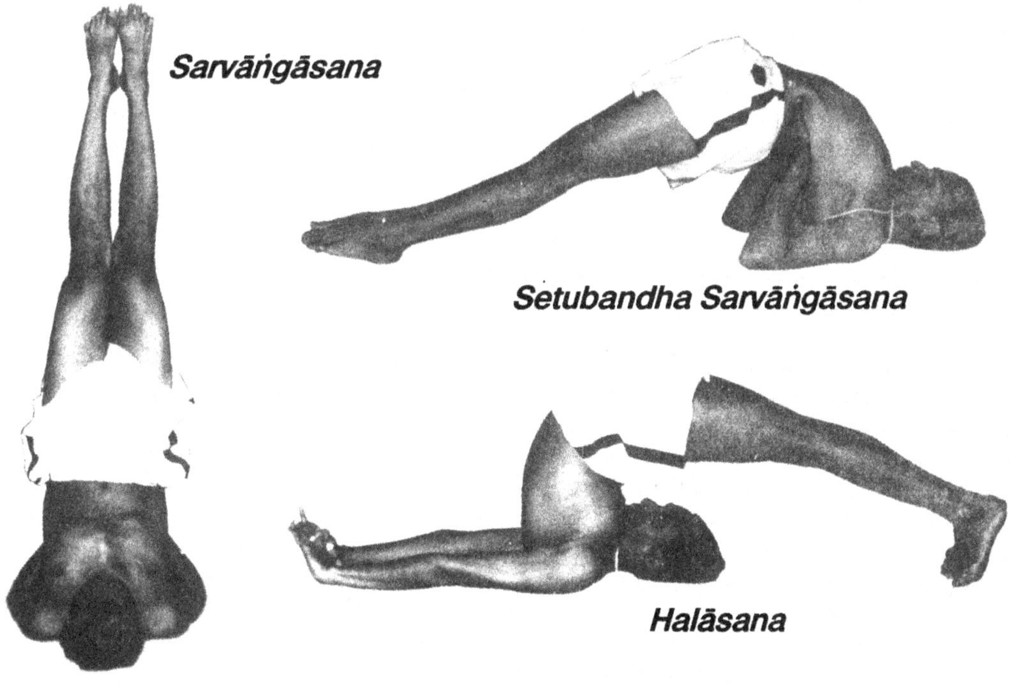
Sarvāṅgāsana
Setubandha Sarvāṅgāsana
Halāsana

Plate n. 21c – Intelligence of the head and heart (cont.)

the *āsana* is my God. The moment I ridicule that art, then what respect have I got? We have to decide whether the art is important or the individuals are important. If we do not cultivate individualism, I think yoga will grow very well.

Q.- One of the problems, I think, is that there seem to have been some teachers that have not stayed close to your teaching.

It is said, you cannot fool all the people, all the time, is it not? You can fool only one, once in a while. Do you mean to say I could not have adopted into my system all these simple methods that are going on today? To make name and fame some are saying that they have found out something new. This is the reason for some to stay away. Yoga has become a saleable product. Under the name of yoga, people do anything that they want. Consumers have to be careful.

When you have learned from Yehudi Menuhin, would you like to go to an ordinary teacher to learn violin and give his name? Why then in yoga? They put ten names of yoga teachers and people think, "Oh, he must have got a lot of knowledge from so many people". This is your intellectual defect which has created the problem. You think that by going to many teachers you may develop more intelligence, you may grasp some more points. You do not become intelligent by gathering knowledge. The intelligence gets matured by one's own experiment and experience. Know that body has its own factual intelligence. It has to digest before you take somebody's words for action. Many people have adapted my ways but my own students are throwing them out later.

I want you all to come together. Unfortunately I have not one person in the world with whom I can exchange experiences. I am apart; I am alone, but I am not lonely, I am not empty; I am full. Whereas many of you have this opportunity for exchange of thoughts. Instead of taking advantage of this, you just fight with each other as if one knows better than the other.

Really, what a chance you people have to get ideas from each other! If you all exchange, then where is room for friction? All of you have learnt yoga from me. So get together and exchange thoughts so that you all live closer to the art.

Those teachers who learn from me but do not stay close to my teaching, I would say, it is their bad luck. Moreover, there are many who have put less efforts to learn but started teaching since yoga has gained popularity with my earlier efforts. Many use my name because my name adds to their recognition. Humbleness is the key for learning. Those who stay away definitely loose the in-depth that contains in this art and science.

Q.- Do you think having an association would help us come together and share more?

An association is meant to bring one another together to exchange inner experiences, to exchange ideas. From that angle I say it is worth having. Also it's necessary, so that pupils will know who the bonafide teachers are. Nowadays people are using my name though they have never learnt from me, or even from my pupils. They take *Light on Yoga*[1] and say, "I am a student of Iyengar because I follow his book". That is not the right way. In order to stop this we have to have an association where we can come and discuss things as a single family. If we all put aside our personalities and work together, we can bring a big change in the way of living.

Again, the association can question those who teach something else using my name and also it can question if someone does not stay closer to my teaching.

I like to emphasise that the association must act as a co-ordinating unit and not as an authoritative unit.

Q.- In Australia, and I also think in America, people are going to many different places to learn yoga from many different teachers. What is your feeling on that?

My feeling is that unless and until a beginner sticks to one teacher for a long period, one cannot differentiate between the teaching of one teacher and another. Maturity does not come by going to different people. Only doubts increase. It is for publicity's sake one says, "I have been to so and so, so and so, and so on. So I know more". What does one learn in the end? Nil, except pride. One has to be clear with one person, then when one goes to a second person the clarity which one developed earlier will help him to discriminate differences in teaching. But when one is raw, if one listens to ten people, one ends up with raw knowledge only and more confusion. To run after teachers is not a good sign for the pupil.

A base has to be established. Once you have found a reliable teacher, why should you want to search for another? If you have not learned what the first teacher has taught, what is the use of going to a second teacher? When you have exhausted the first person's knowledge, then find a better teacher; there's nothing wrong in that. Or the teacher might tell you, "I have given you all I know, now find out for yourself". This is the right method.

In London I suggested to have a guinea pig class for teachers' training – ten experienced teachers to take it in turns to teach a class. Make notes of all that has been explained. The next time the same *āsana* should be taught by another teacher and so on. Continue for a month. Find

[1] Harper Collins, London.

the variations in explanations; then find out how to connect them. Then this could become the syllabus for other yoga teachers.

I have seen that teachers teach certain points according to their own mobility. This is wrong. You have to teach according to the pupil's mobility. The subject is being approached intellectually whereas the defect in the body is emotional. Suppose, you have a knee pain. It requires intelligence to move and use that aching knee in a proper way. However, the intelligence doesn't feel the pain – the heart does. The knee pain pricks the heart and your emotions surface in the heart. Therefore, while working on that knee you have to move, bend or extend that knee carefully as though that knee is your baby. You cannot be aggressive on the knee. That is how one has to deal with the knee emotionally.

I also know of some very well-known teachers with certain defects in their spine, who are teaching the *āsana* according to those defects. If it were me, I would say, "Unfortunately, I have got this defect, the problem interfered in my tail bone. So don't follow me regarding that defective area. I may feel sorry for my defect but I explain the right way, how it should be for all of you to do. Do not copy me", this is how I say. I request them to do as I say but not to do as I present. Explaining the weakness of mine, I say, "Follow the correct method". *(Laughter).* I would be honest; while others give explanations according to their own bodies – how the energy should move and so on. For me it is wrong teaching. Unfortunately pupils don't question them because they think they are such experienced teachers. In workshops, teachers should express their weaknesses and then guide the new ones.

In India, I would say, "How much did you collect from the brain?", because they remain attached to the teachers emotionally. They accept the teachers' words. Here, I have to inquire, "Did the body catch what was said?". That is the difference. You want to catch everything intellectually, therefore, the teaching comes from the brain and not from the heart. The teaching has to be from heart though the subject has to be known through the brain. The tendency to gather knowledge without deliberation, verification and experience makes people go from one teacher to the other.

As teachers, it is the duty of all of you to give them the feel of experience since yoga is an experiential knowledge.

Don't be carried away by techniques; but study the needs of man to man, and teach. Commune with each other. Give the understanding to those who come to you. One can certainly go to other teachers to further knowledge. But that knowledge should be linked to the basic knowledge. Whereas those who go to other schools and change the methods, should know well that by teaching mixed methods they are not helping but harming the students. The teachers who mix will never be able to solve the physical or mental problems of their students. So my feeling and logical deliberation is that they should first understand one method properly and thoroughly before thinking of going to other teachers.

Q.- As well as the tendency towards going to different teachers, there is also a tendency towards workshops for this and workshops for that. What is your feeling about that?

It is almost identical to the previous question, I do not know whether in these workshops both the teacher and those who attend practise with a religious approach. If they are conducted without a right exchange of knowledge, such workshops are bad in taste. Until the pupils have the grip of what they have learnt and are doing, it's no good going to workshops. The participants should have a grip on the subject. When I say grip, I mean maturity: physical maturity, mental maturity and intellectual grasp as well as tone in the body. If such pupils go to a workshop they understand something, because they have already a foundation. In that foundation, if something is not properly taught, they can question, "No, I am getting this, you are explaining that. So what is the right method?"

There should be scope to learn in workshops – scope to exchange views and to question. If they're not getting a certain feeling, they have to ask, "How to get that feeling?" Then a workshop has a meaning for developing one's maturity.

– *Sharing.* –

Ah, for sharing. There need not be a workshop. As far as I get information, it is not sharing – it is a gathering. In a gathering, there is the tendency to make and take ideas without experiences. So first put into practice on yourself the ideas you make or take and then teach them to others.

Here I want to bring to your notice certain things. You see the workshops are conducted by different teachers and different schools. When you enroll your name to these workshops, the teachers do not know you, your body, mind, capacity, grasp of the subject and behaviour. The teachers teach and you follow. You do not even absorb anything. While learning yoga there is a tremendous involvement of both the teacher and pupils. They too need to understand each other. They have to come close to each other for the benefit of both. This does not happen in workshops. In workshops the teacher pours and students gather.

Yoga is a very tricky subject and there has to be a moulding or blending between the body, intelligence and emotion.

Q.- It seems to me that rather than having a fixed structure of grades of teachers, what you are talking about is having teachers able to come together and formulate some sort of standard. In other words, perhaps a convention of Iyengar Yoga teachers.

Yes, it could be made. I have suggested already in America that they should not have international but national conventions. When many people come to Pune, they should amalgamate and constructively build up a programme from what has been learned here. As I suggest, they should collect ideas from teachers and students, then work out alphabetically simple to complex *āsana* with sequential, progressive teaching points about what can be taken where and how. This will wonderfully build in you all a right background. Then the workshop has meaning.

Amalgamation is important. Once this is established I can see what is missing and make suggestions for improvement. This way you build up by yourselves. I am economising the time and stress of you all provided you take the responsibility of doing the way in which I am asking.

It's a difficult proposition but this is what I suggest; this exchange has come to a standstill as some are complaining that I have interfered regarding holding of workshops. I am suggesting that when local teachers are available, why should others come and hold workshops? Is it to make money or to do devoted service? If one can give more than what the local teachers can impart, it is a different matter. In that case the local teacher has to clarify to the invited teacher where he or she has a blind spot and how he can guide the teacher as well as the pupils to proceed from where they were stuck.

I want the teachers to learn from each other before thinking of workshops. A teacher cannot go from one place to the other place and confuse the students more. Often this is what I see happening.

There are hundreds of teachers in your countries. Why don't they all come together, find out weak points and good points? Learn how to remove the weak points and build up strength and confidence. This cannot become an organisation but one yogic soul.

God gave you what He did not give me. I had no one with whom to exchange views, I myself had to work on my own as if I was of two personalities. So I had to question myself, experiment with and challenge myself. Today instead of exchanging views, many are squabbling among themselves over who is better than whom? If you are better in *Utthita Trikoṇāsana*, the other may be better in the back arch. And you should not consider that the back arch is far superior because you can't do *Utthita Trikoṇāsana*. Exchange good points by collection and correction. Then the spirit of yoga establishes well in you all.

Q.- *Gurujī*, another question which refers to teachers' training as well. It is very obvious to those of us who work with you how your work integrates all the eight limbs of yoga. This is a spiritual practice which we do here; the Institute is a temple. People who come here, and who are open, see this very clearly, but you talked the other day about how, in the West particularly, people use their intellect and get involved in technique. Have you any suggestions for understanding and studying the *sūtras* in the West? It's not part of our culture, the way it is for you.

The *Sūtra* of Patañjali are difficult, they will not convey the depth of understanding very easily. I would prefer people to read epics such as the *Rāmāyaṇa*. Get a background of yoga from this culture. In the *Purāṇa*, each story has a philosophical background. It gives what we call the *saṁskāra*, a sort of spiritual behaviour or life of the *ṛṣī*. Stories are better than just reading philosophy. Each story is full of moral practices. No doubt the *Yoga Sūtra* could help you, but how do you translate them into your practices unless and until you are well equipped to translate the meaning?[1] The *Sūtra* are the cream. But in order to know the cream you should know something gross through the *Purāṇa*: the *Rāmāyaṇa, Mahābhārata, Bhāgavata*. *Rāmāyaṇa* is the life of Rāma, *Mahābhārata* is the historical war in which you come to know how Lord Krishna guides and *Bhāgavata* is full of stories on the life of Lord Krishna. These three books will give a good background for spiritual upliftment. I recommend these books since they give the idea of the ancient culture of yoga and applications of yogic principles at the testing period of life.

Q.- I have observed that a lot of teachers want to do therapeutic work very quickly.

This is not good at all. They don't know about the diseases. They don't know the origin of the problems. They don't know the names of the muscles or the functions of organs. They don't know the symptoms of the disease. I am not speaking about medicines at all but about the cause of the disease.

---

1 The book *Light on the Yoga Sūtras of Patañjali* was published in 1993 (Harper Collins, London), after this interview. Now one may read and study in order to know the connections. Also, the Ramāmaṇi Iyengar Memorial Yoga Institute has brought out an audio casette for students which is in two parts. The Sanskṛt words are broken at euphonic junctions to bring the clarity while reciting.

You have to think that if such and such a source is the cause, then what are the *āsana* to teach in order to give a soothing touch to the affected part of the body. This is needed before you jump into healing. For this the teachers have to know the symptoms and causes of diseases, then study human nature and body functions. After understanding all these they should think how *āsana* have to be done to work effectively on the affected areas for healing and cure. All these aspects need to be known before one goes for therapeutic treatment.

– *It would be dangerous otherwise.* –

That is what I said, don't jump to the sciences of yogic therapy. First take minor cases where, even if you go wrong, the complainant may not suffer for the worst. When you get confidence in handling minor problems, then you learn to tackle a little more complicated ones. Problems are of different natures. If somebody has a heart problem, you cannot teach him standing *āsana*. Then the state of heart gets complicated. In such cases you have to depend on people like us who have some experience in treating. We can guide but one should have innovative and creative sensitivity for precise adjustments. You cannot use different methodology as trials to try things out when a question of life and death is involved. It is important to know how to handle such patients having vital problems.

When I began therapeutic classes I took chances with a great deal of precaution. When I worked with therapeutic problems I moved according to the presentation of their bodies. I used to make them do a little more than they could do in order to have the judgement of introducing *āsana* which they could be capable of doing. That is how I learned. Now just looking at you I can see the maximum you can do, but first I did not know the maximum. I used to ask them, "Can you stretch a little more?" While they were trying I would touch them, and from that touch I would know whether I can proceed further or not. The moment the area refused to move I knew that I should stop. If they co-ordinated, I kept going. The moment the area hit back, I used to hold very firmly, to educate so that at least it may not retard next time. That's how I became a practical doctor.

Therapeutic classes should not be introduced by inexperienced teachers. The teachers should have a special eye for observation. They have to learn to watch the colour of the skin, the expression of the eyes and face, placement of muscles, structure of their bodies, the feel of respiration, the state of the mind, the capacity of doing and being in *āsana* and so forth.

Here, in the medical classes, I concentrate mainly on the bad cases, leaving the light cases to others because I know it will not be dangerous even if they do wrong. But I am there in the class; even the light cases could become dangerous if I were not there. When something happens I am right there. I move quickly from place to place making adjustments and modifying the *āsana*. As these fingers of mine are so much experienced, they naturally move fast and adjust quickly.

Q.- I am interested to know why people start yoga.

Simply because they cannot find relief from any other method. The gateways for human health are the respiratory and the circulatory systems. When you do *Setubandha Sarvāṅgāsana* the lungs expand automatically. In this *āsana*, the breathing process increases indirectly even without

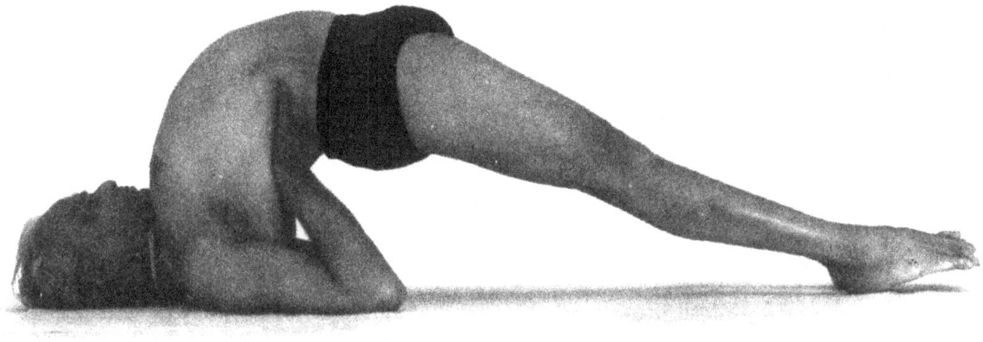

Plate n. 23 – *Setubandha Sarvāṅgāsana*

the knowledge of *prāṇāyāma*. That is why patients find relief as there is no strain. The chemicals of the blood change, which gives them health.

For anything, there is a cause. To come to yoga also there may be a cause in the form of various ailments and pain of the body or mental suffering. Only the religiousness in practice commences later.

First we have to help those who come to yoga to find relief. Then we have to encourage them to get attached to the real art, science and philosophy of yoga and maintain to live in the art. Ninety-nine percent of the people who come are motivated only to get rid of their suffering, and we have to work in that area alone to give them solace. When they come with hope, do not injure them – even if you don't give relief right away. It's all right as long as you keep them safe. In therapeutic classes – this is very important – don't think at once for a cure, but try to minimise their problems. Just minimise, then you are guarding yourself as well as the patient. Though you accept to take the case, sometimes fear inside haunts you. Yet I say that such a fear is very good, because the fear stops you from stretching yourself on the patient too far. You are afraid, so you take the minimum.

I can give quick relief because I know the direction in which each and every cell of the body has to move in the *āsana*. But your knowledge is limited and you should make sure you do not go beyond your limited capacity. Find out how you can help within that capacity. Many people have taken complicated cases just to make a name and fame, and I am dead against it. When something went wrong I have seen them getting scared and fail to put them back on the right track. Is that the way, to play with those who come to you for help? Do not play with the life of others, it is as precious as yours.

Unfortunately some of those who have received advice from me hold on to it, saying, "We can teach for these problems". That is certainly not the way. This is not teachers' exchange. If you know something, you need to pass on that knowledge and not to hold it for yourself. They don't pass this advice on to their co-teachers, and that hurts me. They are building up their own career, saying, "I am very good in this area, I can teach you", because a letter of information, sequence of *āsana* and also the list of danger points of the *āsana* have gone from me. Now I am saying that if there is an organisation, let them pool their questions and send them to me. I will answer the organisation so that everybody will know – nobody can hide. This information should be for the use of all, and not for the advantage of one person. Everybody should know or nobody should know the method.

So I can say that people take to yoga to get rid of pain and they take up the job of teaching yoga because of their freedom from pain and develop pride that they can teach also. The knowledge is meant to share with fellow-teachers so that they too get to understand how to help others.

Q.- Well, that is another example of sharing, isn't it?

Yes. Advice has to be pooled.[1] This is one reason why I wanted associations. The associations have to undertake such work so that I can answer them directly. If the answer is published in their newsletter, everybody will know. I don't mind answering the association which is publishing newsletters so it's an open secret to all.

People may start yoga with good motivation but end up with selfish motives. But if the association of each country takes up such work, it will be beneficial to one and all.

Q.- Perfect, and then it will be clear what you said and it will not be passed on second hand through people who have not understood.

---

[1] B. K. S. Iyengar Yoga Associations are established in every country to propagate the teachings of the author. See pl. n. 2

This is a must now. I am saying that all should approach me through their association. Earlier, I advised the individual teachers. By giving information to individuals, the headaches have increased. Many self-proclaimed experts have arisen on account of that. I never thought that this type of pride would set in, in the teachers.

Q.- Yes, and one of the problems is the one you said about yoga becoming commercial.

Yes. Commercialisation is wrong. This a kind of hoarding and selling. I don't encourage such commercialisation.

One has to live – you cannot teach free of charge. That is understandable. Earn, but give more than you take. Then it is not the commercialisation. That is the real philosophy of yoga.

If I renounce everything, then even if I know the art, who is going to feed me? Some take donations, I take fees. A donation is also commercial in a way. If you ask somebody to give whatever he wants to give as a gift to the *guru*, what is it? Literally, is it not indirectly a fee? They come for a few minutes, and earn more. Here a yoga teacher sweats and earns less. At least we are more true to ourselves by not asking donations but fees. Hence, I say to all my pupils, "I don't mind if you charge. Charge more but give them more than you have taken." Then that is for me right living. It is in one sense a sacrifice. Renouncing is not right living. I have given more so my conscience says, "Yes, I have done my best". I have given more than I have taken, that is all the satisfaction I have. Yoga cannot be taught for nothing. If you say, "Come, it is free", the value of art gets degraded and nobody shows interest in it.

- It's true, isn't it? It's human nature. (Laughter) -

Yes, human nature does that. The higher the price: "Oh, you must be a better teacher."

Today when you were in class, I was there practising. When I had finished I came to explain *Sālamba Śīrṣāsana* to you. Until then I did not, even though I had seen lots of mistakes; I was involved in my own practice so I said to myself, "Keep quiet, when I finish, I will explain to her". In five minutes what I explained and corrected in you is equal to ten years of your practice.

- It's true. (Laughter) -

Some people come here for three weeks and go away saying they have learnt many things, but they don't come back. If they come back, well and good. Next time they become sober. The first time when they come they are not at all sober. They think they are already far ahead, so they go with pride. Such people commercialise such a beautiful and auspicious art. If they come three or four times their pride changes into humbleness to learn more and more. For us the teaching becomes easier, since sober brain absorbs the knowledge with humbleness.

You can observe this soberness in all my senior pupils. They catch my teachings easily, they understand me easily. The beginners come with pride. They have done very well with so many advanced senior students of mine, but they forget that I am the seniormost teacher for all these senior teachers. *(Laughter)*

Q.- Have you thought of writing a short piece that could go into all the newsletters?

Well, this all should go. For example, something which appears in your paper, could be reproduced in *Dīpikā* of England; England can reproduce from your questions what is common to all. I am telling them all, please share these good points so there can be no misunderstanding. It's good to communicate with each other, so please reproduce those articles which are good. In your magazine[1] you give permission to reprint your articles with acknowledgement. So this way you grow and yoga grows.

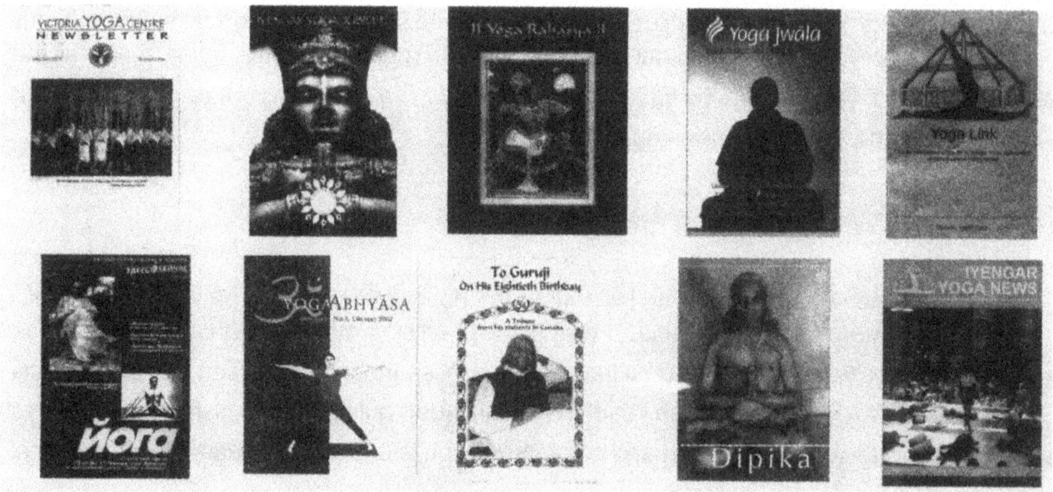

Plate n. 24 – Some newsletters and magazines of Iyengar Associations

[1] Mr. Iyengar speaks here of the Yoga Centre of Victoria Newsletter.

MR. IYENGAR MEETS THE "BRITISH WHEEL OF YOGA"*

Q.- Do *cakra* really exist? Or are they just a convenient system to explain our emotions and temperaments in the light of experience at certain levels?

Suppose someone does not know anything about the human body, and when the doctor says that the glands do exist in the body, will an innocent person say that since he has not seen the glands, he does not believe their existence, or will he accept the doctor's words and accept their existence? I am counter-questioning you, I hope you understand me. As the glands are not visible, do you not trust what the medical scientists say? Similarly, why are you doubting the words of the yogis who had inner vision to explain as well as write on *cakra?* It is easy to put a question, but the question should have a great deal of educative values for the listeners, too.

Cakra are there, but cannot be seen by the physical eyes. The books say that they are invisible, sacred and secret, and on account of this the doubt has arisen. Yoga is a science. According to yoga texts, the plexus, the glands, are outside the spinal column and the *cakra* are inside the spinal column. I hope you understand me. They are the feeding centres to the glands, the seven chambers of the plexus and seven glands. This outer body is explained physiologically by medical science, the causal body or *kāraṇa śarīra* is explained by the yogic science. All accomplished yogis have explained *cakra* after experiencing their functions like the hormone glands which are beyond the physiological field. *Cakra* too is beyond physical, physiological and mental fields but they are close to the spiritual field. As the doctors dissect the dead body with surgical instruments to see through, the yogis dissected their own bodies consciously and could feel the *cakra*.

The *Upaniṣads* say we have about seventy-two thousand nerves. And each nerve has seventy-two thousand branches. So if you multiply seventy-two thousand into seventy-two thousand, you will get an idea of the nervous system as a whole. Medical science says that if the

* These questions were asked of Mr. Iyengar at a public gathering with over 700 students of the British Wheel of Yoga and followers of Mr. Iyengar's method. The meeting was organised by the Bharatya Vidya Bhavan of London, to further the understanding of each other's views. Published in *Yoga Today,* vol. 9, no. 7, November 1984, and no. 8, December 1984.

nervous system is cut and joined together, it is about six thousand miles in length. As such, if these seventy-two thousand times seventy-two thousand are connected together, then you can get the length. And these seventy-two thousand nerves originate from the *kaṇdasthāna*, below the navel the place which is situated between *svādhiṣṭhāna cakra* and *nābhi cakra* according to their studies.

Similarly hundred and one nerves start from the inner core of the heart. From each of these, seventy-two nerves branch of. However, out of a hundred and one nerves, only one nerve is known as *citrā nāḍī*, that splits into two parts. One part moves upwards towards the crown of the head and the other part moves downwards towards the generative organs.

So this one nerve, *citrā nāḍī*, which starts from the very source of our being belongs to the causal body or *kāraṇa śarīra* that moves from the heart, which has no branches at all and penetrates through the gates of the *suṣumṇā*.[1] You are all told that *suṣumṇā* is the seat of *kuṇḍalinī*. But the *Upaniṣads*, like *Chāndogya* and others,[2] will give you detailed information that *suṣumṇā* is just a gateway for the *citrā nāḍī* since it goes through *suṣumṇā*. It is the *citrā nāḍī* alone that is connected to the *sahasrāra* – the crown of the head, and not the *suṣumṇā*. So, when the perfect master yogi takes his vital and conscious energy through the *citrā nāḍī* by breaking the gates of the *suṣumṇā*, then the energy, what you call *kuṇḍalinī*, flows through *citrā nāḍī* and not *suṣumṇā*. In the early days, this energy was not called *kuṇḍalinī*, *kuṇḍalinī* is the new terminology – it was called *agni* in those days. *Sūrya*, *candra* and *agni* are the three important nerves in the human system. So the *agni* or the divine fire was carried through *citrā nāḍī*, and that divine fire was finding divine chambers inside the spinal cord. These divine chambers are known as *cakra*. As they are inside, it is not possible for an ordinary human being to understand, feel or experience them. Only those who have reached that exalted state of *samādhi* can experience and explain, and not others. That is all I can say about it.

These invisible *cakra* have a great bearing on both intellectual and emotional temperaments of the human beings. The energy which exists in us in the form of the physical, vital, mental, intellectual, sexual, spiritual and cosmic finds its root in the *cakra*. As such *cakra* play a major role in the life of human beings on the energetic and intellectual planes. So one cannot limit them just on the experience of emotions and temperament levels.[3]

---

1 See *Aṣṭadaḷa Yogamālā*, vol. 2, section II, *Vīṇādaṇḍa*, pp. 170 -173.

2 *Yogaśikhopaniṣad*, V.27, and *Shiva Samhitā*.

3 See also *Aṣṭadaḷa Yogamālā* vol 2, "Physiology and Cakra", pp. 174 -181.

Q.- In *Light on Yoga* no restriction is mentioned regarding the practice of *Kapālabhāti* and *Bhastrikā* for women. Why therefore in *Light on Prāṇāyāma* are these two *prāṇāyāma* banned? Can you give us a physiological reason for this, please?

Please re-read those sections on *Bhastrikā* and *Kapālabhāti*, they are not banned but cautioned. If you read yoga texts, *Upaniṣads, Gheraṇḍa Samhitā, Haṭhayoga Pradīpikā, Śiva Samhitā*, they say that if you do *Matsyendrāsana* your *kuṇḍalinī* awakens, if you do *Bhastrikā* your *kuṇḍalinī* awakens, if you do *Kapālabhāti* your *kuṇḍalinī* awakens. Then tell me which one does not awaken? They say that *kuṇḍalinī* awakens even in *Paśchimottānāsana*.[1] Have you read it or not? I do not know. Yet, I say "Yes!" This is the reason why doubts set in for those who are not in touch with the texts.

Why preference only to *Kapālabhāti* and *Bhastrikā*? Why not the others? Because that is the easiest and the grossest method that is taught though it is not the safest. When people do jogging they say, "I feel very fresh". In fact, the slow body and dull brain feel this freshness. After jogging their head becomes very hot, their breathing becomes heavy, and their heart pumps faster. Excitement comes in jogging. Similarly, the same kind of excitement, namely, invigoration and exhilaration, occurs in *Bhastrikā* and *Kapālabhāti*.

The effects of *āsana* or *prāṇāyāma* or *mudrā* are written in all the authoritative texts, mentioning that the *kuṇḍalinī* will be awakened by the practice of *Paśchimottānāsana, Siddhāsana, Bhastrikā, Khecarī* and so forth. In short it means that one needs to practise all *āsana, prāṇāyāma, bandha, mudrā* in order to awaken the *daivi śakti* – the divine power or *kuṇḍalinī*. If every text recommends something or the other to awaken *kuṇḍalinī*, which one to be taken would be a big question mark. The texts give me the teaching that one has to make all efforts to do everything that the texts say as a whole.

When a person is suffering from heart trouble, is it good for him to do jogging, running, climbing steps? Is it good for him to do *Bhastrikā, Kapālabhāti*? One has to think about what is irritating and what is soothing. There is a difference between the irritative and stimulative states. Therefore some warnings have to be given, care has to be taken. Some guidance should be there to who should be doing and who should not be doing.

Now, coming to the point, let me tell you. When I wrote *Light on Yoga*, I wrote it to introduce yogic science to one and all. You do not see any other book before *Light on Yoga* which gives so many *āsana* and *prāṇāyāma* in detail. When I wrote *Light on Prāṇāyāma*,[2] I specified certain things clearly. Yet, as far as *Bhastrikā* and *Kapālabhāti* are concerned, I have said that women and particularly pregnant women should avoid them. Of course I don't know in

---

[1] *Yogaśikhopaniṣad*, I.112.

[2] Both *Light on Yoga* and *Light on Prāṇāyāma* are published by Harper Collins, London.

your country whether they ask or not, but in my country they ask though they are very shy. By doing *Bhastrikā* and *Kapālabhāti*, what happens to the breast? They become loose due to force, and hang down. Then they come to you or me to ask the reason and solution. Definitely a few came with a worried mind and said, "I don't know, my breast has fallen down. What to do? My husband wants to divorce me." *(Laughter.)*

So, no doubt yoga is spiritual, but at the same time we need to caution people for what purpose we are teaching *Bhastrikā* and to whom we are teaching. So keeping this in my mind, knowing very well what type of questions have come to me in my years of teaching, I have brought in *Light on Prāṇāyāma*. If women blast vigorously in *Bhastrikā* or *Kapālabhāti*, though less likely to happen in *Kapālabhāti*, the prolapse of abdominal organs or the uterus can happen, the breasts may sag. I have not banned these two *prāṇāyāma*, but I have cautioned. If women suffer from heavy bleeding, either menorrhagia or metrorrhagia, of course, I will not allow them to do these practices. So discrimination is essential. In both these *prāṇāyāma* the exhalation is done rapidly, with force. One should use the discriminative intelligence on the sound of breath. If the tone changes and the practitioner continues to blast, it affects the position of the breasts as well as the abdominal organs. It may also cause prolapse of the uterus. Therefore, it is harmful to women in general and pregnant, menstruating women in particular, as well as women ageing when they lose the control over the urinary bladder.

Anyway, as the question has been raised, let me explain further in detail in my *Light on Prāṇāyāma* book. I have given *Nāḍī Śodhana prāṇāyāma* at the end. The others have all brought it in the very beginning. I have explained all others nasal or digital *prāṇāyāma* earlier to sequences of *Nāḍī Śodhana*. Why did I put it at the end? Because I constructed the *prāṇāyāma* from the gross to the subtle, stage by stage. That is the difference as far as my practice and others' practices are concerned. I do it every day, not just a few minutes but I am in it. For many yoga is in their pockets. I am sorry for using such language. I never wrote for making money but to give the best with a religious and spiritual touch.

Knowing very well that *Nāḍī Śodhana*, being complicated and ultimate *prāṇāyāma*, it requires a very skilful adjustment of the finger-tips on the nose to produce the proper sound or *svara*, hence I described this at the end. *Nāḍī Śodhana prāṇāyāma* is a very subtle *prāṇāyāma*. Here, you have to trace the *prāṇa-nāḍī* so that the *prāṇa* is carried through the right channel to reach the avenues in a right direction.

A flautist with holes on the flute or a violinist with four strings on the violin produces the finest type of sound. There is a skill in the movement of the arm holding the bow. The finger movements are skilful. Even the breath control for the flautist is important. Similarly, you have to know, having two nostrils, how to adjust the tip of fingers on the walls of the nose in order to produce proper sound of the breath while doing the *prāṇāyāma*.

Prāṇāyāma is known as *nāda brahman.* It is not just a breathing exercise. You have to listen to the sound. For instance, listen to the sound of breath in *Ujjāyī.* You attend to the sound in the nostril second to second in *Ujjāyī,* you realise the sound is very rough and strong as well. In the *Nāḍī Śodhana prāṇāyāma* the sound is very minute and subtle. Therefore it is very essential to adjust the tips of the fingers on the nose. Your finger should be tapping the skin of your nose moment to moment skilfully to get the right route and correct sound. That is why I have put this *prāṇāyāma* at the end, mentioning it as the most complex *prāṇāyāma.*

Prāṇāyāma is not merely breathing or expanding the chest. It is the study of the sound. There is a difference between the sound of *Ujjāyī prāṇāyāma* and *Nāḍī Śodhana prāṇāyāma.* There is a difference between the sound of inhalation and exhalation in each *prāṇāyāma.* That is why I said *prāṇāyāma* is *nāda brahman. Nāda* means sound, *brahman* is the all-pervading, supreme, infinite Being. The continuous process of inhalation and exhalation which produces a type of sound is known as a *mantra* called *soham.* So the respiration is a continuous *japa* of the *mantra* called *soham.* Inhalation produces sound which is similar to *sa...* meaning, He – the *brahman,* and exhalation produces sound which is similar to *aham...* meaning, I – pointing at the soul. The process of *prāṇāyāma* which is based on inhalation and exhalation is nothing but the *japa* of *soham mantra.* However, the *soham japa* becomes subtler in *Nāḍī Śodhana prāṇāyāma* compared to *Ujjāyī prāṇāyāma.* You need to tune your nostrils, respiratory system and nervous system in order to produce proper, subtle, refined sound. As there is difference between a master musician and the amateur, you will find a difference between *Nāḍī Śodhana* and *Ujjāyī.* In order to know this difference one has to practise meticulously.

However the others have said that *Nāḍī Śodhana* is the simplest of all *prāṇāyāma.* This indicates the ignorance of the practitioner, who lacks experience. One has to practise to a great extent in order to have the depth of experience so that one can say which can fit in exactly, in a particular situation, and which is suitable in a particular condition.

Which *āsana* exactly fit in at what time also has to be known. So, considering all this, I definitely said that *Bhastrikā* and *Kapālabhāti* only trigger the brain, but not the rest of the body. A dull and sluggish person, or a person who is inert, mentally lazy, does *Kapālabhāti* and *Bhastrikā* for a few minutes, it is very very good. But if one continues to do so for a longer time, it is harmful. Some teachers advise their students to do a hundred cycles of these types of *prāṇāyāma* on each side and people do that without questioning. How many of you observe the first sound and the last sound of *Bhastrikā?* Is it mechanical or is it dynamic? Doing a hundred blasts is mechanical. Doing those hundred strokes without changing the sound is dynamic. Do we observe each stroke? When the sound changes and the quality disappears, know very well that it is harmful to the brain as well as abdominal organs. The metallic sound that you get in the first stroke does not continue, then it means that the lungs cannot produce that sound. So what is the use of doing *Bhastrikā* when the same quality of the first stroke is not maintained? The moment that healthy sound is lost, know that you have to stop that *prāṇāyāma* then and there.

In *prāṇāyāma*, if you are inhaling, observe the first sound and when you finish observe the last sound. If there is a variation, you have done only with the mechanical will without savouring the depth of that breath. The fragrance of the breath has to be felt, whether it is *Bhastrikā, Kapālabhāti, Nāḍī Śodhana, Sūrya Bhedana, Chandra Bhedana* or any type of *prāṇāyāma*. If the body is sound, your lungs are strong, you can do *Nāḍī Śodhana prāṇāyāma* and *Ujjāyī prāṇāyāma*. But if you have emphysema, asthma, bronchitis, I would like to know whether you can do *Bhastrikā* like a healthy man. Find out for yourselves. Why could *Ujjāyī* be given to those who have these problems instead of *Bhastrikā* and *Kapālabhāti*? Because *Bhastrikā* and *Kapālabhāti* are strenuous *prāṇāyāma*, whereas *Ujjāyī* is soothing and energising.

And now I come to the point of *āsana*. You all say, if I teach a little complicated *āsana*, I am too strong. "Iyengar is too strong, he goes very fast." But what about you people who teach *Bhastrikā* and *Kapālabhāti* without teaching them the simple *prāṇāyāma* such as *Ujjāyī*? In fact, the methods, the steps and the gradations of each *āsana* and *prāṇāyāma* have to be known. So if you study the gradations there will be no mistakes or misunderstandings between what I say and the doubt which you have, provided you study each time. Sir, I hope I have cleared your doubts.

Unfortunately, the question has come from a male and not a female. A male cannot experience the female body. Yet, as a man you can experience your physiological body. The lungs, the brain, the generative organs are physiological organs. Spine is a physiological part. The nerves carry the physiological function. There will be a tremendous strain on them. *Bhastrikā* and *Kapālabhāti* will be disturbing the area. The exhalation breath in *Bhastrikā* and *Kapālabhāti* exerts the brain when prolonged or done wrongly. These *prāṇāyāma* pump and push the abdominal organs down. This can cause displacement and bring unwanted strain on ovaries and uterus. The pregnant women may get discharge or have miscarriage. Women may suffer from white discharge. Are these not the disturbances in the physiological functioning? People, whether men or women, who have hypertension should not do these as the blood pressure shoots up. Men having hernia whether it is hiatus, umbilical or inguinal have to avoid strenuous actions.

Q.- Mr. Iyengar, why do you advocate such extreme prohibitions? I have some trouble with fluid in the middle ear and according to your book I should do no *Kapālabhāti* or shoulder stands. My ear problem is related to breathing problems caused by a deviated septum and comes as a feeling of constriction in the throat; I can feel the pressure put on the ears and am aware of the need for caution, but I have found a limited practice of *Kapālabhāti* very helpful for breathing and likewise the shoulder stand for the throat though it gives pain in the ear. Thanks to Mr. Iyengar's strictures, however, I cannot help feeling a little concerned as to whether I should be practising these things.

The question is so long that the man who has to answer forgot everything what was said in the beginning. The question was like an essay; this was not a question at all. First of all it was said "the strictest prohibition". What are those prohibitions? What are such extreme prohibitions? I myself don't know, unless it is expressed. My dear friend, I have written in my books on yoga a few cautions as it is a book which imparts indirect teaching and know that it has to be read by thousands of people. When a pupil is doing without the direct guidance from a teacher and a teacher is involved in the art of teaching, should I give some warnings or not? That's the first question. Who will be responsible if the pus oozes from ears with the practice of *Bhastrikā* and *Kapālabhāti?* Warnings are meant so that the one who practises without the guidance from the teacher can judge.

Then the person has said: how many books have said not to do, not only Mr. Iyengar's? All the researchers in the field of yoga have also talked of what are the things prohibited for practice. If one has ear pain or nose pain, have they not said not to do *Bhastrikā, Kapālabhāti?* So it is a general statement. Since thousands of people may be reading the book, they may be trying, so naturally one has to guard them. I think somewhere I have said that if you don't know or understand, go to your teacher and learn. All these are mentioned there in the book. They are not extreme prohibitions even for your itching or fluid in the ear. You say that you are doing *Sālamba Sarvāṅgāsana*, which is helping your throat. Luckily your structure may be very good. But you say that *Sālamba Sarvāṅgāsana* gives more ear pain. Suppose I take that *Sālamba Sarvāṅgāsana* just now and lessen your pain in the ear, will you accept it? So, from the practical point of view and being face to face as a teacher, I can help you in relieving both of your problems by direct teaching, but to guide in a book is risky as one may not understand the right way of doing *the āsana*. So warnings are given.

If you insert your fingers into the inner holes of the ears, they are circular. When you do *Sālamba Śīrṣāsana* - head balance - and *Sālamba Sarvāṅgāsana* - shoulder balance -, if that circular portion of the inner ear is kept in the right circular position, then the pain, the itching disappears immediately and the sense of running of pus in the ears diminishes. If they take an oval shape in head balance or the shoulder balance or the plough pose *(Halāsana)*, then these *āsana* are not a cure for the above irritations. If you insert your finger and they go deep in, then that is the sign of a healthy presentation, and if the fingers do not go deep into the ears, that is the sign of bad practice. If the inner ears are properly balanced, in *Śīrṣāsana* - the inversions -, the itching and running stops. Fortunately the woman who put the question has a long neck. Stand up, please. *(She stands and everyone watches her neck.)*

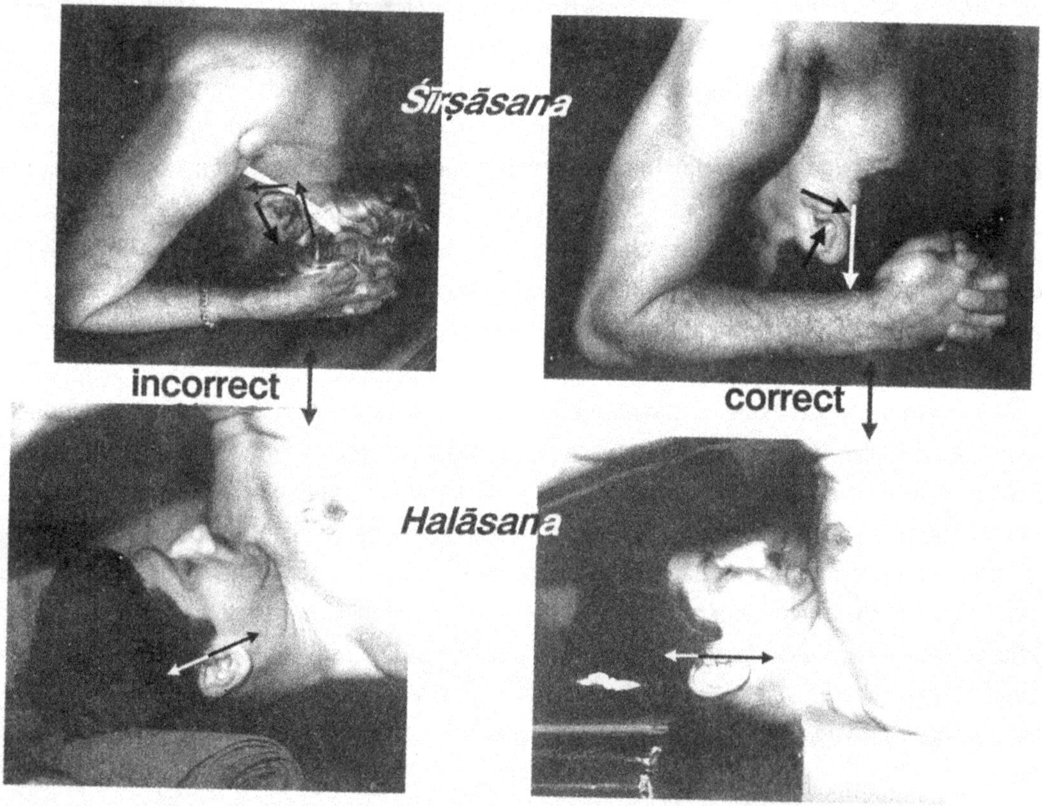

Plate n. 25 – Correct and incorrect ear position in *Śīrṣāsana* and *Halāsana*[1]

[1] It is not possible to illustrate the correct ear position with the fingers placed. However when observing from outside the line of the ear gives an indication if the ear position is correct. When the ear is, exactly perpendicular in *Śīrṣāsana*, and horizontal in *Halāsana* it indicates that there is more space in the inner ear and therefore less pressure).

Can you see her side neck? It is long. But if my friend Dim has got a short neck and if he does *Sālamba Sarvāṅgāsana* with ear pain, he will have excruciating pains in the ears because of the anatomical structure. Again in her case the ear problem is related to breathing problem. It is because of deviated septum. *Bhastrikā* and *Kapālabhāti* are not prohibited for these problems. In fact, they are helpful under certain conditions.

Hence these things come under direct teaching, not through a book. A book is just a guide. The lady said that she did it by following the techniques given in my book *Light on Yoga,* though I said not to do it, and she found much relief. From this you gauge how much *Light on Yoga* helped her though the instructions are general. If my book has helped her so much, then if I guide her directly, can you measure the relief I can give her?

One has to analyse the pain. After analysing the pain while doing *Śīrṣāsana*, if her right ear, as that woman said, is paining and left ear is neither paining nor itching, she has to question herself why is it itching in this ear, why is it not in the other ear? This way one has to analyse. After analysing this pain notice whether the pain is existing on the other side, then watch the structure of the body on that side and the body on the other side. Compare and learn and reach out to the violent part, i.e., the painful part, and transform that part into passivity; make that non-painful part active, then you learn to balance activity and passivity evenly. This is known as analysis and practice. It is not analysis in thinking. You can't solve the problem by thinking, but by acting correctly.

You cannot think on factual things. If my right hand is longer and left hand shorter, and if my right hand stretches more and left hand stretches less, analysis has to start immediately between the right and the left hands. Observe the feel of movement on the extended side to that of the other where there is no movement: outwardly it appears as a non-violent action, whereas it is a violent action inwardly. By this way you learn that you are violent by overstretching and murdering the cells, while on the other side, you are killing them without using them. This is the sign and science of understanding *hiṁsā* and *ahiṁsā*, and when you balance both the sides evenly, then these words 'violence' and 'non-violence' do not leave imprints on the mind. To bring balance between overstretch on one side and understretch on the other side is what Patañjali describes regarding *ahiṁsā* in *yama*.

Q.- Mr. Iyengar, why do you recommend that during *prāṇāyāma* one should hold *Jālandhara bandha* all the time during the in and out breath as well as retention? This is how your teachers teach it and they do not seem to have the answer.

My dear friend, have you read my *Light on Prāṇāyāma* book?

– No. –

Then please read it.

If you have read my *Light on Yoga*, have I not said that you can do *Ujjāyī prāṇāyāma* lying down in *Śavāsana* without *Jālandhara bandha?* It needs common sense to understand why *Jālandhara bandha* is essential in *prāṇāyāma* while sitting. *Haṭhayoga Pradīpikā* speaks in detail about the practice of *prāṇāyāma.* It says that while you are holding the breath – *antara kuṁbhaka* – after inhaling – *pūraka,* it is essential to do *Jālandhara bandha;* and after exhalation it is easy to learn *Uḍḍīyāṇa bandha.*[1] This is the meaning of the *śloka* of *Haṭhayoga Pradīpikā.*

The *śloka* conveys that the *Jālandhara bandha* is to be done at the end of *pūraka, Uḍḍīyāṇa bandha* at the end of exhalation; what does it convey to an ordinary person? It is like Patañjali saying, "Pleasures breed desire, sorrow leads to malice".[2] What is to be done? Patañjali did not say do this or that. He only shows and explains where pleasure and pain lead to. One leads to desire, the other leads to malice. In order not to be caught in the desires or malice what have you to do? He wants you to find out the ways so that your pleasures and sorrows do not breed desires or aversions. Obviously, both the pleasures and sorrows have to be studied and controlled since their breeding ground is in want of knowledge. Similarly, *Haṭhayoga Pradīpikā* says to do *Jālandhara bandha* after inhalation – *pūraka* –, and *Uḍḍīyāṇa bandha* after exhalation – *recaka.* Nothing has been said of what to do while in *pūraka* or *recaka.* Now observe, has the text said to do *Uḍḍīyāṇa* after inhalation? Has it said remove the chin from the chin lock – *Jālandhara bandha* – after exhalation? We do not see that sentence in any yoga texts. As such, one should not be carried away by the literal translation but to understand the non-disturbing factor of mind and body throughout the chain of *prāṇāyāma* practice, wherein the cycles of *pūraka, antara kuṁbhaka, recaka* and *bāhya kuṁbhaka* are involved.

---

1 *Pūrakānte tu kartayo bandho Jālandharābhidhaḥ I*
kumbhakānta rechakādau kartavyastūḍḍiyānakaḥ II (*H.Y.P.,* 2.45) – "do *Jālandharā bandha* (chinlock) while at the time of internal retention and *Uḍḍīyāṇa bandha* at the time of external retention".

2 *Sukha anuśayī rāgaḥ* (*Y.S.,* II.7) and *Duḥkha anuśayī dveṣaḥ* (*Y.S.,* II.8)

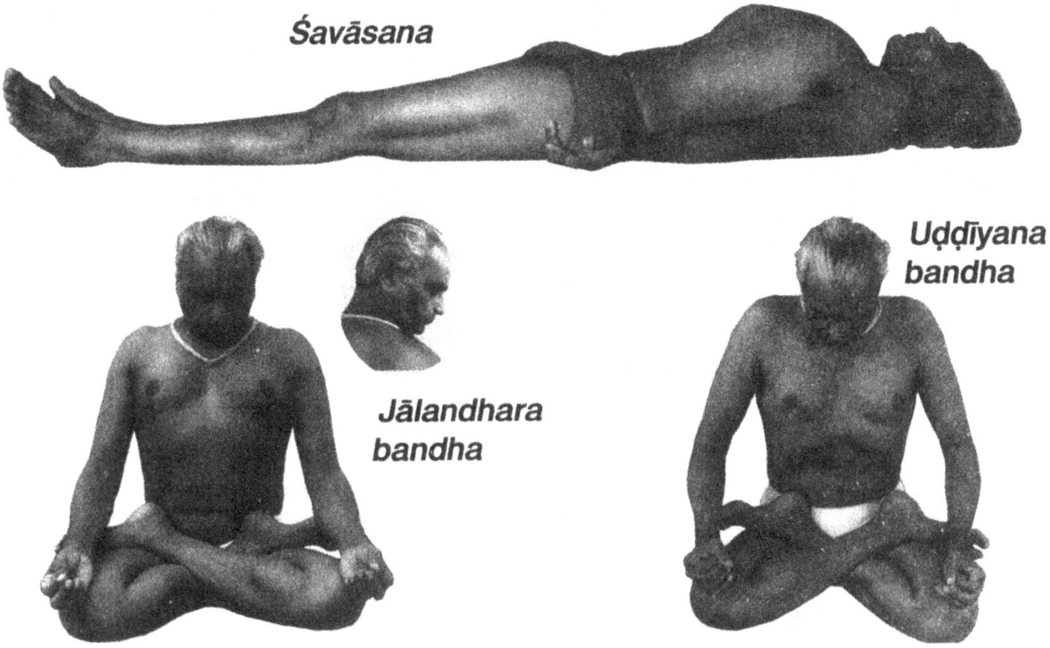

Plate n. 26 – *Śavāsana, Jālandhara bandha & Uḍḍīyāna bandha*

In 1975, when there was a yoga convention at Panchgani near Pune, a paper on *prāṇāyāma* was read by a scientist, who had done research work on *prāṇāyāma*, about *pūraka kuṁbhaka* and *recaka kuṁbhaka*. I was the Chairman for that session and they have not answered the questions I raised then, but the same paper is read over and over in all conferences. It is now ten years and everybody says that as a scientist, there must be some truth in it. According to this scientist whether one does *Jālandhara bandha* or not, the effect of retention is the same. I asked the scientist, "What is the effect of *kuṁbhaka* on the brain cells with *Jālandhara bandha* and without *Jālandhara bandha*." He said, "I have not tried that." Then, how did he come to the conclusion? He is pleased because he is a scientist. I am not a scientist, I am just an ordinary practitioner, so what I say has no meaning at all. When you do *Jālandhara bandha* you are not putting any extra strain on the brain while retaining the breath. If you hold the breath without *Jālandhara bandha* your eyes turn red, your ears get blocked, a load of tension is felt in the electrical nerves of the brain. With *Jālandhara bandha* these loads of strain are not felt on the brain. The load is shifted from the brain to the chest. This is a simple guide given for the student to do the *kuṁbhaka* with *Jālandhara bandha*. While doing *kuṁbhaka*, one has to know whether the lungs hold the breath or the brain. This difference is learnt in *Jālandhara bandha*. *Kuṁbhaka* with *Jālandhara bandha* takes off unnecessary strain and stress, both on the neurological body and the psychological body.

In *prāṇāyāma*, the observer and the observed are the lungs. The brain – the seat of the intellect – has to kept as a steady witness to help the *citta* – the seat of the mind and heart – act as an observer and guide to regulate the flow of energy without any feeling of strain and sees that the attention sets in. For this reason the brain needs to be kept neutral. This passivity is achieved by doing *Jālandhara bandha*, which automatically makes the brain become reflective and pensive.

In *prāṇāyāma* practice, it is the *citta* – the area of the heart and mind – which creates and receives space in the lungs to absorb the *prāṇa* – the energy – . If the head is held up then the brain gets disconnected from the *citta*, and loses its contact with the lungs. This non-contact of the intelligence of the head with the heart not only brings unnecessary strain on the body and mind, but loses the right judgement of the sound and measure of the inbreath, out breath and retention. Hence, keeping the head in the *Jālandhara bandha* brings the intelligence close to the breath, the lungs and the mind, or the intelligence of the heart. If the head is held up, how can you think of your trunk, or torso, or calmness in mind? If the chin-lock is done, your attention enters in and penetrates your torso and also releases the stress in the brain. Therefore, *Jālandhara bandha* is a must throughout the practice of *prāṇāyāma* as it directs the current of energy to flow in the right direction. *Jālandhara bandha* in *kuṁbhaka* helps the *prāṇic* energy not to hit the brain but makes it diffuse towards the torso, spine and lungs. The *Jālandhara bandha* also saves one from hypertension created by *prāṇāyāma* practices. If the head is up, it hardens the brain cells and the blood pressure may go up and tension too may increase. When *prāṇāyāma* is done with *Jālandhara bandha,* one never develops hypertension or hardness in the brain cells. There is no compulsion that one has to do *Jālandhara bandha* in normal breathing since the normal breath remains confined to its allotted area that is the diaphragmatic region.

If my pupils teach *Jālandhara bandha* in normal breathing, I say they are wrong. In the beginning it is better to keep the head down as much as one can, so that the nerves of the brain are not stressed while one does preliminary *prāṇāyāma*. *Jālandhara bandha* also has to be learnt gradually. You cannot force the neck down to have a chin-lock when the cervical body is unprepared. If the neck is forced to down, the neck muscles get irritated. To have a firm chin-lock in *Jālandhara bandha*, one needs to have a proper upright extension of the spine and freedom in the chest muscles for extension and expansion. Here the practice of *Sarvāṅgāsana* is very important. In *Sālamba Śīrṣāsana, Uḍḍīyāṇa bandha* occurs on its own, while in *Sālamba Sarvāṅgāsana* the neck muscles at the back are made to elongate to learn *Jālandhara bandha.*

Sālamba Śīrṣāsana gives a good foundation to learn *Uḍḍīyāṇa bandha: Sālamba Sarvāṅgāsana* and *Halāsana* help one to learn *Jālandhara bandha*. When *Sālamba Śīrṣāsana, Sālamba Sarvāṅgāsana* and *Halāsana* are perfectly mastered, *Jālandhara bandha* and *Uḍḍīyāna bandha* come easier and one is fit for *prāṇāyāma* and not by sitting in a comfortable position.

One is fit after *Sālamba Śīrṣāsana, Sālamba Sarvāṅgāsana* and *Halāsana* as the *bandha* form easily on their own. They are gravitational movements and hence one develops these two *bandha* without calling as *Uḍḍīyāṇa* or *Jālandhara bandha.* Nature helps on its own in these *āsana.* It is not at all necessary to think of these *bandha* while one does these *āsana.* While doing *prāṇāyāma* one has to raise the chest and bring the chin down to form a chin lock. Whereas in inverted *āsana* the neck muscles get elongated, the throat gets softened and they in turn reduce any tension in the brain while doing the *prāṇāyāma.*

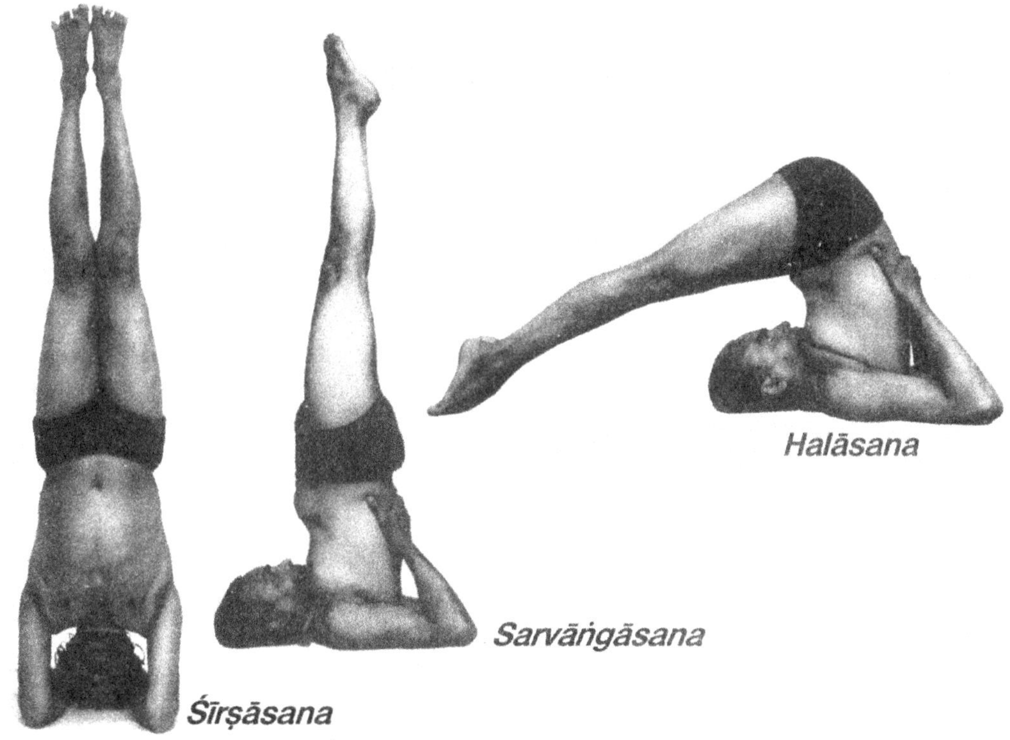

Plate n. 27 – *Śīrṣāsana, Sarvāṅgāsana* and *Halāsana*

Though the yogic texts explain that *Jālandhara* is a must after *pūraka* and *Uḍḍīyāna* after *recaka,* nowhere is it said that one has to raise the head up while doing *pūraka* and *recaka.* It must be understood by this that *Jālandhara* should be maintained throughout the *prāṇāyāma* practice. If one goes on raising the head up and down, where is steadiness and where is concentration? On the contrary, when you keep on raising the head up during inhalation and exhalation and do *Jālandhara bandha* in *antara kumbhaka* and *Uḍḍīyāṇa bandha in bāhya kumbhaka,* it becomes a nuisance every time exercising the head up and down. In long practice, the inhalation breath strains the braincells and inflates them, and in exhalation, the brain cells are squeezed or contracted if done without *jālandhara bandha.* This non-deliberate pressure on the brain affects the electrical cells of the brain. Wrong practice of *prāṇāyāma* can invite all the diseases says the *Haṭhayoga Pradīpikā.*[1]

In order to maintain stability – *sthiratā* – and one-pointed attention – *ekāgratā* –, this moving of the head up and down should not be there in sitting *prāṇāyāma* practices. In *Śavāsana,* as a pillow is used, the head remains restful, and therefore the brain remains quiet. Hence no strain is felt on the head or on the brain.

Q.- Mr. Iyengar, after years of experience with people's bodies, can yoga change for the better the physical shape of the spine? Is there age limitation if so?

Though the questioner is not here, it is a general question and I do not mind answering. Is there an age limit, if I put an ungentlemanly word, for sex? Tell me. Why do people find restrictions to follow the right method? Patañjali guides us: "Friends, be aware, the future is unknown to you. What is in store for the future you do not know. So prepare and buildup defensive force in the body from now on so that the future catastrophes may not touch you."[2] That is why yoga is a preventative healing science as well as a curing science. In the spiritual path the impediments like diseases, anger, carelessness, doing unwanted things, illusive behaviour and so forth, are many. Practice of yoga destroys these impurities and impediments so that the mind is free from the clutches of the body for it to move towards the soul.

Similarly, if the spine is crooked, is it not possible to be straightened by right education and proper alignment of the spine? If a child is walking crookedly in the street, does the mother or the father allow the child to walk in that manner or tell the child to keep the feet straight while walking? Yoga, which is the *guru* for all of us, says if you have got this type of spine do this type of movement. That is why many *āsana* have been traced. It is not that if you do *Sālamba Śīrṣāsana* your spine becomes straight. You have to find out and hit a right *āsana* to get the defective part straight.

---

[1] *Prāṇāyāmena yuktena sarvarogakṣayo bhavet /*
ayuktābhyāsayogena sarvaroga samudbhavaḥ // (*H.Y.P.,* II.16)
Through the proper practice of *prāṇāyāma* all diseases are vanquished. Wrong practice of *prāṇāyāma* brings upon the practitioner all sorts of diseases.

[2] *Heyaṁ duḥkham anāgatam* (*Y.S.,* II.16). The pains which are yet to come can be and are to be avoided.

Haṭhayoga Pradīpikā says that whether one is young or of ripe age, diseased or invalid, he is fit to practise yoga.[1] What more do you want? As far as the physical shape of spine is concerned, know well that the journey of the body from birth is to ascend progressively till death. Body deteriorates. Our duty is to check and minimise its deterioration and decay. So when the shape of the spine changes, it is good to practise yoga to stop from further de-forming. When I have helped people with scoliosis, lordosis, kyphosis and protected them from further deterioration, is it not enough proof? Friend, instead of putting a question and getting satisfied with my answer, remember that those who are affected by spinal deformity have to put tremendous effort with intelligence to make it straight. Only effort brings fruit and not theoretical answers. See that no effort goes wasted. Make an effort for these problems to gain the benefit. You have to earn health by perspiration. You cannot earn health by inspiration alone.

Q.- What are your views on the noticeable increase in vandalism and the particularly violent nature of many young people today, and the apparent lack of respect for the feeling of others?

In the society good and bad move together. If there is vandalism, who is responsible for it? The yoga practitioner, the yoga teacher, or the parents, or the society of ours? You allow such things to happen and when they go beyond a certain point, you may call it danger point, then you brand it as vandalism. We are responsible for the children becoming like that.

Let us bear in mind that the responsibility is ours, and not the children's. Let us not give our opinion about the younger generation. They are missing something. It is our bounden duty of yours and mine to fill that gap. Because we don't fill that gap, violence has taken place. If there is a gigantic tree and if you want the gigantic tree to turn to your side, what happens to the branches if you force your strength on them? The branches break, is it not? If you trim a sapling to the direction you want, what happens to that sapling? It grows according to your wishes, does it not? The children are like saplings. It is our duty to train and nourish them, and not sit here for answers.

You and I are both responsible for that violent vandalism in the youngsters. As such we have to give them constructive ideas, methods to develop a healthy balanced state of body and mind. Some years ago in London, in one of the schools, young children were addicted to psychedelic drugs. One of my pupils was teaching yoga to those children. They were so happy

[1] *Yuvā vṛddho'tivṛddho vā vyādhito durbalo'pi vā /*
abhyāsāt siddhimāpnoti sarvayogeṣvatandritaḥ // (*H.Y.P.*, I.64) – Any person who practises all aspects of yoga untiringly attains success even if he is young, old, very old, sick or weak.

after some months of practice that they never missed their yoga classes. I am not saying "bull stories". It happened in the centre of London and the students forgot that they were addicted to drugs. The headmistress of that school became jealous of my pupil because she became very popular. Due to personal jealousy, the yoga classes were stopped. Within a few days the very same children were caught by the police and those children gave a statement that they had left off when they were practising yoga, and as the yoga teacher was not coming they could not get that tranquil state of feeling, so they went back to the old habit.

Now tell me, why should we not accept the truth and experiment yoga on children? Yoga teachers are here, not in small numbers. How to tap and exhilarate their minds through the art of yoga is important. You need to choose the proper sets of *āsana*. If you make them do for instance *āsana* like *Paśchimottānāsana*, they become dull. This state is worse than a disease. In *āsana* one should know how to keep them alert, active, and how to connect their ears and the eyes to the brain. It is also necessary to see that they do not become introverted. Such *āsana* are quite different. So if one can handle them with complicated balancing *āsana* and *āsana* of backward extensions, they sense the exhilarating feeling. One has to create interest in them to learn.[1]

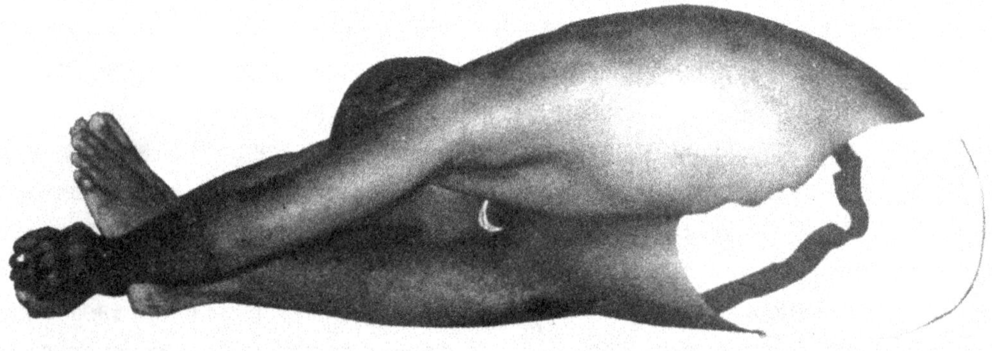

Plate n. 28 - *Paśchimottānāsana*

If I use that word "difficult or complicated *āsana*", you have to excuse me, since you think *āsana* should be non-violent, and for you non-violent means non-painful to your body. You want easy-going *āsana*. You do not know that by introducing simple *āsana* to children you are making them dull and that is violence on them. Though Patañjali uses the word *ahiṁsā* he also says that the yogi should be as hard as a diamond.[2]

[1] See *Aṣṭadaḷa Yogamālā* vol 3, section VI "Yoga in Schools", and *The Tree of Yoga* (Harper Collins, London).
[2] *rūpalāvaṇyabalavajra saṁhananatvāni kāyasaṁpat* (III.47).

This means that one has to have tremendous expressions of firmness in handling children towards the healthy way of living. To cut the diamond you have to use the diamond. Similarly, to stop this state of aggressive violence in children, a constructive type of vehemence has to be shown. When I teach such youngsters, I make them do *Viparīta Cakrāsana*, which is difficult, but creates inner force and strength for transformation from their destructive violence into a constructive ambition. Yoga teachers should lovingly challenge them in the right direction by performing themselves, which creates a will in them to make an effort with determination. This determination is the turning point in their lives.

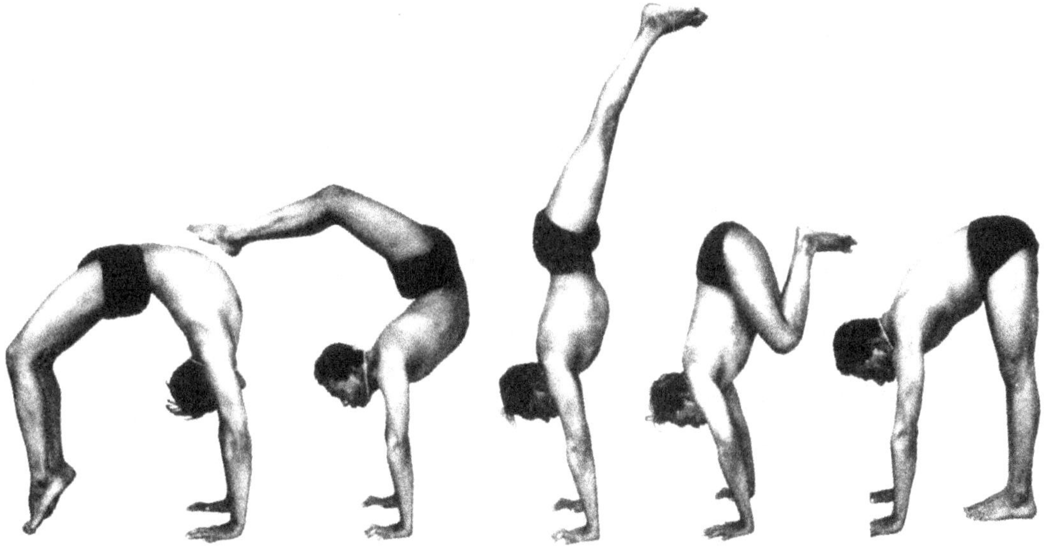

Plate n. 29 – *Viparīta Cakrāsana*

The right and apt adaptation of yoga is the key for changing their behavioural attitudes. If I ask such youngsters to do *Śavāsana*, then I create in their minds a devil's workshop! They will be a hundred percent empty, they will see the world's image at a different angle and violence will crop up in them. Then they will use their energy destructively instead of constructively.

If you know how to use their sword of destructive vandalism as a key, without telling them that you are using it in their practice of yoga, then you are building a constructive method in them. Therefore, the responsibility is not on children alone, but on all of us. In order to improve them we have to think what to do and what to give. They do not need spiritual discourse but a mental approach and physical valour. So select those *āsana* which develop that right pattern of valour by your example of presentation, so that they realise what is strength and what is courage. Engage their minds in a right thing. Build up methods for such types with good idioms to become friendly and good teachers.

Q.- Mr Iyengar, In the month of May Sarah Kennedy asked you to do a television programme the same day as you arrived from India. Well, the programme was *Sixty Minutes*, with Sarah Kennedy. Unfortunately the camera concentrated too much on your head while you were doing head stand. Nevertheless it was very impressive and in the best T.V. tradition of sensationalism, making people who know nothing about yoga believe that yoga means standing on one's head. However, what really surprises me was that you put Sarah into the head stand without enquiring, as far as we know, about her physical condition, spine, neck, heart, etc. It gave the impression that anyone can do it or be put into the head stand regardless of the physical condition.

My friend, it is similar to the previous question. Is yoga meant for the evolved ones only or can we not take yoga even to a man on the street, who knows nothing about the value of yoga? When I was asked to appear on T.V, the crew was so nervous that they could not even keep silent for half a minute. They were so tense and they asked me,

- *What are you going to perform?* -

I said, whatever they want. They said,

- *The duration of shooting is only three minutes* -

(Earlier they had said that the duration would be five minutes). Oh! I said, three minutes is not enough time.

However, they told me to come four hours before. I said, "It is ridiculous to come four hours before for a few minutes programme."

Now, imagine the tension of those people when I said so.

I said, "I will come half an hour before and whatever you want to rehearse I will do, but remember I may not repeat in the same way as you actually see in the rehersal."

They made me wait and wait, coming to the artist's room every second:

- *Mr. Iyengar, now you will be called, now you will be called.* -

I was just laughing and they were all under tension. They called me once and said,

- *No, no, no, still time.* -

When I went to the platform before I was to appear they told me to finish in one and a half minutes. Imagine which yogi would have shown tolerance and patience. Tell me which yogi would have agreed to show for one and a half minutes. Yet I showed something in one and a half minutes. Anybody else would have gone out with disgust and anger. Because I am a devotee of yoga, I made use of one and a half minutes to show at least a few leaves from the tree of yoga. Then they told me,

- You have to make also a non-initiate to do something. -

They wanted the interviewer to be initiated; they discussed that she has her broadcasting machine on her hips; she can't lie down on her back.

I said, "That's all right, I will try some other *āsana* which she can do without inconvenience".

Her trousers were very tight, so she was not able to stretch her legs apart.

I said, "It's all right", and asked her what she wanted to do.

- Can you take Śavāsana? -

"I can take her into *Śavāsana* but you were afraid of the mike which might get damaged by lying on the back".

While they were hesitating and wasting time I said, "If you want continuity, within this limited time, then I can do *Śīrṣāsana* - head balance, and show variations in that one *āsana*, and I showed seven or eight variations in *Śīrṣāsana*."

The crew members said it was okay. But what were they doing? They were taking only my face. It was, technically, unsound. I did lots of variations in head balance to attract the people towards yoga within that time. I turned both legs to the side - *Parśva Śīrṣāsana*, I scissored my legs - *Parivṛttaikapāda Śīrṣāsana*, I brought one leg down - *Ekapāda Śīrṣāsana*, I did cross legs - *Ūrdhva Padmāsana*. What can I do if they showed my head only? It is not my fault.

When I came down from *Sālamba Śīrṣāsana*, they wanted the interviewer in head balance, with her mike and the recorder, the directors were in a quandary. Seeing this, I took her to head balance and pushed the mike into her hip pocket, so that it might not fall. I continued from where I stopped. That's all. I showed how to do the head balance. How can I speak of philosophy of yoga in one minute? How many words can one use in that one minute? Action was important and not words. While I was on my head, I was talking throughout. My friend, that's all I could do. Beyond that I could not do anything. *(Applause.)*

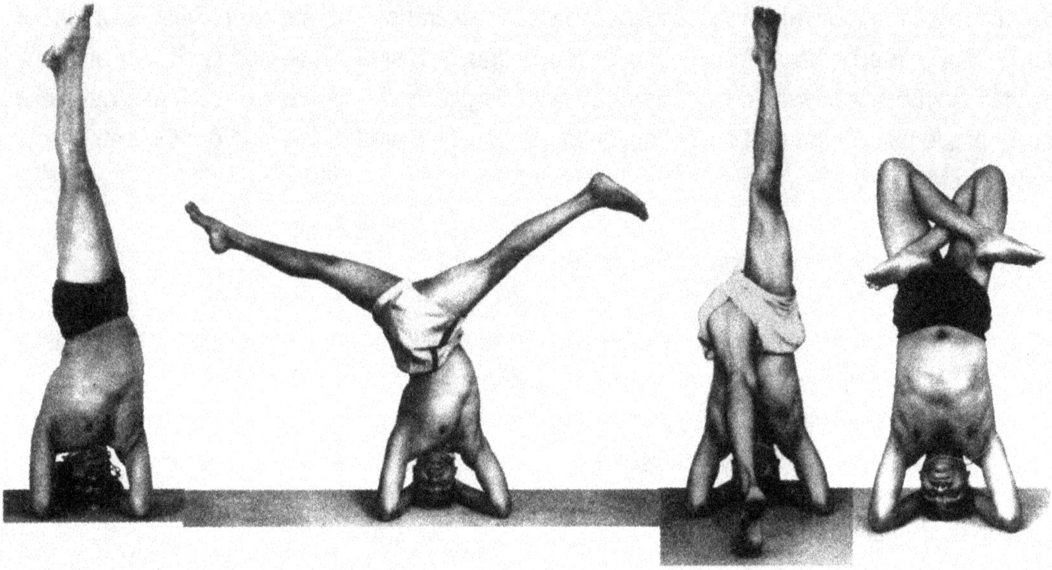

Plate n. 30 – Variations in *Śīrṣāsana*

Regarding my taking her to head balance, I am not a novice. I am a teacher of yoga for decades. With such vast experience if I do not know when to take and when not to take, and whom to take, then I cannot be a teacher of yoga at all. Even if her physical condition was bad, I would have taken in such a way that it did not injure her.

My dear friend, will you permit me to narrate an episode that occurred in my life? You have heard of the late Queen Mother of Belgium. She was eighty-four years old when I met her. I have not seen in my life a more courageous pupil than her, though I have taught men like J. Krishnamurti, Yehudi Menuhin, and so on and so forth. Here was a woman who had a heart problem and was under the care of a cardiac specialist. She had heart problems and blood pressure. She invited me to teach her head balance. I am not a mad cap to make people stand on their heads – but I know when to take a risk and when not to take risk, that's my job. To start with I made her do some standing poses like I teach beginners. I finished for the day and said let us see tomorrow.

"You have not made me stand on my head", she said.

Her bones were brittle and her neck was shaking, I said that I would take the head balance a little later. She refused to leave the room, saying, "Take head balance or go back to your esteemed pupil Yehudi Menuhin who sent you to me. My house is open for you to go!".

I said, "My dear friend, I want to know your blood pressure, the conditions of your heart, your arterial function".

She asked me, "Have you faith in yoga?"

I said, "Yes."

Then she said, "If you have faith in yoga you have no business to ask such things. Would you put me in headstand or not? That's all I want".

I asked, "Have you the courage to stand on your head?"

"I have the courage", she said.

Then I accepted her challenge and lifted her legs. The moment I straightened her legs in head balance, she became unconscious. Which teacher has the courage when such things happen? She was completely unconscious, but I did not bring her down, and I did not place her head on the floor. I formed a cup shape on my two feet and placed her head between the arches of the feet to observe her vibrations and reactions. She was there for sometime with no movements. I did not bring her down. After some time her head moved on my feet. I thanked God, as she regained her consciousness, I asked her how she felt.

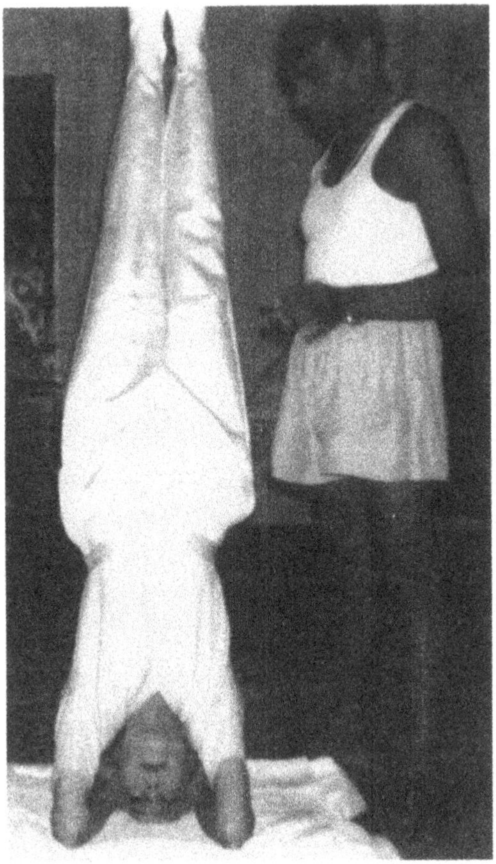

Plate n. 31 – Queen Mother of Belgium in *Sālamba Śīrṣāsana*

She said, " Where am I?"

I said, "You are on your head."

She feebly said, " Was I unconscious?"

I said, "Just a little. Now wait and feel."

She said, " My head is on your feet." I said, "Yes, Madame, you are standing on my feet, now you will touch the ground."

Then I slipped her head from the feet on to the floor after a minute in the head balance I brought her down. I asked her whether she was happy doing the head balance. She was overjoyed that she could do *Śīrṣāsana*. Then I told her, "You have got blood pressure. As you had the courage to do, I had the courage to take." Afterwards she continued with no problems as I had to take other *āsana* to bring the pressure down to make her do *Sālamba Śīrṣāsana* – head balance.

So it depends upon the situation. You cannot take anyone at anytime. If you know that something is going wrong in the head balance, you should know what to do before and after, and how to adjust. If you do not know, then I say, "Do not touch at all."

I know the reactions of *Śīrṣāsana*, when the pressure increases, or why the eyes become red and, by the grace of yoga, I know how to take them so that such things do not happen again.